308
Current Topics
in Microbiology
and Immunology

Editors

R.W. Compans, Atlanta/Georgia
M.D. Cooper, Birmingham/Alabama
T. Honjo, Kyoto · H. Koprowski, Philadelphia/Pennsylvania
F. Melchers, Basel · M.B.A. Oldstone, La Jolla/California
S. Olsnes, Oslo · P.K. Vogt, La Jolla/California
H. Wagner, Munich

T. Honjo and F. Melchers (Eds.)

Gut-Associated Lymphoid Tissues

With 24 Figures and 5 Tables

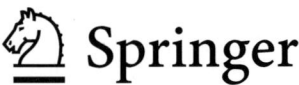

Tasuku Honjo, MD, Ph.D.
Department of Immunology
and Genomic Medicine
Kyoto University
Graduate School of Medicine
Yoshida, Sakyo-ku
Kyoto 606-8501 Japan
e-mail: honjo@mfour.med.kyoto-u.ac.jp

Fritz Melchers
Biozentrum, Department of Cell Biology
University of Basel
Klingelbergstr. 50–70
4056 Basel
Switzerland
and
Max Planck Institute for Infection Biology
Campus Charité
Schumannstrasse 21–22
10117 Berlin
Germany
e-mail: Fritz.melchers@unibas.ch

Cover Illustration by S. Fagarasan (this volume)

Library of Congress Catalog Number 72-152360

ISSN 0070-217X
ISBN-10 3-540-30656-0 Springer Berlin Heidelberg New York
ISBN-13 978-3-540-30656-6 Springer Berlin Heidelberg New York

This work is subject to copyright. All rights reserved, whether the whole or part of the material is concerned, specifically the rights of translation, reprinting, reuse of illustrations, recitation, broadcasting, reproduction on microfilm or in any other way, and storage in data banks. Duplication of this publication or parts thereof is permitted only under the provisions of the German Copyright Law of September, 9, 1965, in its current version, and permission for use must always be obtained from Springer-Verlag. Violations are liable for prosecution under the German Copyright Law.

Springer is a part of Springer Science+Business Media
springeronline.com
© Springer-Verlag Berlin Heidelberg 2006
Printed in Germany

The use of general descriptive names, registered names, trademarks, etc. in this publication does not imply, even in the absence of a specific statement, that such names are exempt from the relevant protective laws and regulations and therefore free for general use.

Product liability: The publisher cannot guarantee the accuracy of any information about dosage and application contained in this book. In every individual case the user must check such information by consulting the relevant literature.

Editor: Simon Rallison, Heidelberg
Desk editor: Anne Clauss, Heidelberg
Production editor: Nadja Kroke, Leipzig
Cover design: design & production GmbH, Heidelberg
Typesetting: LE-TEX Jelonek, Schmidt & Vöckler GbR, Leipzig
Printed on acid-free paper   SPIN 11560203   27/3150/YL – 5 4 3 2 1 0

This volume is dedicated to Jon Cebra,
a pioneer of the gut immunology field
who died recently.

Preface

The intestine is the front line of the confrontation between pathogens and the immune system. However, it is also important to emphasize that we have a symbiotic relationship with innumerable bacteria in the intestine. In the gastrointestinal tract of mammals the lower intestine harbors around 1,000 species of anaerobic and aerobic bacteria, in densities up to 10^{12}/ml in the distal small intestine, the cecum, and the colon. A single layer of epithelial cells of the intestine protects the internal organs of the mammalian host from these bacteria. Below these epithelial cells the gut-associated lymphoid tissues (GALT), organized in Peyer's patches, cryptopatches, and isolated lymphoid follicles, as well as isolated, dispersed single cells in the epithelial layer (intraepithelial lymphocytes) and lamina propria, are composed of T lymphocytes, B lymphocytes, Ig-secreting plasma cells, and antigen-presenting cells such as dendritic cells. The importance of the gut barrier is striking, if we consider that in humans the epithelial surface, behind which the immune system faces and senses the endogenous bacteria, is estimated to be as large as a basketball court. Perhaps not surprising then, the gut contains approximately half of all lymphocytes of our immune system. Colonization of the intestine with the flora of commensal bacteria induces the development of the GALT, which in turn responds by the development of IgA-secreting plasma cells. Dimeric and multimeric IgAs can traverse the epithelial layer and are released in the gut lumen, where they bind bacteria. It is thought that this IgA contributes to the control of commensal, nonpathogenic bacteria and the containment of the pathogenic strains of bacteria.

Any changes in gut microbiota, especially those by potentially pathogenic bacteria – inducing gastritis and inflammatory bowel disease – must be sensed by the GALT. It is thought that the mucosal immune system interacts with the bacteria in such a way that this permanent infection is, in fact, beneficial for the host – as the bacteria digest food for which the mammalian host has no enzymes and as bacteria provide vitamins. Besides this metabolic function, as perceived from several chapters of this book, the bacterial colonization of gut is seen as an important event that drives maturation of the immune system and maintains/influences its fitness.

This volume assembles some of the recent, exciting advances in our understanding of the evolutionary origin and ontogeny of the GALT components orchestrated in space and time by multiple lineages of cells, for example, of hematopoietic and mesenchymal origins (Finke and Meier; Ivanov, Diehl, and Litman). As discussed by Nahoum and Medzitov, bacteria harbor a wealth of macromolecules, which are recognized by all lymphocytes through pattern-recognition receptors [Toll-like-receptors (TLR)] that sense the bacteria regardless of the specificity of their antigen receptor, that is, T cell receptor and Ig, in a polyclonal fashion. Thus B lymphocytes appear to be guided and function to assemble to GALT structures even when their capacity to produce antigen-specific B cell receptors, namely, Ig, is impaired or absent. Thus the innate parts of the immune system may be important elements in the interactions between gut microbiota and the GALT system.

On the other hand, IgA is the most abundant antibody isotype produced in our body (with 40–60 mg/kg/day), and 80% of the IgA-producing cells are located in gut. Hamburger, Björkman, and Herr show how dimeric IgA, with its Fc portions, interacts with the Fcγ receptors and how IgA-specific proteases and IgA-binding proteins produced by bacteria compete with this transmigration. Hence, bacteria interfere and compete with the transport of IgA through the epithelial layer of the gut – and certain bacteria have the capacity to hijack the IgA-specific transcytosis pathway to invade the mammalian host. Fagarasan shows how essential gut IgA production must be for maintenance of appropriate densities and proper distribution of aerobic and anaerobic bacteria, especially in the small intestine. If IgA is not produced, as in mice defective in IgA production (through AID deficiency) then anaerobic bacteria overgrow aerobic bacteria and, in fact, expand in numbers and to areas normally not colonized by them. Not unexpectedly, and of significant practical consequence, is the observation that the repertoire of antigen receptors, that is, IgA specificities, in the GALT is adapted to the composition of the endogenous bacterial flora (Macpherson).

The T and B lymphocytes of the GALT appear to be selected from the pool of cells originally generated in the primary lymphoid organs, that is, in thymus and bone marrow. They retain, and maybe are even further instructed, to home to, and back to, the mucosal tissues (Mora and von Andrian). A part of them are thought to form the first layer of defense against and – as we would now more optimistically say – for symbiotic interactions with the gut microbiota. These interactions, from the side of the GALT of the host, are clearly guided by both innate and adaptive forms of immunity.

Our exploration, our voyage into this essential part of our body has just begun.

February 2006 *Tasuku Honjo, Fritz Melchers*

List of Contents

Role of the Innate Immune System and Host–Commensal Mutualism 1
    S. Rakoff-Nahoum and R. Medzhitov

Molecular Networks Orchestrating GALT Development 19
    D. Finke and D. Meier

Lymphoid Tissue Inducer Cells in Intestinal Immunity 59
    I. I. Ivanov, G. E. Diehl, and D. R. Littman

Specificity and Plasticity of Memory Lymphocyte Migration 83
    J. Rodrigo Mora and U. H. von Andrian

IgA Adaptation to the Presence of Commensal Bacteria in the Intestine 117
    A. J. Macpherson

Intestinal IgA Synthesis: A Primitive Form of Adaptive Immunity
That Regulates Microbial Communities in the Gut 137
    S. Fagarasan

B Cell Recruitment and Selection in Mouse GALT Germinal Centers 155
    S. Casola and K. Rajewsky

Structural Insights into Antibody-Mediated Mucosal Immunity 173
    A. E. Hamburger, P. J. Bjorkman, and A. B. Herr

Subject Index 205

List of Contributors

(Addresses stated at the beginning of respective chapters)

Bjorkman, P. J. 173

Casola, S. 155

Diehl, G. E. 59

Fagarasan, S. 137
Finke, D. 19

Hamburger, A. E. 173
Herr, A. B. 173

Ivanov, I. I. 59

Littman, D. R. 59

Macpherson, A. J. 117
Medzhitov, R. 1
Meier, D. 19

Rajewsky, K. 155
Rakoff-Nahoum, S. 1
Rodrigo Mora, J. 83

von Andrian, U. H. 83

CTMI (2006) 308:1–18
© Springer-Verlag Berlin Heidelberg 2006

Role of the Innate Immune System and Host–Commensal Mutualism

S. Rakoff-Nahoum · R. Medzhitov (✉)

Howard Hughes Medical Institute and Section of Immunobiology, Yale University School of Medicine, New Haven, CT 06510, USA
ruslan.medzhitov@yale.edu

1	Introduction	2
2	Different Types of Host–Microbial Mutualism	4
3	Host–Microbe Mutualism in Mammals: Benefits and Mechanisms	5
3.1	Metabolism and Energy Utilization	5
3.2	Organ Development	6
3.3	Development of the Mucosal Immune System	6
3.4	Regulation of Host Immune Responses	7
3.4.1	Positive Regulation	7
3.4.1.1	IgA Immune Responses	8
3.4.2	Negative Regulation	8
3.4.2.1	Oral Tolerance	9
3.4.2.2	Regulation of Atopic Allergic Responses	9
3.5	Resistance to Infection with Pathogens	10
3.6	Maintenance of Tissue Homeostasis and Repair	11
4	Innate Immune Recognition of Commensals in Symbiosis in Other Organisms	13
5	Conclusions and Perspectives	13
	References	15

Abstract Host organisms live in intimate contact with indigenous microflora. The interactions between the host and commensal microbiota are highly complex and heterogeneous. A growing body of evidence indicates that commensal symbionts provide many benefits to the host physiology, particularly in the gastrointestinal system. The molecular mechanisms of the mutualistic interactions between the host and commensals are largely unknown but can be due either to bioactivity of the commensals or to the reaction of the host immune system to the commensal-derived products. Recent advances in our understanding of the innate immune system allow re-evaluation of some of the older findings regarding the mechanisms of benefits conferred by microflora. Here we review the examples of the benefits of host–commensal interactions that are due to recognition of commensal microbial products by the host innate immune system.

1
Introduction

All metazoans are engaged in complex interactions with microorganisms. The nature of these interactions can range from highly antagonistic to mutually beneficial and is determined by evolutionary adaptations of the host and the microbial species. Depending on the outcome of the interaction, the microorganisms are referred to as pathogens, if the interaction results in a loss of fitness of the host, or commensals, if the interaction is either beneficial or neutral for the host. It is generally thought that the host immune system protects from infection by pathogens but somehow avoids responding to commensals, as such responses can be detrimental under certain conditions. This view presupposes that there is something fundamentally different in the way the immune system deals with commensals versus pathogens. The problem with this view, however, is that the distinctions between commensal and pathogenic microbes are often arbitrary, as the ability to cause the disease is not always dependent on characteristics intrinsic to the microorganisms. Further complicating the matter is the fact that the receptors used to sense infection by the innate immune system do not discriminate between pathogens and commensals. This raises several important questions regarding the nature of the interactions between commensal microflora and the host innate immune system and the mechanisms that regulate these interactions. Indeed, the failure of mechanisms that regulate intestinal immune responses can lead to a variety of immunopathologies, including the development of inflammatory bowel disease (IBD). Nevertheless, several aspects of metazoan physiology, most notably of the gastrointestinal system, have clearly coevolved with, and are dependent upon, mutualistic interactions with indigenous microflora.

The aim of this review is discuss the benefits of the indigenous microflora on host biology, especially in the intestine. Emphasis is placed on what is known about the mechanisms by which these benefits occur. In particular we highlight evidence that suggests that recognition of microbes by Toll-like receptors (TLRs) plays a role in mediating host–microbe mutualism.

The life histories of plants and animals are replete with mutualistic relationships with the microbial world. Most complex metazoans are colonized with a consortium of microorganisms comprising an indigenous microflora.

In some cases, the host dependence on symbionts can be truly remarkable. In the plant kingdom, infection of legumes, such as soybeans, by the gram-negative *Rhizobium* leads to root nodulation allowing for the fixation of N_2 by the bacteria, thus providing the host plant with selective advantage in soils with nitrogen deficiency (Fisher and Long 1992). The benefits of microbial colonization of insects leads to increased nutritional sources (Dillon and Dillon 2004), protection from infection with enteropathogens (Dillon and Dillon 2004), and increased life span (Brummel et al. 2004). In the symbiosis between *Vibrio fisheri* and the Hawaiian sepiolid squid, *Euprymna scolopes*, colonization leads to postembryonic development of the squid light organ (Nyholm and McFall-Ngai 2004). The commensal microflora also plays a role in the lives of other aquatic animals, as demonstrated in studies of axenically derived zebra fish (Rawls et al. 2004) and of deep sea vent worms (Jeanthon 2000).

Host–microbe interactions play a profound role in the biology of mammals. Mammals are colonized with a diverse and abundant indigenous microflora. It is estimated that 500–1,000 different species of 10^{14} microorganisms may colonize mammals such as rodents and humans, although the number of species is most likely an underestimate (Sonnenburg et al. 2004). Commensal bacteria colonize many organs of the mammal, including the gingiva, oropharynx, skin, and genitourinary and respiratory tracts. However, the greatest density, magnitude, and diversity occur in the gastrointestinal tract, particularly at the large intestine. Since the original observation that microbial colonization plays a role in the physiological development of rodents, 40 years ago (Schaedler et al. 1965), numerous benefits of the indigenous microflora to mammalian biology have been revealed. These benefits range from those affecting metabolism, development, or various organ systems to tolerance to mucosal antigens and resistance to infection (Berg 1996).

There have been three ways in which the role of the commensal microflora in mammalian biology has been assessed. The most common is the comparison of conventionally raised animals with those that are germ-free, reared in positive-pressure isolators after being delivered by sterile Cesarean section. In gnotobiotic studies, germ-free animals are colonized with a known species or group of species of microorganisms. A third, and very different, approach to study the affect of the commensals on host biology is to deplete conventionally raised mice of their microflora with antibiotics. Although this approach has the advantage of being able to assess the effect of the microflora on animals with normal development, a caveat is the inability to determine the effectiveness of the depletion of commensals because of the inability to culture or identify the majority of microfloral species.

2
Different Types of Host–Microbial Mutualism

Despite the enormous benefits of microorganisms in host biology, relatively little is known about the molecular details of host–commensal interactions. Until recently, it was thought that the majority of benefits provided by the microflora were conferred because of the "bioactivity" of commensals. Two well-known examples of this type of benefits are the roles of indigenous symbionts in energy and nutrient utilization and in resistance to infection by pathogens. In the former, bacterial enzymes, such as those that process polysaccharides normally indigestible by host enzymatic machinery, allow for emergent carbon sources. In the latter, the indigenous flora helps to prevent infection by pathogens by production of antimicrobial compounds or competing for niches necessary for infection.

In addition to these contributions to host biology, recent studies have revealed that commensals and the host are engaged in a much more intimate and complex interactions. Both in vitro and in vivo studies using human intestinal epithelial cell lines have revealed a role of nonpathogenic species of bacteria in the regulation of host cell signaling. An unidentified factor produced by nonvirulent *Salmonella* strains was shown to inhibit IκB degradation and NF-κB activation by blocking IκB polyubiquitination (Neish et al. 2000). Recently, the nonpathogenic PhoP[c] *Salmonella* mutant was demonstrated to increase nuclear localization of β-catenin by inhibiting its ubiquitination and proteosomal degradation (Sun et al. 2004, 2005). Kelly et al. have shown that the intestinal symbiont *Bacteroides thetaiotamicron* may regulate the NF-κB pathway by mediating nuclear export of RelA via a PPARγ-dependent mechanism (Kelly et al. 2004).

Elegant studies by Hooper et al. have characterized a system of bidirectional communication between *B. thetaiotamicron* and intestinal epithelial cells (Hooper et al. 1999). In this relationship, the bacteria upregulate the expression of α1.2-fucosyltransferase in the host cell, which leads to the appearance of fucosylated glycans on the ileal epithelium. The bacteria utilize the fucose residue as an energy source, and in addition fucose levels feed into a regulatory operon in which high fucose levels repress the signal to the epithelium stimulating fucosylated glycan synthesis.

Thus nonpathogenic bacteria and intestinal symbionts have the capacity to interact with and modulate NF-κB and β-catenin signaling and metabolic pathways in host cells. NF-κB plays a critical role the inflammatory response, and β-catenin is an essential regulator of intestinal epithelial proliferation and differentiation. Although the physiological role of commensal-mediated regulation of this pathway is not known, it likely contributes to the maintenance of intestinal tissue homeostasis.

Recent studies in mice have revealed that recognition of the indigenous microflora by TLRs, best known for their role in host defense from infection, may be responsible for mediating some of the benefits of colonization by the indigenous microflora (Araki et al. 2005; Cario et al. 2004; Fukata et al. 2005; Pull et al. 2005; Rakoff-Nahoum et al. 2004). TLRs recognize conserved molecular products present on microorganisms. Ten to fifteen different TLRs have been identified in mammals. A number of TLR ligands have been identified so far, including TLR2 ligands lipotechoic acid (LTA) and bacterial lipoprotein (BLP), TLR4 ligand LPS, TLR3 ligand double-stranded RNA, TLR5 ligand flagellin and TLR9 ligand hypomethylated CpG DNA. TLRs signal through at least four adaptor molecules, MyD88, TRIF, TIRAP, and TRAM. Downstream signaling leads to the activation of NF-κB, IRFs, and MAP kinase pathways (Takeda et al. 2003).

3
Host–Microbe Mutualism in Mammals: Benefits and Mechanisms

3.1
Metabolism and Energy Utilization

The metabolic activity of the indigenous gastrointestinal flora has been described as equaling that of the liver (Berg 1996). Among many other abilities, commensals produce short-chain fatty acids (SCFA), synthesize vitamin B12, and deconjugate bile acids. Compared to conventionally raised animals, germ-free animals show defects in vitamin synthesis (including, biotin, folate, and vitamins B and K), bile acid transformation, carbohydrate and fatty acid digestion, synthesis of SCFA, xenobiotic transformation, and other signs of metabolic deficiencies (Berg 1996; Midvedt 1999; Savage 1986). Many of these benefits are indeed mediated by the novel enzymatic bioactivity of the indigenous flora. However, recent studies by Backhed et al. reveal that some of the effects of intestinal symbionts on host metabolism may be due to regulation of host metabolic enzymes (Backhed et al. 2004). Conventionalization of germ-free mice led to adipogenesis and increased insulin resistance, revealing a role of the microflora in positively regulating fat storage. Gene expression analysis revealed that the microbiota suppressed the expression of fasting-induced adipocyte factor (Fiaf) by intestinal epithelium, which was partly responsible for this phenotype. It is not known how colonization leads to the modulation of the expression of this factor by the intestinal epithelium.

3.2
Organ Development

Many organs, including the heart, liver, spleen, and adrenal glands, are undersized in germ-free rodents. Blood volume is decreased in these animals, perhaps leading to the decreased cardiac output and peripheral blood flow observed (Berg 1996; Savage 1977). Germ-free animals compared to those either conventionally raised or colonized with known species of bacteria show many differences in intestinal anatomy and morphology. Germ-free animals have decreased intestinal mass and surface area, thinner villi, and decreased rates of peristalsis. Intestines show compromised development of the vasculature (Stappenbeck et al. 2002) and abnormalities in glycosylation patterns, mucin production, and proliferation and differentiation of epithelial cells (Banasaz et al. 2002; Gordon et al. 1997). It is not currently known how the commensal microflora mediates these developmental changes.

3.3
Development of the Mucosal Immune System

The commensal microflora has a profound effect on the gut-associated lymphoid tissue (GALT). The GALT can be subdivided into three main sections, lymphoid follicles such as Peyer's patches, lamina propria (LP), and intraepithelial (IE) compartments, all of which require the commensal microflora for aspects of normal development (Jiang et al. 2004; Macpherson et al. 2001).

Compared to conventionalized or gnotobiotic animals, those raised under germ-free conditions have smaller, underdeveloped Peyer's patches, which lack germinal centers. Perhaps one of the most striking effects of the commensal microflora on the GALT is the expansion of IgA-secreting plasma cells in the lamina propria and the increased secretion of intestinal IgA that may contribute to the natural antibody pool (Jiang et al. 2004; Macpherson et al. 2001). In rabbits, commensal microflora induce the somatic diversification of the primary antibody repertoire (Lanning and Knight 1998). The number of total $CD4^+$ T cells and the ontogeny of mucosa-associated invariant T cells (MAIT) present in the lamina propria are commensal dependent (Treiner et al. 2003). Germ-free mice show a reduction in $CD8\alpha^+$ $\alpha\beta TCR^+$ T cell numbers in the IEL (Umesaki et al. 1993) compartment, but no difference in $CD8\alpha^+$ $\gamma\delta TCR^+$ T cells (Bandeira et al. 1990).

Given their known role in the immune system, it would seem likely that TLR signals induced by the commensal microflora may be important in the development of the mucosa-associated lymphoid tissue of the intestine. However, in initial analyses of adult animals, mice deficient in MyD88, TLR2, or TLR4 do not show gross abnormalities in the development of Peyer's patches, differences in the morphology of small or large intestinal villi, or phenotype of intraepithelial lymphocytes with regard to αβ vs. γδ TCR and CD4 vs. CD8α surface expression (Iiyama et al. 2003).

However, on further analysis, significant differences were noted in the size of Peyer's patches at 2 weeks of age between TLR4$^{-/-}$, but not TLR2$^{-/-}$, and WT mice (Iiyama et al. 2003), suggesting that TLR4-dependent signaling by ligands present during this early postnatal stage may be important for Peyer's patch development but may be compensated for later by other mechanisms.

A more focused analysis of small intestinal intraepithelial lymphocytes revealed decreased numbers of CD8αα TCRα$^+$ IEL in various strains of mice deficient in TLR4 signaling (Kaneko et al. 2004). Investigation into the mechanism causing this reduction of IEL subset revealed diminished IL-15 expression in isolated intestinal epithelium from TLR4-deficient mice. This suggests that the mechanism of commensal-dependent development of certain subsets of intraepithelial lymphocytes, whether of thymic (Eberl and Littman 2004) or extrathymic (Lefrancois and Olson 1994; Rocha et al. 1994; Saito et al. 1998; Umesaki et al. 1993) origin, may actually be due to constitutive signaling of TLR4 in the intestine induced by the commensal microflora.

Thus in the mouse, TLR-mediated signals are important in various aspects of the development of intestinal lymphoid tissue. It is unknown what role commensal-TLR interactions play in GALT development in humans, given the differential programs of GALT organogenesis between these two species (McCracken and Lorenz 2001).

3.4
Regulation of Host Immune Responses

3.4.1
Positive Regulation

The commensal microflora plays an important role in the induction and regulation of immune responses, both systemically and locally. Germ-free animals show defective induction of peripheral delayed-type hypersensitivity to sheep red blood cells (MacDonald and Carter 1979) and antibody responses to haptenated antigens (Bos and Ploplis 1994; Ohwaki et al. 1977)). In vitro studies of splenic and peritoneal macrophages from germ-free mice showed decreased proliferation, MHC class II expression, and production of IL-1, IL-6, and IL-12 (Nicaise et al. 1998, 1999). Peritoneal macrophages from germ-free rats showed defects in chemotaxis (Jungi and McGregor 1978), whereas those from bronchoalveolar lavage were found to have decreased lysosomal enzyme activity (Starling and Balish 1981). Germ-free mice show decreased lytic activity of natural killer cells (Bartizal et al. 1984). It is not known how the indigenous microflora mediates these functions; however, a role for TLRs is likely given that such TLR signaling is known to activate many of these events.

3.4.1.1
IgA Immune Responses

Association of germ-free animals with known species of commensal bacteria leads to germinal center reactions in Peyer's patches in which B cells become committed to the production of IgA. Studies of the antigen specificity of the IgA revealed that the commensal microflora may be inducing IgA specific to commensal antigens (specific IgA) and also nonspecific IgA, termed "natural IgA" (Bos et al. 2001; Macpherson and Uhr 2004). Analysis of the relative proportions of commensal-specific and natural IgA of the monoassociated germ-free mice demonstrated that the overwhelming majority of IgA was not specific to the commensals. For example, colonization of germ-free mice with SFB results in the production of IgA of which only 1% is antigen specific to the commensal (Talham et al. 1999).

These findings suggest polyclonal activation of the natural B cell pool. TLR ligands, including LPS, are well known to be polyclonal activators of B cells (Andersson et al. 1972; Armerding and Katz 1974). It is thus very likely that ligation of TLRs either directly on B cells or on accessory cells (such as DC) in the intestine, may be responsible for the polyclonal expansion of B cells and production of intestinal IgA on conventionalization of germ-free animals (Fagarasan and Honjo 2003; Jiang et al. 2004). Although the functions of the natural IgA induced nonspecifically by commensals remain unknown and controversial, it is possible that these antibodies function similarly to natural serum IgM [although these are not commensal dependent (Haury et al. 1997), acting as an early defense system, before the induction of an antigen-specific immune response (Baumgarth et al. 1999; Ochsenbein et al. 1999)]. Thus this may be another example in which a commensal dependent benefit to host biology may be mediated by TLR recognition of the indigenous microflora.

3.4.2
Negative Regulation

Commensal microbiota may also be involved in negative regulation of certain types of immune responses. Germ-free animals have been shown to have defects in inducing systemic tolerance to orally administered foreign antigens (Wannemuehler et al. 1982) and in the regulation of atopic response in the intestine (Sudo et al. 1997; Tanaka and Ishikawa 2004).

3.4.2.1
Oral Tolerance

A role of TLRs in inducing systemic tolerance to oral antigens comes from two lines of evidence. Unlike conventionally raised animals, germ-free BALB/c mice given sheep RBC via gastric gavage were able to induce potent systemic immune responses as determined by detection of high frequencies of antigen-specific antibody (IgG, IgM, and IgA)-producing splenocytes on intraperitoneal immunization with antigen. When these germ-free mice were given a single oral dose of LPS, they became hyporesponsive to systemic challenge (Michalek et al. 1982; Wannemuehler et al. 1982). The role of LPS in the induction of oral tolerance was further suggested by similar studies in which tolerance could not be induced in C3H/HeJ (LPS insensitive) compared with C3H/HeN (LPS-sensitive) mice (Kiyono et al. 1982; Mowat et al. 1986). Both the lack of oral tolerance in germ-free mice and the role of LPS in mediating this tolerance were challenged by studies in germ-free and conventionalized C3H/HeJ mice (Moreau and Corthier 1988) using OVA as fed antigen. However, these studies used a high dose of OVA, which is known to induce T cell deletion rather than induction of regulatory T cells (Chen et al. 1995) and may have been the mode of action in experiments using SRBC.

3.4.2.2
Regulation of Atopic Allergic Responses

The "hygiene hypothesis" suggests that the absence of microbial infection may lead to the development of IgE-mediated atopic allergy by Th2-polarized immune responses (Strachan 1989; Umetsu et al. 2002). It is hypothesized that this may occur through the lack of microbial induced Th1 responses and associated with increased Th2 responses, or by a defective generation of immunoregulatory mediators such as regulatory T cells or interleukin-10 (Macpherson and Harris 2004). Evidence that the indigenous microflora may play a role in regulating IgE responses comes from two lines of evidence: studies in germ-free mice showing increased IgE response to antigen (Sudo et al. 1997; Tanaka and Ishikawa 2004) and observations showing the relationship between the composition of the intestinal microflora and the incidence of atopic allergy in animal models and humans (Bjorksten et al. 2001; Kalliomaki and Isolauri 2003; Kirjavainen et al. 2002).

A role for commensal-TLR interaction in the regulation of intestinal atopy was first suggested by studies in which C3H/HeJ mice, compared to BALB/c, showed severe anaphylaxis, antigen-specific IgE, and plasma histamine levels on oral administration of both cow's milk and peanut allergen (PNA) (Morafo et al. 2003). Bashir et al. demonstrated that commensal-TLR signaling was responsible for inhibiting this IgE hyperresponsiveness (Bashir et al. 2004). This was evidenced by increased levels of serum IgE in TLR4-deficient mice compared to WT on oral administration of PNA. Antibiotic depletion of commensals in WT mice phenocopied the high serum levels of IgE seen in TLR4$^{-/-}$ mice and was reversed on feeding the mice with CpG oligonucleotides. Thus it appeared that both TLR4 and TLR9 ligands on commensal microflora were capable of inhibiting the IgE induced by oral allergen. In the intestine, immunostimulatory DNA from probiotic bacteria may act on TLR9 and mediate anti-inflammatory effects in an animal model of colitis (Rachmilewitz et al. 2004). A recent report, however, questions the specificity of immunoregulatory DNA for TLR9, showing that germ-free mice fed nucleic acids devoid of CpG motifs were able to skew intestinal immune responses to a Th1 bias (Sudo et al. 2004).

3.5
Resistance to Infection with Pathogens

Studies in both germ-free animals and those depleted of commensals by antibiotics have revealed a role of the indigenous microflora in providing colonization resistance, which helps to prevent infection of the host by pathogenic microorganisms. In humans, a well-known phenomenon is the diarrhea caused by *Clostridium difficile* overgrowth in the intestine following the use of broad-spectrum antibiotics (Stoddart and Wilcox 2002). In mice, oral administration of antibiotics leads to a decrease in the number of pathogenic organisms, such as *Vibrio* and *Shigella*, required for effective colonization (Freter 1955). Infection studies in germ-free mice have demonstrated the beneficial role of the commensal microflora in protecting the host from intestinal pathogens (Filho-Lima et al. 2000; Hudault et al. 2001)

Passive mechanisms may be particularly operative in colonization resistance to infection by intestinal pathogens. Proposed passive mechanisms of such protection include (a) niche competition, both for nutrients and epithelial attachment sites, (b) production of antimicrobial compounds, such as colicins and microcins, and (c) production of metabolites that may be unfavorable to the growth of intestinal pathogens.

However, recent studies have suggested that the intestinal microflora may stimulate host cells in the intestine to produce antimicrobial factors, and this may be one of the ways in which the flora mediates colonization resistance. Paneth cells located at the base of small intestinal crypts, below the stem cell zone (Brittan and Wright 2002; Marshman et al. 2002), may play an important role in maintaining a sterile environment so as to protect the stem cell niche. These cells contain apically oriented intracellular granules containing numerous factors with known antimicrobial effects such as phospholipase2, lysozyme, α-defensin, and angiogenin 4 (Ouellette 1999). Comparisons of genes induced in the ileum on conventionalization or monospecific association of *B. thetaiotamicron* with germ-free mice identified upregulation of a family of antimicrobial proteins known as angiogenins (Hooper et al. 2001, 2003). In particular, angiogenin 4 (which was specifically expressed in Paneth cells on colonization of germ-free mice) was shown to have potent microbicidal activity against the bacterial intestinal pathogens, *Enterococcus faecalis* and *Listeria monocytogenes*. Interestingly this protein had very limited ability to kill *B. theatiotamicron* itself.

How does the intestinal flora or a symbiont such as *B. thetaiotamicron* induce the production or secretion of antimicrobial factors? Studies performed on isolated intestinal crypts have suggested a role of TLR ligation on Paneth cells in inducing degranulation. Contact with bacteria, both live and dead, has been shown to induce degranulation of Paneth cells (Ayabe et al. 2000). A role for TLRs and NOD proteins in inducing Paneth cell degranulation was suggested by studies showing that degranulation can be induced in isolated small intestinal crypts by various TLR and NOD ligands, such as LPS, LTA, lipid A, and muramyl dipeptide (MDP) (Ayabe et al. 2000). The degranulation results in a release of lysozyme, angiogenin 4 (Hooper et al. 2003) and α-defensins (Ayabe et al. 2000). In addition, intraperitoneal injection of CpG oligonucleotides was shown to result in Paneth cell degranulation and increased expression of cryptdin-1 in isolated intestinal crypts. Consistent with these findings, TLR9 was found to be expressed in Paneth cells of both murine and human small intestine, located mainly at intracellular granules (Rumio et al. 2004).

3.6
Maintenance of Tissue Homeostasis and Repair

The indigenous microflora may be important in maintaining barrier function, epithelial integrity, and wound healing in many organs. Germ-free mice have been shown to be extremely susceptible to nonspecific intestinal epithelial injury (Kitajima et al. 2001; Pull et al. 2005). Ex vivo studies of rat bowel loops revealed that some commensal bacteria (such as *Lactobacillus brevis*), but not others (*Bacteriodes fragilis*, *Escherichia coli*), may maintain epithelial integrity (Garcia-Lafuente et al. 2001). The commensal microflora may also play a role in the maintenance of liver homeostasis after injury (Cornell et al. 1990). In various models, germ-free animals show defective healing after intestinal resection (Okada et al. 1999), skin incision (Okada 1994), tooth extraction (Rovin et al. 1966), and tongue injury (Rovin et al. 1965).

The ability of the indigenous flora to produce (SCFA, which are known to affect various aspects of intestinal epithelial cell biology, perhaps by acting as an inhibitor of histone deacetylase, may be one way in which microbial symbionts confer this benefit to the host (Blottiere et al. 2003; Sanderson 2004).

A new role for beneficial commensal-TLR interactions in protecting the large intestine from injury has recently been suggested (Araki et al. 2005; Cario et al. 2004; Fukata et al. 2005; Pull et al. 2005; Rakoff-Nahoum et al. 2004). Animals deficient in MyD88, TLR2, and TLR4 showed severe mortality, weight loss, and intestinal bleeding and epithelial cell injury (Rakoff-Nahoum et al. 2004). WT mice were rendered susceptible to the epithelial injurious agent DSS when depleted of all culturable commensals by treatment with broad-spectrum antibiotics. The susceptibility of commensal-depleted animals was completely reversed by oral pretreatment with either LPS or LTA (Rakoff-Nahoum et al. 2004). Additional studies in MyD88$^{-/-}$ mice revealed an inability to regenerate colonic epithelial cells after whole body irradiation (Rakoff-Nahoum et al. 2004) and DSS administration (Pull et al. 2005). Together, these studies demonstrated that activation of TLRs by commensal-derived products is essential for protecting the intestinal epithelium from injury and for the induction of tissue repair responses. In vitro studies have recently demonstrated that TLR2 signaling in intestinal epithelium may aid in maintaining epithelial barrier function by increasing tight junction formation (Cario et al. 2004).

A LPS-unresponsive mouse strain (C3H/HeJ) was found to have a defect in hepatocyte proliferation after partial resection compared with LPS-responsive C3H/HeN mice (Cornell et al. 1990). A critical role of TLRs in repair of the liver after injury was further demonstrated in studies using MyD88$^{-/-}$ mice (Seki et al. 2005). As the portal vein contains commensal-derived TLR ligands, such as LPS, this protective effect is likely mediated by commensal product-TLR interactions in the liver.

A series of experiments performed in rats suggested that microflora of the skin may aid in skin wound healing. In experiments originally performed to study the effects of heating scalpels on wounds, the authors revealed a surprising role for *Staphylococcus aureus* in accelerating the healing of epidermal-dermal incisions (Levenson et al. 1983). Further investigation into this phenomenon revealed that this benefit was mediated by *S. aureus* cell wall and specifically by its peptidoglycan (Kilcullen et al. 1998). Thus although in many circumstances, such as in deep tissue wounds, the microflora of the skin may cause infection, pattern recognition of the commensal bacteria of the skin may be important in skin tissue regeneration and repair.

4
Innate Immune Recognition of Commensals in Symbiosis in Other Organisms

Recent investigations in squid and zebra fish indicate that signaling via TLRs (or other pattern recognition receptors) may be involved in mediating host–microbe mutualism in animals other than mammals. Studies in the symbiosis between the bacteria *Vibrio fisheri* and the Hawaiian sepiolid squid, *Euprymna scolopes* have revealed that LPS, peptidoglycan, and tracheal cytotoxin may be responsible for various aspects of light organ development (Foster et al. 2000; Koropatnick et al. 2004; Nyholm et al. 2002). The microbial flora of the zebra fish digestive tract was found to induce a widespread host gene expression program (Rawls et al. 2004). Fifty-nine of the 212 genes upregulated on microbial colonization of zebra fish were shared with those induced on introduction of commensals to mice, revealing an evolutionarily conserved response to the intestinal microflora. These include genes involved in many biological processes such as epithelial proliferation, nutrient metabolism, and innate immunity. It is not known whether TLRs are responsible for the recognition of symbionts or symbiont-derived products in either squid or zebra fish. Homologs of TLR and TLR signaling intermediates have recently been identified in zebra fish (Jault et al. 2004; Meijer et al. 2004). One report has shown that LPS may decrease glutathione-S-transferase activity in these fish, decreasing the detoxification of cyanobacteria-derived toxins (Best et al. 2002); however, the role that this activity and LPS-zebra fish interactions may have on other aspects of zebra fish biology is unknown.

5
Conclusions and Perspectives

Complex metazoans coexist with different types of microorganisms ranging from overt pathogens to beneficial symbionts. This co-existence requires that the host (a) be able to mount protective immune responses to potential pathogens, (b) allow for the mutualist microbes to confer benefit to host biology, (c) prevent constitutive immune responses to the indigenous microbes that would cause immune-mediated pathology, and (d) prevent opportunistic infections caused by endogenous pathogens (components of the indigenous microflora).

A predominant theory has been that anatomic compartmentalization fulfills these four conditions. According to this hypothesis, symbionts are confined to living outside of the host by a physical barrier. This barrier simultaneously prevents both recognition by the host immune system and consequent immunopathology and also opportunistic infection by the indigenous flora.

On infection with a pathogen, virulence factors enable the pathogen to traverse this barrier. It is thought that this desequestration allows for recognition of the microbe by the host immune system and the induction of host defense responses.

However, as discussed in this review, many of the benefits conferred by the indigenous microflora do not simply occur by passive means and indeed could not occur if there was strict compartmentalization between the host and their symbionts. In many instances, activation of host cell signaling is required. Furthermore, we have highlighted evidence to suggest that many of the benefits conferred by symbiotic microorganisms occur through recognition of commensals by the TLRs. It is this same family of receptors that are known to be responsible for orchestrating host defense responses to microbial pathogens. Thus it appears that TLRs do not distinguish between pathogenic and nonpathogenic microbes on the basis of their ligand specificity.

A future challenge will be to determine how the four conditions of host–microbe interactions outlined above may be fulfilled given that recognition of microbes by TLR is involved both in protection from microbial pathogens and in mediating the benefits of colonization with symbiotic bacteria. It appears that active regulatory mechanisms, in addition to physical barriers such as anti-inflammatory cytokines, may be instrumental in setting a threshold of the immune response of host organisms to their indigenous flora. How these factors modulate TLR signaling and allow for the induction of both TLR-mediated host defense to pathogens and homeostatic interactions with the flora, while simultaneously preventing commensal-induced immunopathology, is unknown.

TLRs are thought to have evolved to protect the host from microbial pathogens. However, as illustrated by many examples discussed in this review, TLR-mediated recognition of commensals is also highly beneficial to the host. Therefore, both TLR-mediated recognition of pathogens and TLR-mediated recognition of commensals have their own benefits that would provide selective advantage to the host. This implies that either one of the two functions of TLRs could have evolved on its own right. Thus the question arises as to which of the two functions has been the primary driving force in the evolution of the TLR family and which was the secondary adaptation. As discussed at the beginning of this text, the distinctions between commensals and pathogens are not absolute and static, but rather relative and dynamic. It is likely, therefore, that TLRs have evolved to detect microorganisms and to induce responses ranging from inflammatory and antimicrobial to tissue protective and reparative. Which type of response would dominate in any particular situation is likely determined by multiple variables, including microbial strategy of host colonization.

References

Andersson J, Sjoberg O, Moller G (1972). *Eur J Immunol* **2,** 349–53.
Araki A, Kanai T, Ishikura T, Makita S, Uraushihara K, Iiyama R, Totsuka T, Takeda K, Akira S, Watanabe M (2005). *J Gastroenterol* **40,** 16–23.
Armerding D, Katz DH (1974). *J Exp Med* **139,** 24–43.
Ayabe T, Satchell DP, Wilson CL, Parks WC, Selsted ME, Ouellette AJ (2000). *Nat Immunol* **1,** 113–8.
Backhed F, Ding H, Wang T, Hooper LV, Koh GY, Nagy A, Semenkovich CF, Gordon JI (2004). *Proc Natl Acad Sci USA* **101,** 15718–23.
Banasaz M, Norin E, Holma R, Midtvedt T (2002). *Appl Environ Microbiol* **68,** 3031–4.
Bandeira A, Mota-Santos T, Itohara S, Degermann S, Heusser C, Tonegawa S, Coutinho A (1990). *J Exp Med* **172,** 239–44.
Bartizal KF, Salkowski C, Pleasants JR, Balish E (1984). *J Leukoc Biol* **36,** 739–50.
Bashir ME, Louie S, Shi HN, Nagler-Anderson C (2004). *J Immunol* **172,** 6978–87.
Baumgarth N, Herman OC, Jager GC, Brown L, Herzenberg LA (1999). *Proc Natl Acad Sci USA* **96,** 2250–5.
Berg RD (1996). *Trends Microbiol* **4,** 430–5.
Best JH, Pflugmacher S, Wiegand C, Eddy FB, Metcalf JS, Codd GA (2002). *Aquat Toxicol* **60,** 223–31.
Bjorksten B, Sepp E, Julge K, Voor T, Mikelsaar M (2001). *J Allergy Clin Immunol* **108,** 516–20.
Blottiere HM, Buecher B, Galmiche JP, Cherbut C (2003). *Proc Nutr Soc* **62,** 101–6.
Bos NA, Jiang HQ, Cebra JJ (2001). *Gut* **48,** 762–4.
Bos NA, Ploplis VA (1994). *Eur J Immunol* **24,** 59–65.
Brittan M, Wright NA (2002). *J Pathol* **197,** 492–509.
Brummel T, Ching A, Seroude L, Simon AF, Benzer S (2004). *Proc Natl Acad Sci USA* **101,** 12974–9.
Cario E, Gerken G, Podolsky DK (2004). *Gastroenterology* **127,** 224–38.
Chen Y, Inobe J, Marks R, Gonnella P, Kuchroo VK, Weiner HL (1995). *Nature* **376,** 177–80.
Cornell RP, Liljequist BL, Bartizal KF (1990). *Hepatology* **11,** 916–22.
Dillon RJ, Dillon VM (2004). *Annu Rev Entomol* **49,** 71–92.
Eberl G, Littman DR (2004). *Science* **305,** 248–51.
Fagarasan S, Honjo T (2003). *Nat Rev Immunol* **3,** 63–72.
Filho-Lima JV, Vieira EC, Nicoli JR (2000). *J Appl Microbiol* **88,** 365–70.
Fisher RF, Long SR (1992). *Nature* **357,** 655–60.
Foster JS, Apicella MA, McFall-Ngai MJ (2000). *Dev Biol* **226,** 242–54.
Freter R (1955). *J Infect Dis* **97,** 57–65.
Fukata M, Michelsen KS, Eri R, Thomas LS, Hu B, Lukasek K, Nast CC, Lechago J, Xu R, Naiki Y, Soliman A, Arditi M, Abreu MT (2005). *Am J Physiol Gastrointest Liver Physiol* **288,** G1055–65.
Garcia-Lafuente A, Antolin M, Guarner F, Crespo E, Malagelada JR (2001). *Gut* **48,** 503–7.
Gordon JI, Hooper LV, McNevin MS, Wong M, Bry L (1997). *Am J Physiol Gastrointest Liver Physiol* **273,** G565–70.

Haury M, Sundblad A, Grandien A, Barreau C, Coutinho A, Nobrega A (1997). *Eur J Immunol* **27,** 1557–63.
Hooper LV, Stappenbeck TS, Hong CV, Gordon JI (2003). *Nat Immunol* **4,** 269–73.
Hooper LV, Wong MH, Thelin A, Hansson L, Falk PG, Gordon JI (2001). *Science* **291,** 881–4.
Hooper LV, Xu J, Falk PG, Midtvedt T, Gordon JI (1999). *Proc Natl Acad Sci USA* **96,** 9833–8.
Hudault S, Guignot J, Servin AL (2001). *Gut* **49,** 47–55.
Iiyama R, Kanai T, Uraushihara K, Ishikura T, Makita S, Totsuka T, Yamazaki M, Nakamura T, Miyata T, Yoshida H, Takeuchi O, Hoshino K, Takeda K, Ishikawa H, Akira S, Watanabe M (2003). *Scand J Immunol* **58,** 620–7.
Jault C, Pichon L, Chluba J (2004). *Mol Immunol* **40,** 759–71.
Jeanthon C (2000). *Antonie Van Leeuwenhoek* **77,** 117–33.
Jiang HQ, Thurnheer MC, Zuercher AW, Boiko NV, Bos NA, Cebra JJ (2004). *Vaccine* **22,** 805–11.
Jungi TW, McGregor DD (1978). *Infect Immun* **19,** 553–61.
Kalliomaki M, Isolauri E (2003). *Curr Opin Allergy Clin Immunol* **3,** 15–20.
Kaneko M, Mizunuma T, Takimoto H, Kumazawa Y (2004). *Biol Pharm Bull* **27,** 883–9.
Kelly D, Campbell JI, King TP, Grant G, Jansson EA, Coutts AG, Pettersson S, Conway S (2004). *Nat Immunol* **5,** 104–12.
Kilcullen JK, Ly QP, Chang TH, Levenson SM, Steinberg JJ (1998). *Wound Repair Regen* **6,** 149–56.
Kirjavainen PV, Arvola T, Salminen SJ, Isolauri E (2002). *Gut* **51,** 51–5.
Kitajima S, Morimoto M, Sagara E, Shimizu C, Ikeda Y (2001). *Exp Anim* **50,** 387–95.
Kiyono H, McGhee JR, Wannemuehler MJ, Michalek SM (1982). *J Exp Med* **155,** 605–10.
Koropatnick TA, Engle JT, Apicella MA, Stabb EV, Goldman WE, McFall-Ngai MJ (2004). *Science* **306,** 1186–8.
Lanning DK, Knight KL (1998). *Curr Top Microbiol Immunol* **229,** 45–57.
Lefrancois L, Olson S (1994). *J Immunol* **153,** 987–95.
Levenson SM, Kan-Gruber D, Gruber C, Molnar J, Seifter E (1983). *Arch Surg* **118,** 310–20.
MacDonald TT, Carter PB (1979). *J Immunol* **122,** 2624–9.
Macpherson AJ, Harris NL (2004). *Nat Rev Immunol* **4,** 478–85.
Macpherson AJ, Hunziker L, McCoy K, Lamarre A (2001). *Microbes Infect* **3,** 1021–35.
Macpherson AJ, Uhr T (2004). *Science* **303,** 1662–5.
Marshman E, Booth C, Potten CS (2002). *Bioessays* **24,** 91–8.
McCracken VJ, Lorenz RG (2001). *Cell Microbiol* **3,** 1–11.
Meijer AH, Gabby Krens SF, Medina Rodriguez IA, He S, Bitter W, Ewa Snaar-Jagalska B, Spaink HP (2004). *Mol Immunol* **40,** 773–83.
Michalek SM, Kiyono H, Wannemuehler MJ, Mosteller LM, McGhee JR (1982). *J Immunol* **128,** 1992–8.
Midvedt T (1999). Microbial Functional Activities. *In* "Probiotics, Other Nutritional Factors, Intestinal Microflora" (L. a. Y. Hanson RH, ed.), pp. 79–96. Lippincott-Raven, Philadelphia.
Morafo V, Srivastava K, Huang CK, Kleiner G, Lee SY, Sampson HA, Li AM (2003). *J Allergy Clin Immunol* **111,** 1122–8.
Moreau MC, Corthier G (1988). *Infect Immun* **56,** 2766–8.

Mowat AM, Thomas MJ, MacKenzie S, Parrott DM (1986). *Immunology* **58,** 677–83.
Neish AS, Gewirtz AT, Zeng H, Young AN, Hobert ME, Karmali V, Rao AS, Madara JL (2000). *Science* **289,** 1560–3.
Nicaise P, Gleizes A, Sandre C, Forestier F, Kergot R, Quero AM, Labarre C (1998). *Scand J Immunol* **48,** 585–91.
Nicaise P, Gleizes A, Sandre C, Kergot R, Lebrec H, Forestier F, Labarre C (1999). *Eur Cytokine Netw* **10,** 365–72.
Nyholm SV, Deplancke B, Gaskins HR, Apicella MA, McFall-Ngai MJ (2002). *Appl Environ Microbiol* **68,** 5113–22.
Nyholm SV, McFall-Ngai MJ (2004). *Nat Rev Microbiol* **2,** 632–42.
Ochsenbein AF, Fehr T, Lutz C, Suter M, Brombacher F, Hengartner H, Zinkernagel RM (1999). *Science* **286,** 2156–9.
Ohwaki M, Yasutake N, Yasui H, Ogura R (1977). *Immunology* **32,** 43–8.
Okada M (1994). *Surg Today* **24,** 347–55.
Okada M, Bothin C, Kanazawa K, Midtvedt T (1999). *Br J Surg* **86,** 961–5.
Ouellette AJ (1999). *Am J Physiol Gastrointest Liver Physiol* **277,** G257–61.
Pull SL, Doherty JM, Mills JC, Gordon JI, Stappenbeck TS (2005). *Proc Natl Acad Sci USA* **102,** 99–104.
Rachmilewitz D, Katakura K, Karmeli F, Hayashi T, Reinus C, Rudensky B, Akira S, Takeda K, Lee J, Takabayashi K, Raz E (2004). *Gastroenterology* **126,** 520–8.
Rakoff-Nahoum S, Paglino J, Eslami-Varzaneh F, Edberg S, Medzhitov R (2004). *Cell* **118,** 229–41.
Rawls JF, Samuel BS, Gordon JI (2004). *Proc Natl Acad Sci USA* **101,** 4596–601.
Rocha B, Vassalli P, Guy-Grand D (1994). *J Exp Med* **180,** 681–6.
Rovin S, Costich ER, Fleming JE, Gordon HA (1965). *Arch Pathol* **79,** 641–3.
Rovin S, Costich ER, Fleming JE, Gordon HA (1966). *J Oral Surg* **24,** 239–46.
Rumio C, Besusso D, Palazzo M, Selleri S, Sfondrini L, Dubini F, Menard S, Balsari A (2004). *Am J Pathol* **165,** 373–81.
Saito H, Kanamori Y, Takemori T, Nariuchi H, Kubota E, Takahashi-Iwanaga H, Iwanaga T, Ishikawa H (1998). *Science* **280,** 275–8.
Sanderson IR (2004). *J Nutr* **134,** 2450S-2454S.
Savage DC (1977). *In* "Microbial Ecology of the Gut" (R. T. J. a. B. Clark T, ed.), pp. 277–310. Academic Press.
Savage DC (1986). *Annu Rev Nutr* **6,** 155–78.
Schaedler RW, Dubs R, Costello R (1965). *J Exp Med* **122,** 77–82.
Seki E, Tsutsui H, Iimuro Y, Naka T, Son G, Akira S, Kishimoto T, Nakanishi K, Fujimoto J (2005). *Hepatology* **41,** 443–50.
Sonnenburg JL, Angenent LT, Gordon JI (2004). *Nat Immunol* **5,** 569–73.
Stappenbeck TS, Hooper LV, Gordon JI (2002). *Proc Natl Acad Sci USA* **99,** 15451–5.
Starling JR, Balish E (1981). *J Reticuloendothel Soc* **30,** 497–505.
Stoddart B, Wilcox MH (2002). *Curr Opin Infect Dis* **15,** 513–8.
Strachan DP (1989). *BMJ* **299,** 1259–60.
Sudo N, Aiba Y, Oyama N, Yu XN, Matsunaga M, Koga Y, Kubo C (2004). *Int Arch Allergy Immunol* **135,** 132–5.
Sudo N, Sawamura S, Tanaka K, Aiba Y, Kubo C, Koga Y (1997). *J Immunol* **159,** 1739–45.

Sun J, Hobert ME, Duan Y, Rao AS, He TC, Chang EB, Madara JL (2005). *Am J Physiol Gastrointest Liver Physiol.*, in press.
Sun J, Hobert ME, Rao AS, Neish AS, Madara JL (2004). *Am J Physiol Gastrointest Liver Physiol* **287,** G220–7.
Takeda K, Kaisho T, Akira S (2003). *Annu Rev Immunol* **21,** 335–376.
Talham GL, Jiang HQ, Bos NA, Cebra JJ (1999). *Infect Immun* **67,** 1992–2000.
Tanaka K, Ishikawa H (2004). *Histol Histopathol* **19,** 907–14.
Treiner E, Duban L, Bahram S, Radosavljevic M, Wanner V, Tilloy F, Affaticati P, Gilfillan S, Lantz O (2003). *Nature* **422,** 164–9.
Umesaki Y, Setoyama H, Matsumoto S, Okada Y (1993). *Immunology* **79,** 32–7.
Umetsu DT, McIntire JJ, Akbari O, Macaubas C, DeKruyff RH (2002). *Nat Immunol* **3,** 715–20.
Wannemuehler MJ, Kiyono H, Babb JL, Michalek SM, McGhee JR (1982). *J Immunol* **129,** 959–65.

Molecular Networks Orchestrating GALT Development

D. Finke (✉) · D. Meier

Center for Biomedicine, Developmental Immunology,
Department of Clinical and Biological Sciences (DKBW),
University of Basel, Mattenstrasse 28, 4058 Basel, Switzerland
Daniela.Finke@unibas.ch

1	Evolution of Gut-Associated Lymphoid Tissue	20
1.1	Phylogenetic Development of Lymphoid Compartments	20
1.2	Inductive Sites for Mucosal Immune Responses	23
1.2.1	Peyer's Patches	23
1.2.2	Alternative Sites for Immune Responses	25
2	Control of Gut-Associated Fetal Lympho-Organogenesis	26
2.1	Mesenteric LN Formation: From Vasculature to Lymph Sacs	26
2.2	Lymphoid Tissue Inducer Cells	28
2.3	PP Anlage Formation and Mesenchymal Cell Differentiation	29
2.4	Isolated Lymphoid Follicles	31
3	Signaling and Transcription Factors Altering the Development of Secondary Lymphoid Organs	32
3.1	Mutations Affecting GALT and LN Development	32
3.2	Genes Regulating the Development of Lymphoid Tissue Inducers	34
3.3	Mutations Affecting Spleen but Not LN and PP Development	35
4	Role of Receptor/Ligand Interactions Between Fetal Hematopoietic and Mesenchymal Cells	36
4.1	TNF Family Members	36
4.2	IL-7 and IL-7R Signaling Pathway	40
4.3	Chemokines and Adhesion Molecules	42
5	Conclusions	44
References		44

Abstract During evolution, the development of secondary lymphoid organs has evolved as a strategy to promote adaptive immune responses at sites of antigen sequestration. Mesenteric lymph nodes (LNs) and Peyer's patches (PPs) are localized in proximity to mucosal surfaces, and their development is coordinated by a series of temporally and spatially regulated molecular events involving the collaboration between hematopoietic, mesenchymal, and, for PPs, epithelial cells. Transcriptional control of cellular differentiation, production of cytokines as well as adhesion molecules are mandatory for organogenesis, recruitment of mature leukocytes, and lymphoid tissue organization. Similar to fetal and neonatal organogenesis, lymphoid tissue neoformation can occur in adult individuals at sites of chronic stimulation via cytokines and TNF-family member molecules. These molecules represent new therapeutic targets to manipulate the microenvironment during autoimmune diseases.

Abbreviations

Ag	Antigen
BM	Bone marrow
CP	Cryptopatch
DC	Dendritic cell
GC	Germinal center
FDC	Follicular dendritic cell
GALT	Gut-associated lymphoid tissue
HEV	High endothelial venule
ICAM-1	Intercellular adhesion molecule 1
IEL	Intraepithelial lymphocytes
Ig	Immunoglobulin
IKK	Inhibitor of κB kinase
ILF	Isolated lymphoid follicle
IL	Interleukin
LN	Lymph node
LT	Lymphotoxin
mAb	Monoclonal antibody
MAdCAM-1	Mucosal addressin cellular adhesion molecule 1
NALT	Nasopharynx-associated lymphoid tissue
NF-κB	Nuclear factor-κB
NIK	Nuclear factor-κB-inducing kinase
NK	Natural killer cell
PNAd	Peripheral node addressin
PP	Peyer's patch
RORγ	Retinoic acid-related orphan receptor γ
TNF	Tumor necrosis factor
TRAF6	TNF receptor-associated factor 6
TRANCE	Tumor necrosis factor-related activation-induced cytokine
VCAM-1	Vascular cell adhesion molecule 1
VEGF	Vascular endothelial growth factor
WT	Wild type

1
Evolution of Gut-Associated Lymphoid Tissue

1.1
Phylogenetic Development of Lymphoid Compartments

With the development of adaptive immunity, the requirement of specialized organs for antigen (Ag) presentation, clonal expansion of T and B lymphocytes, and affinity maturation of B lymphocytes has evolved. Such secondary (immune response-generating) lymphoid organs have B and T cell compartments and are found in all jawed vertebrates. The capacity to form germinal centers (GCs) after immunization and hence, efficient production of high-affinity antibodies (Abs) is a major advantage of secondary lymphoid organs, which are found in endotherms such as aves and mammalians. In this review, we summarize current knowledge on the development of organized GALT such as PPs and isolated lymphoid follicles (ILFs), as well as the organogenesis of mesenteric lymph nodes (LNs).

Already in Agnatha (e.g., jawless fish), primitive lymphoid tissue composed of accumulating lymphocytes and plasma cells is found in the intestinal lamina propria (Good et al. 1966). On close examination, Agnatha do not possess true secondary lymphoid organs but rather develop structures resembling phylogenetic precursors of bone marrow (BM) and thymus (Zapata et al. 1995). Spleen and gut-associated lymphoid tissue (GALT) are the major secondary lymphoid organs whose presence can be traced throughout vertebrate phylogeny. In vertebrates, these organs can possess both hematopoietic and immune response function. The oldest vertebrate group having secondary lymphoid organs is cartilaginous fish (e.g., shark). Sharks develop a GALT and a spleen, which is divided into two distinct areas, the white pulp and the red pulp. Secondary lymphoid organs in sharks are not as organized as in mammals (Flajnik et al. 2003). After immunization, lymphocyte accumulation can occur resembling GCs. Affinity maturation and Ag-driven hypermutation of immunoglobulins (Ig) are detectable in cartilaginous fish (Dooley and Flajnik 2005). B cells producing pentameric IgM Abs in sharks may reflect an equivalent to B1/marginal zone B cells in mammals, because they are strongly induced on stimulation with T-independent Ags (Shankey and Clem 1980). Considering that cartilaginous fish are the most ancient vertebrates possessing secondary lymphoid organs, the recently reported presence of memory B cell responses in sharks underlines the importance of these organs in adaptive immunity (Dooley and Flajnik 2005). Higher amphibians can display a spleen, GALT, and lymphomyeloid nodes in the neck and upper thoracic region, providing sites of lymphoid cell accumulation and Ag trapping. These structures are clearly different from LNs but may represent phylogenetic precursor structures. Primitive lymphoid organs in amphibians lack GCs (Manning and Horton 1982).

LN development occurs far later in evolution than GALT formation, suggesting a necessity of additional lymphoid compartments in higher developed organisms (Table 1). An additional explanation may be that the innate immune system is sufficient to mount a protective host defense in earlier vertebrates. Lymphoid follicles found in reptiles are histologically very different from

Table 1 Phylogenesis of GALT and LN development

	GALT	LN	T/B zone	GC
Agnatha	–	No	No	No
Cartilaginous fish (shark)	+	No	Not before 5 months old	Primitive cell cluster
Bony fish (carp)	+	No	Poorly developed	Primitive cell cluster
Amphibians (*Xenopus*)	+	No	No	Primitive cell cluster
Reptiles (python)	+	(+)	No	FDC-like cells
Aves (chicken)	+ Bursa	+	+	+
Mammalia (mouse)	+	+	+	+

mammalian LNs and appear to filter blood and lymph. Accumulation of T and B cells in the spleen of reptiles and aves is heterogeneous, and full segregation into T and B cell zones is only found in mammals. Although cell clusters resembling GCs were already found in cartilaginous fish, and follicular dendritic cell (FDC)-type resembling cells were described in reptiles, clear GCs containing FDCs were only found in aves and mammals. In mammals, unlike primary hematopoietic organs such as BM and thymus, secondary lymphoid organs are the major sites of immune responses. Altogether, an increasing architectural complexity and specification occurs in lymphoid tissue of higher vertebrates, with LNs occurring only in endothermic vertebrates such as aves and mammals (Zapata and Amemiya 2000).

Adaptive immune responses are only generated if diverse subpopulations of leukocytes are recruited to sites of Ag sequestration. Migration is coordinated by chemokines, a superfamily of specialized cytokines, which directly trigger chemokine receptors expressed by various leukocytes. In vertebrates, the most conserved chemokine receptor is CXCR4, which is even found in Agnatha (Huising et al. 2003; Kuroda et al. 2003). Characterization of mice deficient for CXCR4 or the corresponding chemokine CXCL12 (SDF-1) have revealed that this chemokine receptor-ligand pair is mandatory for organogenesis and fetal hematopoiesis (Nagasawa et al. 1996; Tachibana et al. 1998). CXCR4 is involved in regulating the migration of fetal hematopoietic progenitor cells to primary lymphoid organs (Wright et al. 2002). Analysis of homologous sequences in other species have demonstrated that CXCR4 is the earliest known chemokine receptor found in vertebrates having similar functions to the homolog in mammals (Braun et al. 2002; Liang et al. 2001). Genomic analysis revealed that numerous chemokine/chemokine receptor sequences are found in early vertebrates. However, studies on the significance and function of these chemokines are still lacking, mostly because of the lack of the appropriate specific detection reagents.

1.2
Inductive Sites for Mucosal Immune Responses

1.2.1
Peyer's Patches

The GALT is composed of first, lymphoid organs representing inductive sites for IgA-mediated B cell and for T cell responses and second, the intraepithelial and lamina propria region reflecting effector sites of mucosal immune responses. The intestinal lymphoid organs are not connected to afferent lymphatics but instead locate below a characteristic epithelium, the follicle-associated epithelium (FAE), harboring "microfold" M cells that can transport luminal Ags to lymphoid follicles. The specification of M-cell-containing FAE is regulated via lymphoepithelial cell interactions (El Bahi et al. 2002; Kerneis et al. 1997; Rumbo et al. 2004). Organized GALT are the sites where both IgA^+-commited B cells and memory IgA^+ B cells are generated (Brandtzaeg et al. 2001; Csencsits et al. 1999; Shikina et al. 2004; Wu et al. 1997a).

The most prominent follicles in the intestinal mucosa are PPs located on the antimesenteric wall of the small intestine (Fig. 1A, B). Dependent on the species, their development is completed prenatally or postnatally (Azzali 2003; Makala et al. 2002). In humans, PPs occur more frequently in the ileum than in the jejunum (Makala et al. 2002). The number and size of PPs increase from birth to adolescence, reach a maximum at puberty, persist at particular places of the small intestine, and decrease in size on further aging (Cornes 1965). Although microbial content of the gut may influence the size of PPs, their numbers and positions remain constant. The molecular mechanism of PP formation during ontogeny is discussed in Sect. 2.3. Like other secondary lymphoid organs, the PP microarchitecture is organized in B cell follicles and interfollicular T cell zones (Fig. 2). Similar to LNs, the B cell follicles contain FDCs and small numbers of follicular $CD4^+$ T cells. The interfollicular T zone contains T lymphocytes, $CD11c^+CD11b^-CD8\alpha^+$ dendritic cells (DCs), macrophages and high endothelial venules (HEVs). Circulating lymphocytes enter mucosal lymphoid tissue via HEVs, which consist of cuboidal endothelial cells and express the mucosal addressin cell adhesion molecule 1 (MAdCAM-1). Both $\alpha 4\beta 7$ integrin and L-selectin expressed by lymphocytes

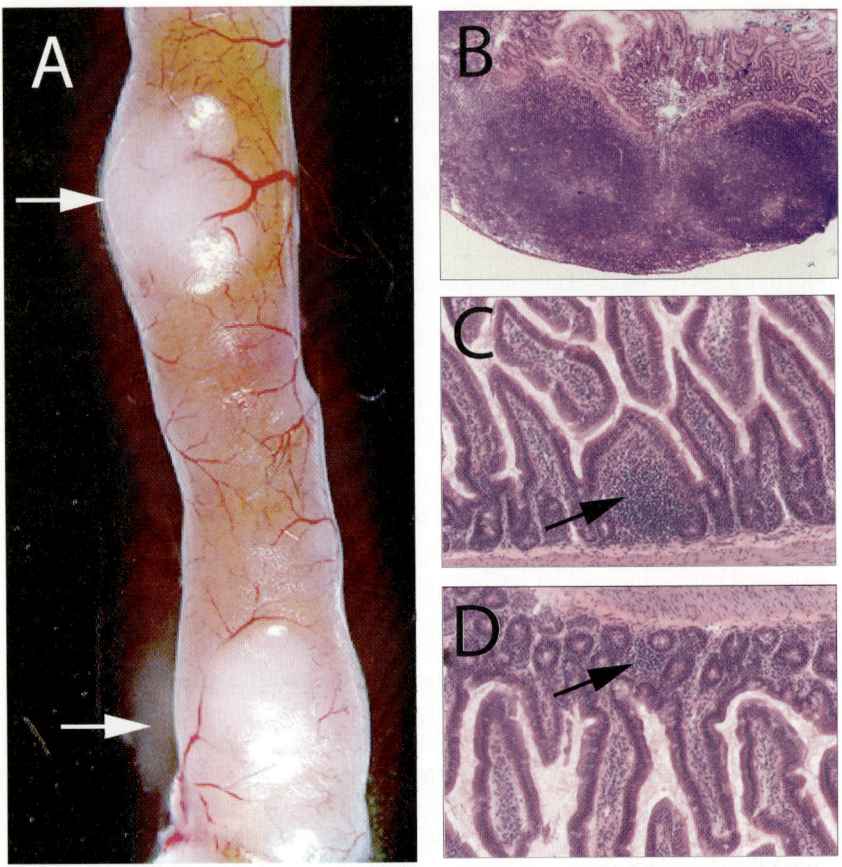

Fig. 1A–D Organized GALT in adult mice. PPs in the small intestine (**A**) and hematoxylin-eosin (HE) staining of frozen sections of PPs in small intestine (**B**). ILF (**C**) and CP (**D**) localized in the small intestine

can bind to MAdCAM-1 and allow migration to the GALT. The subepithelial $CD11c^+CD11b^+CD8\alpha^-$ DCs are localized in close contact to M cells to uptake and process Ags (Iwasaki and Kelsall 2000). Moreover, the intestinal epithelium contains intraepithelial $CD11c^+CD11b^-CD8\alpha^-$ DCs, which can uptake luminal Ags through direct sampling from the lumen (Niess et al. 2005; Rescigno et al. 2001). The lymphatic vessels emerge from lymphoid sinuses draining the serosa and transporting Ags and Ag-loaded DCs via efferent lymphatics to the mesenteric LNs. After Ag exposure, mucosal lymphocytes leave the inductive site and home to mucosal effector sites. PP DCs play a critical role in priming T cells to home back to the intestine (Mora et al. 2003).

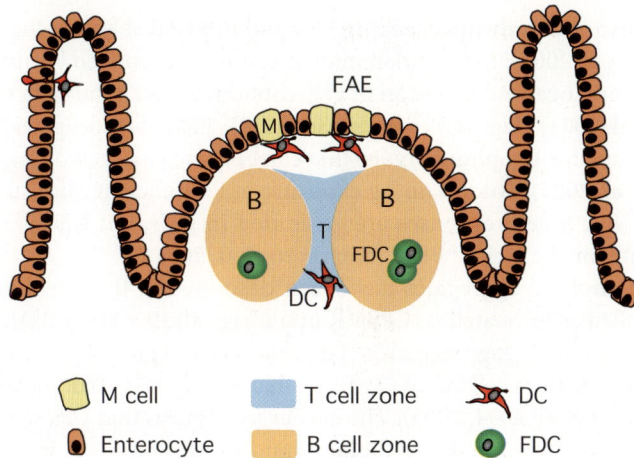

Fig. 2 Schema of the PP and its functional compartments. Below an M-cell-containing FAE, B cell follicles harboring FDCs and T cell zones are localized. DC subsets are found in the epithelium, in the subepithelial region below the FAE and in the T cell zones

1.2.2
Alternative Sites for Immune Responses

Consistent with an essential role of secondary lymphoid organs in adaptive immune responses, splenectomized mice lacking LNs and PPs because of a mutation in the *aly/aly* allele have a severe defect in primary immune responses to a variety of microorganisms (Karrer et al. 1997; Miyawaki et al. 1994), Ags (Rennert et al. 2001), and allografts (Lakkis et al. 2000). When mucosal LNs are removed in normal mice, the spleen can partially replace the function of the LNs, indicating that compartments of primary immune responses are highly dynamic. Similarly, the BM can compensate for the lack of LNs and generate primary immune responses to blood-borne Ags (Feuerer et al. 2003; Tripp et al. 1997). In PP-deficient animals, mucosal immune responses and oral tolerance are still observed, leading to the concept that mesenteric LNs may serve as an alternative site for the induction of immune responses (Spahn et al. 2001; Yamamoto et al. 2000). In addition, inducible lymphoid tissues exist that can replace conventional secondary lymphoid organs during adaptive immune responses. For example, in lymphotoxin (LT) α-deficient mice lacking most LNs, protective immune responses to influenza virus followed by viral clearance result from the formation of induced bronchus-associated lymphoid tissue (iBALT) (Moyron-Quiroz et al. 2004). Perivascular accumulation of leukocytes may be an additional inducible compartment in the lung found during immune responses not only in normal mice but also in *aly/aly* mice lacking LNs and PPs (Pabst and Tschernig 2002; Yasumizu et al. 2000). In the small intestine, multiple isolated lymphoid follicles (ILFs) are localized below an M cell-containing FAE (Hamada et al. 2002; Lorenz et al. 2003) (Fig. 1C) (see also Sect. 2.4). There is strong evidence that ILFs are inducible lymphoid organs that can become enlarged on Ag exposure (Lorenz et al. 2003). Studies on Ag exposure in PP-deficient mice suggest that protective IgA B cell responses are generated in ILFs, but ILFs cannot fully compensate for the lack of PPs (Yamamoto et al. 2004).

Other lymphoid aggregates have been described in the intestinal wall of rodents called cryptopatches (CPs) (Kanamori et al. 1996) (Fig. 1D). CPs were shown to harbor lineage-negative lymphoid cells expressing c-kit (CD117), the receptor for stem cell factor (SCF) but have otherwise striking similarities to ILFs (Pabst et al. 2004, 2005). The earlier hypothesis that CPs represent the sites of extrathymic T cell development and of generation of intraepithelial T cells (IEL) was recently challenged by several studies demonstrating that IEL were thymus derived (Eberl and Littman 2004; Guy-Grand et al. 2003; Pabst et al. 2005). In contrast to mice, CPs are not found in humans, whereas ILFs and lymphocyte aggregates within the muscularis mucosa have been described (Brandtzaeg and Pabst 2004).

An additional component of the gut immune system are colonic lymphoid patches and ILFs in the large intestine (Kweon et al. 2005; Owen et al. 1991). The cellular architecture of these organs seems to be similar to that of PPs and ILFs of the small intestine (Kweon et al. 2005). In colitis models, the generation and hypertrophy of colonic lymphoid patches has been described, indicating a role in adaptive immune responses (Dohi et al. 1999; Spahn et al. 2002).

GALT architecture is not fully developed at birth and needs further maturation to become a specific niche for a functional mucosal adaptive immune system. In mesenteric LNs, the formation of cortex and medulla as well as segregation into B and T cell compartments develop during the first week after birth (Cupedo et al. 2004a). GCs as well as FDC networks are not fully established before 1–2 weeks after birth (Balogh et al. 2002; Pihlgren et al. 2003).

2
Control of Gut-Associated Fetal Lympho-Organogenesis

2.1
Mesenteric LN Formation: From Vasculature to Lymph Sacs

Although mesenteric LNs do not belong to GALT, they represent inductive sites for immune responses to mucosal Ags. The earliest morphologically detectable signs of LN anlagen are groups of capillaries forming the lymph sacs at specific embryonic locations (Lewis 1905; Sabin 1909). The nature of signals that leads to the typical localization of LNs at sites of vascular junctions remains to be defined. One basic concept is that lymphatic vessels are derived from primitive veins. In mice, the first sign of a lymphatic competency is the expression of the endothelial hyaluronan receptor 1 LYVE-1 by a few endothelial cells at E9–9.5 (Oliver 2004). The polarized expression of the homeobox gene Prox 1 in the cardinal vein indicates lymphatic cell-type specification (Wigle et al. 2002; Wigle and Oliver 1999) and conveys endothelial budding from fetal veins by E10.5 leading to sprouting of endothelial cells and formation of lymph sacs. Prox 1 appears to be required to program a population of endothelial progenitor cells into lymphatic endothelial cells. Interleukin (IL)-3 has been recently identified as a soluble factor able to induce the expression of Prox-1 and podoplanin, an additional lymphatic endothelial marker, in human endothelial cells (Groger et al. 2004). Lymph sacs do not develop until elevated levels of vascular endothelial growth factor C (VEGF-C) expression are found in surrounding mesenchymal cells. The corresponding receptor VEGFR3, also known as Fms-like tyrosine kinase 4 (Flt4), is widely expressed on endothelial cells but becomes restricted to the lymphatic endothelium during late development (Kaipainen et al. 1995). The lymphatic specification is accompanied by repression of genes that have been associated with the blood vascular endothelial phenotype (Hong et al. 2002). The separation of lymphatic vessels from the parental vein requires expression of two signaling molecules: SLP-76 and Syk (Abtahian et al. 2003). These proteins are expressed by circulating hematopoietic cells. Mice that have a deletion of these genes have abnormal blood-lymphatic fusions, resulting in hemorrhage and arteriovenous shunting. The exact mechanism of how BM-derived cells contribute to the separation of the two vascular systems remains unknown. The final patterning and maturation of lymphatic endothelial cells requires the expression of angiopoietin-2, neuropilin-2, podoplanin, and secondary lymphoid chemokine (SLC), also known as CCL21 (Breiteneder-Geleff et al. 1999; Gale et al. 2002; Gunn et al. 1998; Kriehuber et al. 2001; Schacht et al. 2003; Yuan et al. 2002). By E15.5, the formation of the lymphatic vascular network is complete. Lymphoid organ anlagen form as a result of invagination of mesenchymal stroma into developing lymph sacs. The lymphoid stroma contains reticular cells, fibroblasts, and endothelial cells. Finally, fetal hematopoietic cells colonize the developing LN anlage, inducing further stromal cell differentiation and tissue maturation.

2.2
Lymphoid Tissue Inducer Cells

CD45$^+$CD4$^+$CD3$^-$ cells are among the earliest hematopoietic cells colonizing the fetal (E13.5) LN anlagen, spleen, stomach, and intestine (Adachi et al. 1997; Mebius et al. 1997; Yoshida et al. 1999). Apart from CD4, these cells are negative for lymphoid, myeloid, or erythroid lineage markers. They can

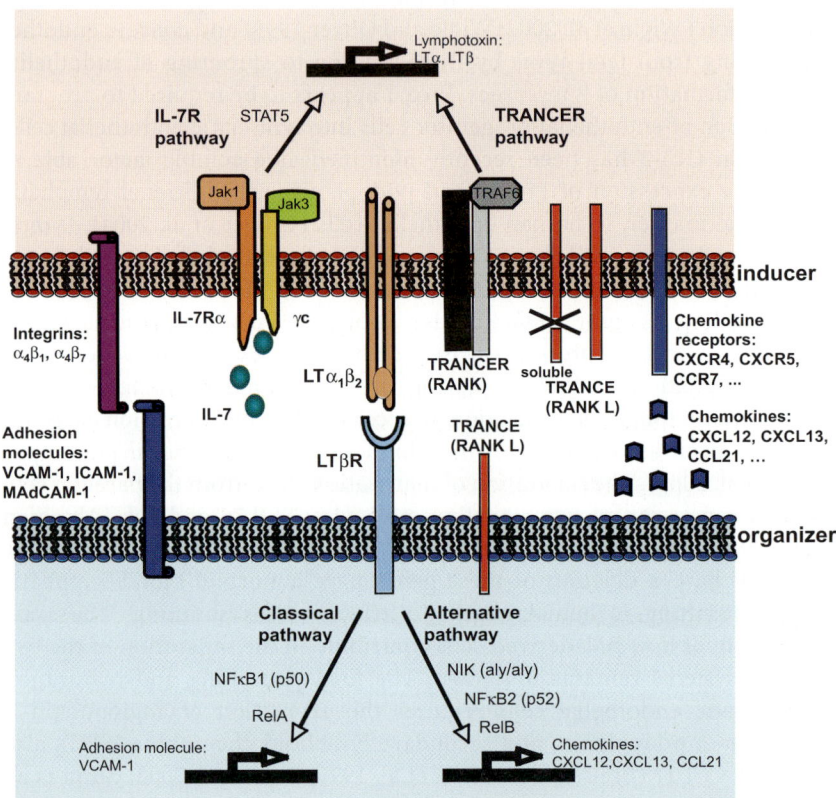

Fig. 3 Schema of the molecular crosstalk between hematopoietic inducer and mesenchymal organizer cells. Inducer cells express LTα$_1$β$_2$, IL-7R, TRANCER, and TRANCE. In addition, integrins (α4β1, α4β7) and chemokine receptors (e.g., CXCR4, CXCR5, CCR7) are found on the surface of inducer cells. The IL-7R or TRANCER signaling pathway can trigger LT expression by the inducer cells. The organizer cells produce the corresponding receptors and ligands, respectively. They express LTβR, TRANCE, and IL-7 and produce adhesion molecules (VCAM-1, ICAM-1, MAdCAM-1) as well as chemokines (CXCL12, CXCL13, CCL21). Signaling via the classic NF-κB1 and NF-κB2 pathway induces gene expression of adhesion molecules and chemokines

be generated from a fetal liver cell subset expressing IL-7 receptor α (IL-7Rα, CD127) and α4β7 integrin (Mebius et al. 2001; Yoshida et al. 2001). IL-7Rα$^+$ progenitor cells colonize peripheral sites before they start to express CD4, as both IL-7Rα$^+$CD4$^+$ and IL-7Rα$^+$CD4$^-$ cells are found in developing lymphoid organs (Yoshida et al. 1999). We and others have shown that fetal or neonatal CD45$^+$CD4$^+$CD3$^-$ cells adoptively transferred into PP-deficient mice are able to restore PP and nasopharynx-associated lymphoid tissue (NALT) development (Finke et al. 2002; Fukuyama et al. 2002). Moreover, in mice, which are unable to generate these cells during development, PPs, LNs, and NALT are not formed (Eberl et al. 2004; Sun et al. 2000; Yokota et al. 1999) (see also Sect. 3.2). The normal splenic architecture in these mutant mice demonstrates that lymphoid tissue inducer cells are not involved in splenic T/B segregation or marginal zone development. Nishikawa and colleagues have termed CD45$^+$CD4$^+$CD3$^-$ cells *inducer cells* collaborating with mesenchymal *organizer cells* in LN and PP development (Nishikawa et al. 2003) (Fig. 3). Inducer cells express α4β1 and α4β7 integrin but are negative for L-selectin (Finke et al. 2002; Mebius et al. 1998). The firm adhesion of inducer and organizer cells needs the activation of α4β1 integrin expressed by the inducer cells via an "inside-out" signal (Finke et al. 2002). Inducer cells express LTα$_1$β$_2$, tumor necrosis factor (TNF)-related activation-induced cytokine receptor (TRANCER, RANK, OPG, TNFRSF11A), TRANCE (RANKL), IL-7Rα, and various chemokine receptors (e.g. CXCR4, CXCR5, and CCR7) (for review, see Finke 2005). LTαβ expression by the inducer cells is critical for the formation of clusters of both CD45$^+$CD4$^+$CD3$^-$ inducer and VCAM-1$^+$ organizer cells (see also Sect. 4.1). The engagement of IL-7R or, alternatively, TRANCER plays an important role in lymphoid organ development, as both signaling pathways stimulate the production of membrane LTα$_1$β$_2$ by the inducer cells.

2.3
PP Anlage Formation and Mesenchymal Cell Differentiation

Visceral mesoderm in vertebrates differentiates into a complex array of cell types, including the smooth muscle layers of the intestine, endothelial cells, and stromal cells. VCAM-1$^+$ MAdCAM-1$^+$ ICAM-1$^+$ stromal cells found in PPs and LNs were termed organizer cells because of their capacity to establish lymphoid tissue compartments and to induce the recruitment of mature lymphocytes via chemokines (Adachi et al. 1997; Nishikawa et al. 2003; Yoshida et al. 1999). The organizer cells express mesenchymal marker such as PDGFRα and PDGFRβ (Hong et al. 2002). Dependent on the expression levels of adhesion molecules, two different types of mesenchymal cells were described in mesenteric or peripheral LNs of newborn mice (Cupedo et al. 2004b).

The two populations express different levels of the homeostatic chemokines CXCL13, CCL19, and CCL21, suggesting that they may differ in the capacity to recruit mature lymphocytes. The initial mesenchymal specification of organizer cells in developing mesenteric LNs and PPs is independent of LTαβ, as single VCAM-1$^+$ organizer cells are found in the fetal gut of LTα-deficient mice (Finke et al. 2002). PP organogenesis proceeds through distinct steps that have been identified histologically. The earliest sign of PP anlage formation are clusters of VCAM-1$^+$ LTβ-R$^+$ mesenchymal cells forming at day 15 of gestation, which appear from the cranial to caudal axis of the small intestine (Adachi et al. 1997). The clustering of mesenchymal cells requires cell-to-cell contact with fetal hematopoietic cells expressing LTα$_1$β$_2$. Hashi and colleagues could show that cluster formation is detectable even in *scid/scid* mice, indicating that this process proceeds independently of mature lymphocytes (Hashi et al. 2001). Ligation of LTβR on the stromal cells leads to activation of two nuclear factor-κB (NF-κB) signaling pathways followed by production of homeostatic chemokines (CXCL12, CXCL13, CCL19, CCL21), proinflammatory chemokines (CCL4, CCL5, CXCL9, CXCL10), adhesion molecules (VCAM-1, MAdCAM-1, ICAM-1, PNAd), IL-7, and TRANCE (Dejardin et al. 2002; Drayton et al. 2003; Ngo et al. 1999; Nishikawa et al. 2000). Similarly, the FAE starts to become specified, to express CCL20 in a LTα$_1$β$_2$-dependent manner (Rumbo et al. 2004) and to recruit cells expressing the corresponding receptor CCR6 such as subepithelial DCs and diverse subsets of memory T cells (Cook et al. 2000; Ebert and McColl 2002; Liao et al. 1999). In addition to CCL20, CCL9 is specifically expressed by the FAE but not by the villus enterocytes (Zhao et al. 2003). Mice lacking CCL9 have a severe reduction of CD11b$^+$ DCs in the subepithelial dome indicating an important role of CCL9 for recruitment of DCs. HEVs forming in the developing PP express MAdCAM-1 and PNAd (Hashi et al. 2001). MAdCAM-1 is the ligand for α4β7 integrin and leukocyte homing receptor L-selectin and is known to function predominantly in the mucosa (Butcher and Picker 1996), but is also transiently expressed in developing peripheral LNs (Mebius et al. 1996). Mature lymphocytes enter the developing PPs via HEV around E18.5. B220$^+$ B cells and CD3$^+$ T cells are diffusely distributed before compartmentalization into B and T cell zones occurs during the first week after birth.

By comparing PP development with formation of other organs, it is likely that morphogens and growth factors are mandatory for the initial differentiation of the mesenchymal cells. During ontogeny, gut morphogenesis occurs through epithelial-mesenchymal cell interactions and is controlled by signaling pathways involving the fibroblast growth factor (FGF), Wnt, bone morphogenetic protein (BMP)/transforming growth factor (TGF-β), Sonic Hedgehog (Shh), and Notch ligands (Finke and Kraehenbuhl 2001).

These morphogens are developmental regulators providing positional information and organizing pattern formation (Christian 2000). Foxl1, a member of the winged helix/forkhead family of DNA binding proteins, is expressed by mesenchymal cells of the developing gut and is required for the control of gastrointestinal proliferation and differentiation (Kaestner et al. 1997). Importantly, in Foxl1$^{-/-}$ mice, a delay in fetal PP development was reported that was correlated with reduced responsiveness of mesenchymal cells to LTαβ as revealed by the downmodulation of LTβR in the fetal gut (Fukuda et al. 2003).

2.4
Isolated Lymphoid Follicles

ILFs are small, solitary follicles localized below a FAE at the antimesenteric site of the small intestine (Hamada et al. 2002) (Fig. 1C). In addition, ILFs are found in the large intestine of mice (Kweon et al. 2005; Owen et al. 1991). Small intestinal ILFs are generated in T- and B cell- deficient mice (RAG-2$^{-/-}$, μm$^{-/-}$, TCRβ$^{-/-}$, IL-7Rα$^{-/-}$, *nu/nu*$^{-/-}$), indicating that they develop independently of mature lymphocytes (Hamada et al. 2002). They are absent in neonatal intestines but can be identified 1 or 4 weeks after birth in BALB/c or C57BL/6 mice, respectively (Hamada et al. 2002). The question of whether ILFs are secondary lymphoid organs or inducible lymphoid structures that are assembling de novo at sites of chronic Ag stimulation was investigated in germ-free mice (Hamada et al. 2002; Lorenz et al. 2003). Whereas Hamada and colleagues reported the presence of ILFs in germ-free BALB/c mice, Lorenz et al. could not find mature ILFs in germ-free C57BL/6 animals (Hamada et al. 2002; Lorenz et al. 2003). The discrepancy between the two studies might be explained by the use of different mouse strains and detection methods or by the fact that small B cell assemblies were not considered as ILFs in one of the studies. These data demonstrate that ILFs can develop in the absence of external stimuli but, depending on mouse strain, can proceed through several histological maturation steps before Ag stimulation in adult mice can enlarge the structures. In this regard, it was shown that alterations in the bacterial flora by antibiotic treatment prevented ILF hyperplasia that was induced by the deficiency of activation-induced cytidine deaminase (Fagarasan et al. 2002).

There is a debate about the developmental and functional relationship of ILFs and PPs. Treatment of BALB/ c mice during gestation with anti-IL-7Rα monoclonal Abs (mAbs) or LTβR-Ig fusion protein disrupted PP but not ILF development, arguing for different requirements of PP and ILF organogenesis during ontogeny (Hamada et al. 2002). However, in C57BL/6 mice with a deletion of IL-7Rα, LTα or in mice with the *aly/aly* mutation, ILFs in adult animals were strongly reduced in number or even absent (Hamada et al. 2002). These diverse results may be explained by either the different mouse strains used in this study or by the lower efficiency of in utero administration of Ig compared to genetic deletion of the target genes. Several arguments speak in favor of the hypothesis that ILFs represent "immature-type" PPs. First, both PPs and ILFs are localized at the antimesenteric border and are enriched in the distal part of the small intestine. Second, they are overlaid by an M cell-containing epithelium. Third, they have a similar architecture containing B cells, T cells, GCs, and VCAM-1$^+$ stromal cells. Fourth, LTβR signaling controls both PP and postnatal ILF development in small and large intestine (Hamada et al. 2002; Kweon et al. 2005) (see also Sect. 4.1). A number of mutant mice lacking PP macroscopically retain solitary intestinal follicles, which are detectable only by microscopy analysis. Further studies are required to elucidate the relationship of ILF and PP ontogeny in the gastrointestinal tract. For example, it will be important to test whether genes exist that exclusively affect the development of ILFs but not PPs.

3
Signaling and Transcription Factors Altering the Development of Secondary Lymphoid Organs

3.1
Mutations Affecting GALT and LN Development

One of the most important signals mediating lympho-organogenesis is the ligation of LTβR on stromal cells by membrane-bound LT$α_1β_2$, expressed by hematopoietic cells. Activation of LTβR triggers two NF-κB signaling pathways (Dejardin et al. 2002) (Fig. 3). The classic (canonical) NF-κB activity consists of the p50-RelA heterodimer (NF-κB1) and requires the inhibitor of κB kinase (IKK)γ and IKKβ subunits of the IKK complex (Weih and Caamano 2003). The alternative pathway involves phosphorylation of the precursor molecule p100 (subunit of NF-κB2) by the NF-κB-inducing kinase (NIK) and IKKα.

A mouse strain with a spontaneous, autosomal recessive single gene mutation, termed alymphoplasia (*aly*), was characterized by the absence of LNs and PPs, disorganized splenic and thymic architecture, and immunodeficiency (Miyawaki et al. 1994; Shinkura et al. 1996). The origin of the defect is a point mutation within NIK that retains catalytic activity (Shimizu et al. 1999). The precise function of NIK was uncovered by the generation of NIK-deficient mice (Yin et al. 2001). NIK is involved not only in the LTβR but also in the CD40, BAFF-R, and to some extent the toll-like receptor signaling cascade (Weih and Caamano 2003). Interestingly, *aly/aly* mice have normal expression levels of most adhesion molecules in the spleen and intestine, although MAdCAM-1$^+$ cells are absent from the spleen (Koike et al. 1997). In addition, ligation of the LTβR was shown to induce a normal increase in VCAM-1 mRNA levels in *aly/aly* cells, although VCAM-1 protein levels were not induced (Dejardin et al. 2002; Matsumoto et al. 1999). Some homeostatic chemokines (CCL21) were normally expressed, whereas others were reduced or absent (CCL19, CXCL13) (Fagarasan et al. 2000). Therefore, the severe phenotype of *aly/aly* mice may not exclusively rely on a defective LTβR-signaling in stromal cells. Supporting this idea, NIK was shown to be involved in the chemokine signaling pathway of hematopoietic cells, causing an intrinsic migratory defect of *aly/aly* lymphocytes (Fagarasan et al. 2000).

Studies in mice with mutations in individual Rel/NF-κB family members have demonstrated that both NF-κB1 and NF-κB2 signaling pathways are critical for PP and LN organogenesis and formation of lymphoid tissue architecture, although NF-κB1-deficient mice show a milder phenotype. RelB (NF-κB2-subunit)-deficient mice lack all LNs (Weih et al. 1995). PPs are barely detectable in RelB$^{-/-}$, NF-κB2$^{-/-}$, and IKKα$^{-/-}$ mice, whereas in NF-κB1$^{-/-}$ mice, LNs are normal, although PPs appear to be reduced in size and number (Matsushima et al. 2001; Paxian et al. 2002; Weih and Caamano 2003; Yilmaz et al. 2003). Weih and colleagues could show that the production of B cell follicle-forming chemokines such as CXCL13 by stromal cells was impaired in the absence of functional RelB (Weih et al. 2001). RelA (NF-κB1-subunit)-deletion is lethal in mice at E15 because of TNF receptor (TNFR)I-mediated apoptosis in hepatocytes. To circumvent this problem, Alcamo and colleagues have generated RelA-TNFRI-double-deficient mice. Whereas TNFRI$^{-/-}$ mice generate small PPs, RelA$^{-/-}$TNFRI$^{-/-}$ mice completely lack peripheral and mucosal LNs and PPs because of a defect in stromal cells (Alcamo et al. 2002). Importantly, both RelA$^{-/-}$TNFRI$^{-/-}$ mice and RelB$^{-/-}$ mice have normal numbers of lymphoid tissue inducer cells, indicating that functional NF-κB pathways are dispensable for the generation of the fetal hematopoietic cells but crucial for mesenchymal cell specification during LN and PP development.

NKX homeodomain proteins are members of the transcription factors implicated in controlling cell type specification, growth, and proliferation. A vertebrate member of the NK-2 class of homeobox genes is NKX2.3, found in midgut and hindgut mesoderm and spleen (Pabst et al. 1997). In mice, targeted deletion of the NKX2.3 gene leads to abnormal gut development, primarily in the distal part of the small intestine (Pabst et al. 1999). Depending on the genetic background, occasional asplenia was found in the NKX2.3-deficient mice. All mutant mice were shown to have morphological defects in the spleen and to lack marginal zones and expression of MAdCAM-1, a target gene of NKX2.3 transactivation, in secondary lymphoid organs (Pabst et al. 2000; Wang et al. 2000). The reduction of MAdCAM-1 expression was not a consequence of loss of FDCs, as normal numbers of FDC-M1$^+$ cells could be detected in the white pulp (Wang et al. 2000). PPs were macroscopically absent, and only by histological analysis were small PPs with reduced follicle number occasionally found (Pabst et al. 2000; Wang et al. 2000). Segregation into T and B cell zones occurred normally in rudimentary PPs and in LNs except in mesenteric LNs, where T cells were abnormally found in the cortical area of the LN. Obviously, the complexity of the phenotype of mutant mice requires additional investigations to better understand the role of NKX2.3 for PP organogenesis and mesenteric LN organization.

The common γ chain (γc) of the IL-2 family receptors (IL-2, IL-4, IL-7, IL-9, and IL-15) is linked to a Janus family tyrosine kinase JAK3. In IL-7Rα-, JAK3-, and γc-deficient mice, only mesenteric and occasionally brachial and axillary LNs were found, whereas inguinal, popliteal, sacral, and iliac LNs as well as PPs were undetectable. GCs were not found in secondary lymphoid organs (Adachi et al. 1998; Cao et al. 1995; Park et al. 1995). These data indicate that the IL-7R-signaling pathway is mandatory for PP and some LN organogenesis as well as GC formation (see also Sect. 4.2). Importantly, NALT development occurs independently of IL-7R, LTβR, and NIK signaling, providing evidence for a differential regulation of mucosal lymphoid tissue formation (Fukuyama et al. 2002).

3.2
Genes Regulating the Development of Lymphoid Tissue Inducers

Little is known about the origin and the developmental regulation of CD45$^+$CD4$^+$CD3$^-$ lymphoid tissue inducer cells. They are found in normal numbers in RAG-deficient, *scid*, or athymic *nude* mice indicating first, that they develop independently of RAG recombination and second, that they do not require a functional thymus for their generation (Mebius et al. 1997). However, they are barely detectable in mice lacking the basic helix-loop-helix inhibitor Id2 (Yokota et al. 1999). Id2 plays a crucial role in lineage commitment and cell specification of hematopoietic cells and was found to be expressed in lymphoid tissue inducer cells of normal mice (Yokota et al. 1999). Consistent with the lack of CD45$^+$CD4$^+$CD3$^-$ lymphoid tissue inducer cells, Id2$^{-/-}$ mice failed to develop PPs and LNs. In contrast, splenic architecture with marginal zone and germinal center formation was completely normal, clearly demonstrating that CD45$^+$CD4$^+$CD3$^-$ lymphoid tissue inducer cells are dispensable for the maturation of splenic architecture.

The retinoic acid-related orphan receptor (ROR)γt belongs to a family of nuclear hormone receptors regulating development and differentiation (Mangelsdorf et al. 1995). RORγt has been detected only in double-positive (DP) $CD4^+CD8^+$ thymocytes and $CD45^+CD4^+CD3^-$ lymphoid tissue inducer cells (Sun et al. 2000) and was shown to have an anti-apoptotic function in DP thymocytes through the expression of the anti-apoptotic factor Bcl-xL. Deletion of RORγt interrupts the development of LNs and PPs while retaining the organogenesis of spleen and NALT (Eberl et al. 2004; Harmsen et al. 2002; Kurebayashi et al. 2000; Sun et al. 2000). The failure to generate LNs and PPs was accompanied by the absence of $CD45^+CD4^+CD3^-$ cells in these mice (Eberl et al. 2004; Sun et al. 2000). For more detailed information, see the chapter by Ivanov et al. in this volume.

The *Ikaros* gene, a member of the kruppel family of zinc finger DNA-binding proteins, is required for the development of early hematopoietic progenitor cells (Georgopoulos et al. 1994). Mice carrying an Ikaros mutation fail to develop mature T, B, and NK cells and DCs (Wang et al. 1996; Wu et al. 1997b). In addition, these mice show defective peripheral LN and PP formation (Georgopoulos et al. 1997; Wang et al. 1996). One explanation could be that, through the early block of hematopoiesis, lymphoid tissue inducer cells are not generated in these mice, although this hypothesis remains to be tested.

3.3
Mutations Affecting Spleen but Not LN and PP Development

Several studies in vertebrates have indicated that the spleen develops from the dorsal mesogastrium in close proximity to the pancreas. Therefore, the ontogeny of the spleen is clearly different from that of LNs and PPs. Nevertheless, studies on the origin of asplenia can help to understand common rules in mesenchymal cell differentiation during secondary lymphoid organ formation. In mice having a deletion of *Hox11* gene, which encodes a homeobox-like DNA-binding protein, normal spleen organogenesis occurs until E11.5, but by E13.5 the spleen anlage has almost completely disappeared (Dear et al. 1995; Roberts et al. 1994). The early differentiation of mesenchymal cells as well as the capacity for recruitment of hematopoietic cells is clearly not affected. However, cell maintenance and further differentiation are inhibited in the absence of Hox11, clearly demonstrating that induction and maintenance of organ formation are differentially regulated (Kanzler and Dear 2001). It is possible that $Hox11^{-/-}$ mesenchymal cells lack factors such as adhesion molecules required for cellular aggregation and retention. *Bapx1* gene, the mouse homologue of *Drosophila* "bagpipes" and *Capsulin*, a basic helix-loop-helix transcription factor gene, are required for Hox11 expression, reflected by the absence of a spleen in gene-deleted mice (Lettice et al. 1999; Lu et al. 2000; Tribioli and Lufkin 1999). Other mutations were described affecting the early steps of spleen formation before the invasion of hematopoietic progenitor cells (Herzer et al. 1999; Searle 1964; Sock et al. 2004; Suto et al. 1995). Thus, different genes are required for the early and late steps of secondary lymphoid organ development.

4
Role of Receptor/Ligand Interactions Between Fetal Hematopoietic and Mesenchymal Cells

4.1
TNF Family Members

Members of the TNF/TNFR superfamily play a major role in multiple pathways that orchestrate lymphoid organogenesis, activation, differentiation, and survival (Locksley et al. 2001). Both TNFα and LTα can be secreted as homotrimers and signal via either TNFRI (TNFR55) or TNFRII (TNFR75) (Weih and Caamano 2003). LTβ is a type II integral membrane-bound protein that can form a heterotrimer with LTα. $LT\alpha_1\beta_2$ heterotrimer binds to the LTβR. Several members of the TNF/TNFR family have been implicated in peripheral LN and PP induction and organization of the splenic architecture. LTβR is ubiquitously expressed (e.g., stromal cells, HEVs, DCs, monocytes, DP thymocytes), whereas the corresponding ligand $LT\alpha_1\beta_2$ is restricted to hematopoietic cells in lymphoid organs and the intestine (Browning and French 2002; Gommerman and Browning 2003). $LT\alpha_1\beta_2$ expressed by the CD4$^+$CD3$^-$ inducer cells triggers LTβR expressed by stromal cells and, in the case of FAE development, by epithelial cells. In mice lacking LTβ on B cells, LNs and PPs occur normally (Tumanov et al. 2002), indicating that CD4$^+$CD3$^-$ inducer cells are the major population triggering LTβR signaling in stromal cells during ontogeny. This is a critical step for PP and LN organogenesis demonstrated by analysis of mutant mice in which the LTβR or LTα is deleted (Table 2). LTβR$^{-/-}$ and LTα$^{-/-}$ mice completely lack PPs, solitary follicles (ILFs, CPs) in the small intestine, and LNs, although the presence of small rudimentary mesenteric LN anlagen at birth was reported in LTα$^{-/-}$ mice (Fu et al. 1997a). In contrast, LNs and PPs, although reduced in size and number, develop in TNFRI$^{-/-}$ or TNFRII$^{-/-}$ mice (Erickson et al. 1994; Neumann et al. 1996; Pasparakis et al. 1997; Pfeffer et al. 1993; Rothe et al. 1993), and in TNF$^{-/-}$ mice, LNs and PPs develop normally (Pasparakis et al. 1996). Rennert and colleagues could show that treatment of mice with a fusion protein blocking LTβR engagement prevented LN and PP development in a temporally and spatially coordinated manner (Rennert et al. 1996). Conversely, in utero injection of agonist Abs specific for LTβR was able to restore LN development in LTα$^{-/-}$ mice (Rennert et al. 1998). Approximately 75% of LTβ$^{-/-}$ mice retain the capacity to form mesenteric LNs, a phenotype that is rarely found in LTα$^{-/-}$ mice (Alimzhanov et al. 1997). This observation, together with the occasional formation of rudimentary mesenteric LNs and cervical LNs in LTα$^{-/-}$ mice, indicates an incomplete penetrance of the gene deficiency (Banks et al. 1995; De Togni et al. 1994). In contrast to gene targeting of LTβR in mice leading to the complete absence of all LNs and PPs (Futterer et al. 1998), in utero inhibition of LTβR by injecting an antagonist receptor fusion protein was insufficient to block organogenesis of all LNs. The development of mucosa-draining LNs such as mesenteric, cervical, sacral and lumbal LNs occurred normally, although PPs and some peripheral LNs were absent in LTβR-Ig-treated mice (Rennert et al. 1996, 1997, 1998). Only the combination of both inhibition of LTβR and TNFRI-signaling was sufficient to completely abrogate organogenesis of all LNs. Obviously, fusion protein-treatment is less efficient than gene silencing and hence, other ligands triggering TNFRI such as TNFα or LTα$_3$ may surpass fusion protein-mediated inhibition of LTβR-signaling during mesenteric LN development. Evidence for functional synergism of TNFRI and LTβR ligands is further given by crossing LTβ$^{-/-}$ mice onto the TNFRI-deficient background, resulting in loss of mesenteric LNs, in addition to the loss of PPs and peripheral LNs (Koni and Flavell 1998) (Table 2). The consequence of inhibiting either the LTβR or the TNFRI signaling pathway on the organization of the GALT was studied in adult mice (Yamamoto et al. 2004). Histological analysis showed that in LTβR Ig- but not TNFRI Ig-treated mice, the follicle formation and segregation into T- and B cell zones was completely disrupted in mesenteric LNs, and the number of FDCs was severely reduced. Furthermore, the average number of PPs in LTβR-Ig-treated mice was reduced from 6–10 visible PP to 2–4, confirming the critical role of LTβR even after birth (Dohi et al. 2001). Taken together, signaling pathways through LTβR but not TNFRI are mandatory for the maintenance of mesenteric LNs and PPs in adult mice.

LIGHT is a second ligand for LTβR. Although normal LN development occurs in the absence of LIGHT, combined immune defects such as in LIGHT$^{-/-}$LTβ$^{-/-}$ mice result in a more severe phenotype than LTβ$^{-/-}$ mice. This is similar to the effect of combined deletion of TNFRp55 and LTβ, suggesting that several TNF family members and both LTβR and TNFR can contribute to secondary lymphoid organ formation (Kuprash et al. 1999; Scheu et al. 2002; Wang et al. 2002; Wang et al. 2001).

Table 2 Organized GALT and MLN development in mutant mouse strains

Mutant mouse strains	GALT PP	Solitary follicles	MLN	Reference
TNF family members and adapters				
$LT\alpha^{-/-}$	–	–	–[1]	De Togni 1994, Banks 1995, Hamada 2002
$LT\beta^{-/-}$	–	–	+[2]	Koni 1998, Alimzhanov 1997, Papst 2005
B $LT\beta^{-/-}$	+	nd	+	Tumanov 2002
$LT\beta R^{-/-}$	–	–	–	Futterer 1998, Lorenz 2003
$LIGHT^{-/-}$	+	nd	+	Scheu 2002
$LIGHT^{-/-} LT\beta^{-/-}$	–	nd	–[1]	Scheu 2002
$TNF^{-/-}$	+	nd	+	Pasparakis 1996
$TNF^{-/-} LT\beta^{-/-}$	–	nd	+	Kuprash 1999
$TNFRI^{-/-}$	(+)[3]	–	+	Neumann 1996, Pasparakis 1997, Lorenz 2003
$TNFRI^{-/-} LT\beta^{-/-}$	–	nd	–	Koni 1998
$TNFRII^{-/-}$	+	(+)[3]	+	Erickson 1994, Lorenz 2003
$TRANCE^{-/-}$	+	nd	–	Kong 1999, Kim 2000
$TRANCER^{-/-}$	+	nd	–	Dougall 1999
$TRAF6^{-/-}$	+	nd	–	Naito 1999
NFκB pathway				
aly/ aly$^{-/-}$	–	–	–	Miyawaki 1994, Hamada 2002
$NIK^{-/-}$	–	nd	–	Yin 2001
$NF\text{-}\kappa B1^{-/-}$	(+)[3]	nd	+	Paxian 2002
$RelA^{-/-} TNFR\text{-}1^{-/-}$	–	nd	–	Alcamo 2002
$NF\text{-}\kappa B2^{-/-}$	–	nd	+	Paxian 2002, Yilmaz 2003
$IKK\alpha^{-/-}$	–	nd	–	Matsushimi 2001
$RelB^{-/-}$	–	nd	–	Weih 1995
IL-7R pathway				
$IL\text{-}7^{-/-}$	–[4]	(+)[3]	+	Laky 2000, Nishikawa 2003
$IL\text{-}7R\alpha^{-/-}$	–	(+)[3]	+	Adachi 1998, Hamada 2002, Luther 2003
$\gamma c^{-/-}$	–	nd	+	Cao 1995
$Jak3^{-/-}$	–	nd	+	Park 1995
$STAT5^{-/-}$	–[4]	(+)[3]	+	Kang 2004
Gene regulatory factors				
$Id2^{-/-}$	–	nd	–	Yokota 1999
$ROR\gamma^{-/-}$	–	nd	–	Sun 2000, Kurebayashi 2000

Table 2 (continued)

Mutant mouse strains	GALT PP	Solitary follicles	MLN	Reference
IKAROS$^{-/-}$	−	nd	−	Georgopoulos 1994, Wang 1996
NKX2.3	−	(+)³	+	Wang 2000, Pabst 2000
Chemokines and chemokine receptors				
CXCR5$^{-/-}$	−¹	nd	+	Forster 1996
CXCL13$^{-/-}$	−¹	nd	+	Ansel 2000
CXCL13$^{-/-}$ IL-7R$\alpha^{-/-}$	−	nd	−	Luther 2003
CCR7$^{-/-}$	+	nd	+	Forster 1999
CXCR5$^{-/-}$ CCR7$^{-/-}$	−¹	nd	+	Ohl 2003a
Plt/plt	+	nd	+	Nakano 1998

Organized GALT is composed of PPs and solitary aggregates (ILFs, CPs) in the small intestine. + normal; − undetectable; nd not detectable; 1) occasionally; 2) 75% have mesenteric LNs; 3) strongly reduced number; 4) VCAM-1$^+$ cell cluster present

TRANCER, a member of the TNFR superfamily, was described as osteoclast differentiation factor (Lacey et al. 1998). Importantly, TRANCER is expressed by lymphoid tissue inducer and CD45$^+$ hematopoietic cells (Kim et al. 2000). In fetal and adult mice, the corresponding ligand TRANCE is found in lymphoid organs such as BM, thymus, spleen, LNs, and PPs, whereas in humans, TRANCE expression is highly restricted to LNs (Lacey et al. 1998). Kim and colleagues could show that, in LNs of fetal mice, TRANCE is expressed by lymphoid tissue inducer cells (Kim et al. 2000). Targeted deletion experiments revealed that TRANCE is essential for mesenteric and peripheral LN development except for cervical LNs (30% of TRANCE$^{-/-}$ mice examined) but is dispensable for PP development (Kim et al. 2000; Kong et al. 1999; Wong et al. 1997). This was also confirmed by studies in TRANCER$^{-/-}$ mice, which show a complete lack of LNs but only a slight reduction in size and number of PPs (Dougall et al. 1999). Similarly, mice lacking TRAF-6, the signal transducer of TRANCER, had a defect in LN organization (Naito et al. 1999). As TRANCE and TRANCER are expressed by the inducer cells, it is possible that the receptor engagement occurs in an autocrine manner, although mesenchymal cells may be alternative producers of TRANCE. The effect of recombinant TRANCE was shown to depend on induction of LT$\alpha\beta$ production by the inducer cells (Yoshida et al. 2002). Nevertheless, neither TRANCE overexpression in LT$\alpha^{-/-}$ mice nor agonist anti-LTβR mAb treatment in pregnant TRANCE$^{-/-}$ mice could restore LN organogenesis (Cupedo et al. 2002; Kim et al. 2000)/ indicating that both TRANCE and LTαβ are mandatory for LN development. Interestingly, in TRANCE$^{+/-}$ mice, some peripheral LNs were lacking but mesenteric LN development occurred normally. These results indicate that lymphoid organogenesis may be regulated by threshold-dependent signals and, in the case of mesenteric LNs, stromal cells either require less activation for differentiation or, alternatively, can be stimulated through a combination of TRANCE with alternative factors. Therefore, we propose that the requirements for TNF family ligands are distinct in different secondary lymphoid organs.

Studies on the receptor-ligand interactions during ILF formation have revealed that in utero treatment with either LTβR Ig or TNFRI/II Ig does not inhibit the formation of ILFs (Hamada et al. 2002; Lorenz et al. 2003), and even higher numbers and size of ILF were observed in both small and large intestine (Kweon et al. 2005; Lorenz et al. 2003; Yamamoto et al. 2004). In contrast, mice treated with LTβR fusion protein after birth or mutant mice lacking either LTα or LTβR failed to form ILFs (Lorenz et al. 2003; Yamamoto et al. 2004). Similarly, TNFRI$^{-/-}$ mice were reported to lack ILFs (Lorenz et al. 2003), although blocking of the TNFRI signaling pathway with a fusion protein after birth was less efficient (Yamamoto et al. 2004). In TNFRII$^{-/-}$ mice, ILF numbers were strongly reduced (Lorenz et al. 2003). Taken together, the data demonstrate that ILF formation and maintenance after birth are controlled by LTβR and to a lesser extent by TNFRI/II. Inflammatory signals augmenting TNFα production in the gut may trigger ILF hypertrophy via activation of TNFRI and II. Studies in LTα$^{-/-}$ and LTβR$^{-/-}$ mice have indicated that CP development is abrogated and, similar to PPs and ILFs, specifically depends on membrane-bound LTα$_1$β$_2$ interactions with LTβR. In contrast to PPs or LNs, the adoptive transfer of wild type (WT) BM to adult LTα$^{-/-}$ mice restored ILF and CP development, indicating that these structures were inducible by hematopoietic cells (Fu and Chaplin 1999; Fu et al. 1997b; Lorenz et al. 2003; Taylor et al. 2004). As ILFs are detectable in mice lacking T and B cells, other LTαβ-expressing BM-derived cells must be required for ILF formation. Interestingly, the *aly/aly* mutation did not abrogate CP formation, indicating that alternative pathways could compensate for the mutation in the LTβR-NIK pathway (Taylor et al. 2004).

4.2
IL-7 and IL-7R Signaling Pathway

The IL-7R complex is composed of two subunits, the IL-7Rα chain and the common γ chain (γc) (for review, see Kang and Der 2004). The pleiotropic cytokine IL-7, known to stimulate IL-7R signaling, was identified as an important factor for proliferation and homeostasis of lymphocytes (Fry and Mackall 2002). In mice lacking one of the IL-7R subunits or Jak3, B and T cell development and the formation of PPs were severely disturbed (Adachi et al. 1998; Cao et al. 1995; Park et al. 1995). In embryonic Jak3$^{-/-}$ mice, VCAM$^+$ organizer cells failed to aggregate, although IL-7Rα$^+$ inducer cells were present in the gut, suggesting that inducer cell production and migration to the intestine were not severely affected (Adachi et al. 1998). However, the hematopoietic cells appeared to require an activation signal via IL-7R/Jak3 in order to initiate organizer/inducer cell assembly. Accordingly, the single injection of a blocking anti-IL-7Rα mAb before gestation day 16.5 was sufficient to inhibit the development of PPs (Yoshida et al. 1999). The same mAb was unable to affect LN development or splenic organization, suggesting that IL-7R is dispensable for the development of LNs and maturation of the splenic architecture. In IL-7Rα-, JAK3-, and γc-deficient mice, however, except for mesenteric and occasionally brachial and axillary LNs, inguinal, popliteal, sacral, and iliac LNs as well as PPs were reported to be absent. (Adachi et al. 1998; Cao et al. 1995; Kang et al. 2004; Luther et al. 2003; Park et al. 1995). Mice lacking STAT5, a kinase involved in the IL-7R-signaling-pathway, lack PPs although LN development is normal (Kang et al. 2004). These data indicate that the IL-7R-signaling pathway is mandatory for PP development and the maturation of some LNs. IL-7 was shown to be expressed in the fetal intestine as well as in primary lymphoid organs (Murray et al. 1998). Nishikawa and colleagues reported that fetal intestinal organizer cells can produce IL-7 (Nishikawa et al. 2003). One of the key functions of IL-7 during lymphoid organogenesis is the induction of LTαβ expression by lymphoid tissue inducer cells (Luther et al. 2003; Yoshida et al. 2002). It is conceivable that the availability of cytokines produced by stromal cells varies between the different LNs and the intestine. Other cytokines, such as TRANCE, may compensate for the lack of IL-7R engagement in some but not all LNs. Evidence for the partial redundancy of the IL-7R and TRANCER/TRAF6 signaling pathway come from studies in mice lacking TRAF6, the adapter molecule of the TRANCER signaling pathway. These mice completely lack LNs but have normal PPs. Intraembryonic IL-7 injection at E13.5–14.5 rescued LN genesis, although histological analysis revealed that the LNs still lacked T/B segregation and FDC development (Yoshida et al. 2002). These data suggest that IL-7R signaling is able to replace TRANCER signaling for LN induction but not for maturation into segregated compartments.

Intriguingly, mice double deficient in the IL-7Rα chain and the fms-like tyrosine kinase-3 receptor (flt3 or flk2) are completely deficient in mesenteric LNs and PPs, whereas IL-7Rα or flt3 single-deficient mice have mesenteric LNs (Sitnicka et al. 2003). Flt3, a cytokine receptor expressed on early hematopoietic progenitors, is known to be important for B cell development, and hence flt3$^{-/-}$ mice lack early B cell progenitors (pro-B cells), including common lymphoid progenitors (Sitnicka et al. 2002). The data obtained from double-deficient mice suggest that the two cytokine receptors, flt3 and IL-7R, have a synergistic effect on LN development.

Similar to IL-7R$^{-/-}$ mice, mature PPs are absent in IL-7$^{-/-}$ mice. However, unlike IL-7R$^{-/-}$ mice, IL-7$^{-/-}$ mice can form rudimentary intestinal VCAM-1$^+$ cell clusters at birth (Laky et al. 2000; Nishikawa et al. 2003) (Table 2). IL-7 transgene expression in enterocytes of IL-7$^{-/-}$ mice was able to restore PP size, follicular organization, and CP numbers (Laky et al. 2000). Altogether, these data indicate that although intestinal IL-7 can promote lympho-organogenesis in the gut, additional ligands and receptor pathways may exist that function synergistically to induce PP formation in a threshold-dependent manner. The spatial restriction of IL-7 expression to the fetal gut and to primary lymphoid organs (thymus, BM) may explain why a network of alternative cytokines regulating secondary lymphoid organ development has evolved.

4.3
Chemokines and Adhesion Molecules

Trafficking of mature B and T lymphocytes to lymphoid organs is regulated by homeostatic chemokines (e.g., CXCL12, CXCL13, CCL19, and CCL21) expressed by endothelial and stromal cells (Cyster 2005). One of the intriguing questions that have not been answered yet is how lymphoid tissue inducer cells home to putative sites of LN and PP development. In vitro, inducer cells are responsive to a number of chemokines (CXCL13, CCL19, CCL21) (Honda et al. 2001), but in vivo, expression levels of chemokines in the developing embryo seem to be rather low (Cupedo et al. 2004a). Inducer cells were shown to express mRNA for CXCR5 and CCR7 (Hashi et al. 2001; Mebius et al. 1997), and CXCR4 protein was found on their surface (Finke et al. 2002). These chemokine receptors and their corresponding chemokine ligands CXCL13, CCL19, CCL21, and CXCL12 appear to act simultaneously during lympho-organogenesis. Mice deficient in CXCR5 or CXCL13 lack most PPs and most LNs, except for cervical, facial, brachial, and mesenteric LNs (Ansel et al. 2000; Forster et al. 1996; Ohl et al. 2003b). CCR7$^{-/-}$ or CCL19$^{-/-}$ and CCL21$^{-/-}$ deficient (*plt/plt*) mice have a normal phenotype with respect to secondary lymphoid organ development (Forster et al. 1999; Nakano et al. 1998). However, by combining the ablation of CXCR5 and CCR7, LN organogenesis was almost completely abrogated. Mesenteric LNs were still present, but they had a disturbed architecture most likely due to an impaired migration of B cells (Ohl et al. 2003a). Similarly, combining the deficiency of CXCL13 with the plt mutation caused an occasional block of brachial and axillary LN development, but the mice retained the capacity to form mesenteric LNs. These results display a cooperative function of CXCR5 and CCR7 during LN development. The development of the mesenteric LNs was recently shown to be dependent on at least two pathways acting via CXCR5 and IL-7Rα, because in CXCL13$^{-/-}$ and IL-7Rα$^{-/-}$ double-deficient mice, all LNs including the mesenteric LN were absent (Luther et al. 2003).

Inducer cells were recently reported to have a multiple responsiveness toward either single homeostatic or inflammatory chemokines or toward a combination of chemokines (Luther et al. 2005). These findings indicate that several chemokines exert a synergistic function in lymphoid tissue development. Messenger RNAs for homeostatic chemokines are expressed by VCAM$^+$ organizer cells, emphasizing the molecular feedback loops that can be established between inducer and organizer cells during organogenesis (Cupedo et al. 2004b; Honda et al. 2001; Luther et al. 2003). Ectopic expression of CXCL13, CCL19, or CCL21 under the pancreas-specific RIP promoter caused focal development of lymphoid infiltrates with distinct B- and T cell zones (Luther et al. 2000a, 2000b, 2002). In CXCL13 transgenic mice, CD4$^+$ CD3$^-$ cells were recruited to sites of transgene expression (Luther et al. 2003), confirming earlier studies that after adoptive transfer, the inducer cells migrate to B cell follicles (Mebius et al. 1997). However, the number of inducer cells in the developing mesenteric LNs of CXCL13$^{-/-}$ mice is relatively normal, arguing for additional chemokines regulating lymphoid tissue inducer cell migration (Luther et al. 2003).

Unlike lymphoid tissue inducer cells, B cells upregulate LTαβ expression after the engagement of CXCR5 (Ngo et al. 1999). We recently reported that CXCR5 expressed by lymphoid tissue inducer cells is crucial for the activation of α4β1 integrin expressed by the same cells and that consecutively activated α4β1 integrin can mediate firm adhesion of inducer cells to VCAM-1$^+$ organizer cells (Finke et al. 2002). These data are further supported by the observations that blocking of α4β1 integrin-VCAM-1 interactions during embryogenesis by mAb injection into pregnant mice severely affected the development of PPs in the offspring. This was not a result of inhibiting recruitment of the inducer cells, as normal numbers of inducer cells were present in the gut of both anti-β1-integrin and anti-VCAM-1 mAb-treated mice. Similarly, α4β7 integrin was not mandatory for entry of circulating inducer cells to sites where PPs and LNs develop (Finke et al. 2002; Hashi et al. 2001; Mebius et al. 1998).

5
Conclusions

During evolution, GALT develops from primitive lymphoid cell clusters with both hematopoietic and immune function to organized tissues able to generate highly specific adaptive immune responses. In mice, the cellular interactions between lymphoid tissue inducer cells and mesenchymal organizer cells regulate PP and LN development during ontogeny. The formation of cell clusters triggers a series of signaling events involving adhesion molecules, cytokines, chemokines, and TNF-family member molecules. The activation of integrins via molecular feedback loops appears to be essential for the prolonged cell-to-cell contact between the inducer and the organizer cells. The expression of adhesion molecules and chemokines by organizer cells is induced via LTβR signaling, thus leading to the recruitment and compartmentalization of mature lymphocyte subsets. The inducer cells are the major cell population engaging LTβR on stromal cells via LTαβ. After birth, the maintenance of organized lymphoid tissue is still dependent on signaling via TNF-family receptors, and other lymphoid cells such as B cells and T cells as well as microbial stimuli may trigger lymphoid tissue organization. It is evident that different TNF family member molecules, cytokines, and chemokines have a synergistic function in lympho-organogenesis, and the availability of these factors determines the formation of PPs, mucosa-draining LNs, or peripheral LNs. Similar mechanisms may operate during the neoformation of lymphoid tissue at sites of chronic inflammation.

Acknowledgements We sincerely apologize to all the colleagues whose work has been omitted because of space limitations. We wish to thank Dr. R. Ceredig and the members of the Developmental Immunology Division for critical reading of the manuscript and L. Du Pasquier for discussions and insights into the phylogenetic development of the immune system. DF is supported by grants from the Swiss National Science Foundation, the Walter Honegger Foundation and the Swiss Cancer League. D. Meier is supported by the Wehrenfels Foundation.

References

Abtahian F, Guerriero A, Sebzda E, Lu MM, Zhou R, Mocsai A, Myers EE, Huang B, Jackson DG, Ferrari VA, Tybulewicz V, Lowell CA, Lepore JJ, Koretzky GA, Kahn ML (2003) Regulation of blood and lymphatic vascular separation by signaling proteins SLP-76 and Syk. Science 299:247–251

Adachi S, Yoshida H, Honda K, Maki K, Saijo K, Ikuta K, Saito T, Nishikawa S (1998) Essential role of IL-7 receptor α in the formation of Peyer's patch anlage. Int Immunol 10:1-6

Adachi S, Yoshida H, Kataoka H, Nishikawa S (1997) Three distinctive steps in Peyer's patch formation of murine embryo. Int Immunol 9:507–514

Alcamo E, Hacohen N, Schulte L, Rennert P, Hynes R, Baltimore D (2002) Requirement for the NF-κB family member RelA in the development of secondary lymphoid organs. J Exp Med 195:233–244

Alimzhanov MB, Kuprash DV, Kosco-Vilbois MH, Luz A, Turetskaya RL, Tarakhovsky A, Rajewsky K, Nedospasov SA, Pfeffer K (1997) Abnormal development of secondary lymphoid tissues in lymphotoxin β-deficient mice. Proc Natl Acad Sci USA 94:9302–9307

Ansel KM, Ngo VN, Hyman PL, Luther SA, Forster R, Sedgwick JD, Browning JL, Lipp M, Cyster JG (2000) A chemokine-driven positive feedback loop organizes lymphoid follicles. Nature 406:309–314

Azzali G (2003) Structure, lymphatic vascularization and lymphocyte migration in mucosa-associated lymphoid tissue. Immunol Rev 195:178–189

Balogh P, Aydar Y, Tew JG, Szakal AK (2002) Appearance and phenotype of murine follicular dendritic cells expressing VCAM-1. Anat Rec 268:160–168

Banks TA, Rouse BT, Kerley MK, Blair PJ, Godfrey VL, Kuklin NA, Bouley DM, Thomas J, Kanangat S, Mucenski ML (1995) Lymphotoxin-α-deficient mice. Effects on secondary lymphoid organ development and humoral immune responsiveness. J Immunol 155:1685–1693

Brandtzaeg P, Baekkevold ES, Morton HC (2001) From B to A the mucosal way. Nat Immunol 2:1093–1094

Brandtzaeg P, Pabst R (2004) Let's go mucosal: communication on slippery ground. Trends Immunol 25:570–577

Braun M, Wunderlin M, Spieth K, Knochel W, Gierschik P, Moepps B (2002) *Xenopus laevis* stromal cell-derived factor 1: conservation of structure and function during vertebrate development. J Immunol 168:2340–2347

Breiteneder-Geleff S, Soleiman A, Kowalski H, Horvat R, Amann G, Kriehuber E, Diem K, Weninger W, Tschachler E, Alitalo K, Kerjaschki D (1999) Angiosarcomas express mixed endothelial phenotypes of blood and lymphatic capillaries: podoplanin as a specific marker for lymphatic endothelium. Am J Pathol 154:385–394

Browning JL, French LE (2002) Visualization of lymphotoxin-β and lymphotoxin-β receptor expression in mouse embryos. J Immunol 168:5079–5087

Butcher EC, Picker LJ (1996) Lymphocyte homing and homeostasis. Science 272:60–66

Cao X, Shores EW, Hu-Li J, Anver MR, Kelsall BL, Russell SM, Drago J, Noguchi M, Grinberg A, Bloom ET, et al. (1995) Defective lymphoid development in mice lacking expression of the common cytokine receptor γchain. Immunity 2:223–238

Christian JL (2000) BMP, Wnt and Hedgehog signals: how far can they go? Curr Opin Cell Biol 12:244–249

Cook DN, Prosser DM, Forster R, Zhang J, Kuklin NA, Abbondanzo SJ, Niu XD, Chen SC, Manfra DJ, Wiekowski MT, Sullivan LM, Smith SR, Greenberg HB, Narula SK, Lipp M, Lira SA (2000) CCR6 mediates dendritic cell localization, lymphocyte homeostasis, and immune responses in mucosal tissue. Immunity 12:495–503

Cornes JS (1965) Peyer's patches in the human gut. Proc R Soc Med 58:716

Csencsits KL, Jutila MA, Pascual DW (1999) Nasal-associated lymphoid tissue: phenotypic and functional evidence for the primary role of peripheral node addressin in naive lymphocyte adhesion to high endothelial venules in a mucosal site. J Immunol 163:1382–1389

Cupedo T, Kraal G, Mebius RE (2002) The role of CD45+CD4+CD3- cells in lymphoid organ development. Immunological Rev 189:41–50

Cupedo T, Lund FE, Ngo VN, Randall TD, Jansen W, Greuter MJ, de Waal-Malefyt R, Kraal G, Cyster JG, Mebius RE (2004a) Initiation of cellular organization in lymph nodes is regulated by non-B cell-derived signals and is not dependent on CXC chemokine ligand 13. J Immunol 173:4889–4896

Cupedo T, Vondenhoff MF, Heeregrave EJ, De Weerd AE, Jansen W, Jackson DG, Kraal G, Mebius RE (2004b) Presumptive lymph node organizers are differentially represented in developing mesenteric and peripheral nodes. J Immunol 173:2968–2975

Cyster JG (2005) Chemokines, sphingosine-1-phosphate, and cell migration in secondary lymphoid organs. Annu Rev Immunol 23:127–159

De Togni P, Goellner J, Ruddle NH, Streeter PR, Fick A, Mariathasan S, Smith SC, Carlson R, Shornick LP, Strauss-Schoenberger J (1994) Abnormal development of peripheral lymphoid organs in mice deficient in lymphotoxin. Science 264:703–707

Dear TN, Colledge WH, Carlton MB, Lavenir I, Larson T, Smith AJ, Warren AJ, Evans MJ, Sofroniew MV, Rabbitts TH (1995) The Hox11 gene is essential for cell survival during spleen development. Development 121:2909–2915

Dejardin E, Droin NM, Delhase M, Haas E, Cao Y, Makris C, Li ZW, Karin M, Ware CF, Green DR (2002) The lymphotoxin-βreceptor induces different patterns of gene expression via two NF-κB pathways. Immunity 17:525–535

Dohi T, Fujihashi K, Rennert PD, Iwatani K, Kiyono H, McGhee JR (1999) Hapten-induced colitis is associated with colonic patch hypertrophy and T helper cell 2-type responses. J Exp Med 189:1169–1180

Dohi T, Rennert PD, Fujihashi K, Kiyono H, Shirai Y, Kawamura YI, Browning JL, McGhee JR (2001) Elimination of colonic patches with lymphotoxin βreceptor-Ig prevents Th2 cell-type colitis. J Immunol 167:2781–2790

Dooley H, Flajnik MF (2005) Shark immunity bites back: affinity maturation and memory response in the nurse shark, *Ginglymostoma cirratum*. Eur J Immunol 35:936–945

Dougall WC, Glaccum M, Charrier K, Rohrbach K, Brasel K, De Smedt T, Daro E, Smith J, Tometsko ME, Maliszewski CR, Armstrong A, Shen V, Bain S, Cosman D, Anderson D, Morrissey PJ, Peschon JJ, Schuh J (1999) RANK is essential for osteoclast and lymph node development. Genes Dev 13:2412–2424

Drayton DL, Ying X, Lee J, Lesslauer W, Ruddle NH (2003) Ectopic LT αβdirects lymphoid organ neogenesis with concomitant expression of peripheral node addressin and a HEV-restricted sulfotransferase. J Exp Med 197:1153–1163

Eberl G, Littman DR (2004) Thymic origin of intestinal αβ T cells revealed by fate mapping of RORγt$^+$ cells. Science 305:248–251

Eberl G, Marmon S, Sunshine MJ, Rennert PD, Choi Y, Littman DR (2004) An essential function for the nuclear receptor RORγ$_t$ in the generation of fetal lymphoid tissue inducer cells. Nat Immunol 5:64–73

Ebert LM, McColl SR (2002) Up-regulation of CCR5 and CCR6 on distinct subpopulations of antigen-activated CD4+ T lymphocytes. J Immunol 168:65–72

El Bahi S, Caliot E, Bens M, Bogdanova A, Kerneis S, Kahn A, Vandewalle A, Pringault E (2002) Lymphoepithelial interactions trigger specific regulation of gene expression in the M cell-containing follicle-associated epithelium of Peyer's patches. J Immunol 168:3713–3720

Erickson SL, de Sauvage FJ, Kikly K, Carver-Moore K, Pitts-Meek S, Gillett N, Sheehan KC, Schreiber RD, Goeddel DV, Moore MW (1994) Decreased sensitivity to tumour-necrosis factor but normal T-cell development in TNF receptor-2-deficient mice. Nature 372:560–563

Fagarasan S, Muramatsu M, Suzuki H, Nagaoka H, Hiai H, Honjo T (2002) Critical roles of activation-induced cytidine deaminase in the homeostasis of gut flora. Science 298:1424

Fagarasan S, Shinkura R, Kamata T, Nogaki F, Ikuta K, Tashiro K, Honjo T (2000) Alymphoplasia (aly)-type nuclear factor κB-inducing kinase (NIK) causes defects in secondary lymphoid tissue chemokine receptor signaling and homing of peritoneal cells to the gut-associated lymphatic tissue system. J Exp Med 191:1477–1486

Feuerer M, Beckhove P, Garbi N, Mahnke Y, Limmer A, Hommel M, Hammerling GJ, Kyewski B, Hamann A, Umansky V, Schirrmacher V (2003) Bone marrow as a priming site for T-cell responses to blood-borne antigen. Nat Med 9:1151–1157

Finke D (2005) Fate and function of lymphoid tissue inducer cells. Curr Opin Immunol 17:144–150

Finke D, Acha-Orbea H, Mattis A, Lipp M, Kraehenbuhl J (2002) CD4+CD3− cells induce Peyer's patch development: role of α4β1 integrin activation by CXCR5. Immunity 17:363–373

Finke D, Kraehenbuhl JP (2001) Formation of Peyer's patches. Curr Opin Genet Dev 11:561–567

Flajnik M, Miller K, Du Pasquier L (2003) Evolution of the immune system. In Fundamental Immunology, edited by WE Paul, fifth edition: 519–570

Forster R, Mattis AE, Kremmer E, Wolf E, Brem G, Lipp M (1996) A putative chemokine receptor, BLR1, directs B cell migration to defined lymphoid organs and specific anatomic compartments of the spleen. Cell 87:1037–1047

Forster R, Schubel A, Breitfeld D, Kremmer E, Renner-Muller I, Wolf E, Lipp M (1999) CCR7 coordinates the primary immune response by establishing functional microenvironments in secondary lymphoid organs. Cell 99:23–33

Fry TJ, Mackall CL (2002) Interleukin-7: from bench to clinic. Blood 99:3892–3904

Fu YX, Chaplin DD (1999) Development and maturation of secondary lymphoid tissues. Annu Rev Immunol 17:399–433

Fu YX, Huang G, Matsumoto M, Molina H, Chaplin DD (1997a) Independent signals regulate development of primary and secondary follicle structure in spleen and mesenteric lymph node. Proc Natl Acad Sci USA 94:5739–5743

Fu YX, Molina H, Matsumoto M, Huang G, Min J, Chaplin DD (1997b) Lymphotoxin-α (LTα) supports development of splenic follicular structure that is required for IgG responses. J Exp Med 185:2111–2120

Fukuda K, Yoshida H, Sato T, Furumoto TA, Mizutani-Koseki Y, Suzuki Y, Saito Y, Takemori T, Kimura M, Sato H, Taniguchi M, Nishikawa S, Nakayama T, Koseki H (2003) Mesenchymal expression of Foxl1, a winged helix transcriptional factor, regulates generation and maintenance of gut-associated lymphoid organs. Dev Biol 255:278–289

Fukuyama S, Hiroi T, Yokota Y, Rennert PD, Yanagita M, Kinoshita N, Terawaki S, Shikina T, Yamamoto M, Kurono Y, Kiyono H (2002) Initiation of NALT organogenesis is independent of the IL-7R, LTβR, and NIK signaling pathways but requires the Id2 gene and $CD3^-CD4^+CD45^+$ cells. Immunity 17:31–40

Futterer A, Mink K, Luz A, Kosco-Vilbois MH, Pfeffer K (1998) The lymphotoxin β receptor controls organogenesis and affinity maturation in peripheral lymphoid tissues. Immunity 9:59–70

Gale NW, Thurston G, Hackett SF, Renard R, Wang Q, McClain J, Martin C, Witte C, Witte MH, Jackson D, Suri C, Campochiaro PA, Wiegand SJ, Yancopoulos GD (2002) Angiopoietin-2 is required for postnatal angiogenesis and lymphatic patterning, and only the latter role is rescued by Angiopoietin-1. Dev Cell 3:411–423

Georgopoulos K, Bigby K, Wang M, Molnar J-H, Wu A, Winandy S, Sharpe A (1994) The Ikaros gene is required for the development of all lymphoid lineages. Cell 79:143–156

Georgopoulos K, Winandy S, Avitahl N (1997) The role of the Ikaros gene in lymphocyte development and homeostasis. Annu Rev Immunol 15:155–176

Gommerman JL, Browning JL (2003) Lymphotoxin/light, lymphoid microenvironments and autoimmune disease. Nat Rev Immunol 3:642–655

Good RA, Finstad J, Pollara B, BGabrielsen AE (1966) Morphologic studies on the evolution of the lymphoid tissues among the lower vertebrates. In: Phylogeny of Immunity (RT Smith, RA Good, and PA Miescher, eds)149–170

Groger M, Loewe R, Holnthoner W, Embacher R, Pillinger M, Herron GS, Wolff K, Petzelbauer P (2004) IL-3 induces expression of lymphatic markers Prox-1 and podoplanin in human endothelial cells. J Immunol 173:7161–7169

Gunn MD, Tangemann K, Tam C, Cyster JG, Rosen SD, Williams LT (1998) A chemokine expressed in lymphoid high endothelial venules promotes the adhesion and chemotaxis of naive T lymphocytes. Proc Natl Acad Sci USA 95:258–263

Guy-Grand D, Azogui O, Celli S, Darche S, Nussenzweig MC, Kourilsky P, Vassalli P (2003) Extrathymic T cell lymphopoiesis: ontogeny and contribution to gut intraepithelial lymphocytes in athymic and euthymic mice. J Exp Med 197:333–341

Hamada H, Hiroi T, Nishiyama Y, Takahashi H, Masunaga Y, Hachimura S, Kaminogawa S, Takahashi-Iwanaga H, Iwanaga T, Kiyono H, Yamamoto H, Ishikawa H (2002) Identification of multiple isolated lymphoid follicles on the antimesenteric wall of the mouse small intestine. J Immunol 168:57–64

Harmsen A, Kusser K, Hartson L, Tighe M, Sunshine M, Sedgwick JD, Choi Y, Littman DR, Randall TD (2002) Cutting edge: Organogenesis of nasal-associated lymphoid tissue (NALT) occurs independently of lymphotoxin- (LT) and retinoic acid receptor-related orphan receptor, but the organization of NALT Is LT dependent. J Immunol 168:986–990

Hashi H, Yoshida H, Honda K, Fraser S, Kubo H, Awane M, Takabayashi A, Nakano H, Yamaoka Y, Nishikawa S (2001) Compartmentalization of Peyer's patch anlagen before lymphocyte entry. J Immunol 166:3702–3709

Herzer U, Crocoll A, Barton D, Howells N, Englert C (1999) The Wilms tumor suppressor gene wt1 is required for development of the spleen. Curr Biol 9:837–840

Honda K, Nakano H, Yoshida H, Nishikawa S, Rennert P, Ikuta K, Tamechika M, Yamaguchi K, Fukumoto T, Chiba T, Nishikawa SI (2001) Molecular basis for hematopoietic/mesenchymal interaction during initiation of Peyer's patch organogenesis. J Exp Med 193:621–630

Hong YK, Harvey N, Noh YH, Schacht V, Hirakawa S, Detmar M, Oliver G (2002) Prox1 is a master control gene in the program specifying lymphatic endothelial cell fate. Dev Dyn 225:351–357

Huising MO, Stet RJ, Kruiswijk CP, Savelkoul HF, Lidy Verburg-van Kemenade BM (2003) Molecular evolution of CXC chemokines: extant CXC chemokines originate from the CNS. Trends Immunol 24:307–313

Iwasaki A, Kelsall BL (2000) Localization of distinct Peyer's patch dendritic cell subsets and their recruitment by chemokines macrophage inflammatory protein (MIP)-3α, MIP-3β, and secondary lymphoid organ chemokine. J Exp Med 191:1381–1394

Kaestner KH, Silberg DG, Traber PG, Schutz G (1997) The mesenchymal winged helix transcription factor Fkh6 is required for the control of gastrointestinal proliferation and differentiation. Genes Dev 11:1583–1595

Kaipainen A, Korhonen J, Mustonen T, van Hinsbergh VW, Fang GH, Dumont D, Breitman M, Alitalo K (1995) Expression of the fms-like tyrosine kinase 4 gene becomes restricted to lymphatic endothelium during development. Proc Natl Acad Sci USA 92:3566–3570

Kanamori Y, Ishimaru K, Nanno M, Maki K, Ikuta K, Nariuchi H, Ishikawa H (1996) Identification of novel lymphoid tissues in murine intestinal mucosa where clusters of c-kit+ IL-7R+ Thy1+ lympho-hemopoietic progenitors develop. J Exp Med 184:1449–1459

Kang J, Der SD (2004) Cytokine functions in the formative stages of a lymphocyte's life. Curr Opin Immunol 16:180–190

Kang J, DiBenedetto B, Narayan K, Zhao H, Der SD, Chambers CA (2004) STAT5 is required for thymopoiesis in a development stage-specific manner. J Immunol 173:2307–2314

Kanzler B, Dear TN (2001) Hox11 acts cell autonomously in spleen development and its absence results in altered cell fate of mesenchymal spleen precursors. Dev Biol 234:231–243

Karrer U, Althage A, Odermatt B, Roberts CW, Korsmeyer SJ, Miyawaki S, Hengartner H, Zinkernagel RM (1997) On the key role of secondary lymphoid organs in antiviral immune responses studied in alymphoplastic (aly/aly) and spleenless (Hox11$^{-/-}$ mutant mice. J Exp Med 185:2157–2170

Kerneis S, Bogdanova A, Kraehenbuhl JP, Pringault E (1997) Conversion by Peyer's patch lymphocytes of human enterocytes into M cells that transport bacteria. Science 277:949–952

Kim D, Mebius RE, MacMicking JD, Jung S, Cupedo T, Castellanos Y, Rho J, Wong BR, Josien R, Kim N, Rennert PD, Choi Y (2000) Regulation of peripheral lymph node genesis by the tumor necrosis factor family member TRANCE. J Exp Med 192:1467–1478

Koike R, Watanabe T, Satoh H, Hee CS, Kitada K, Kuramoto T, Serikawa T, Miyawaki S, Miyasaka M (1997) Analysis of expression of lymphocyte homing-related adhesion molecules in ALY mice deficient in lymph nodes and Peyer's patches. Cell Immunol 180:62-69

Kong YY, Yoshida H, Sarosi I, Tan HL, Timms E, Capparelli C, Morony S, Oliveira-dos-Santos AJ, Van G, Itie A, Khoo W, Wakeham A, Dunstan CR, Lacey DL, Mak TW, Boyle WJ, Penninger JM (1999) OPGL is a key regulator of osteoclastogenesis, lymphocyte development and lymph-node organogenesis. Nature 397:315-323

Koni PA, Flavell RA (1998) A role for tumor necrosis factor receptor type 1 in gut-associated lymphoid tissue development: genetic evidence of synergism with lymphotoxin β. J Exp Med 187:1977-1983

Kriehuber E, Breiteneder-Geleff S, Groeger M, Soleiman A, Schoppmann SF, Stingl G, Kerjaschki D, Maurer D (2001) Isolation and characterization of dermal lymphatic and blood endothelial cells reveal stable and functionally specialized cell lineages. J Exp Med 194:797-808

Kuprash DV, Alimzhanov MB, Tumanov AV, Anderson AO, Pfeffer K, Nedospasov SA (1999) TNF and lymphotoxin β cooperate in the maintenance of secondary lymphoid tissue microarchitecture but not in the development of lymph nodes. J Immunol 163:6575-6580

Kurebayashi S, Ueda E, Sakaue M, Patel DD, Medvedev A, Zhang F, Jetten AM (2000) Retinoid-related orphan receptor γ (RORγ) is essential for lymphoid organogenesis and controls apoptosis during thymopoiesis. Proc Natl Acad Sci USA 97:10132-10137

Kuroda N, Uinuk-ool TS, Sato A, Samonte IE, Figueroa F, Mayer WE, Klein J (2003) Identification of chemokines and a chemokine receptor in cichlid fish, shark, and lamprey. Immunogenetics 54:884-895

Kweon MN, Yamamoto M, Rennert PD, Park EJ, Lee AY, Chang SY, Hiroi T, Nanno M, Kiyono H (2005) Prenatal Blockage of lymphotoxin β receptor and TNF receptor p55 signaling cascade resulted in the acceleration of tissue genesis for isolated lymphoid follicles in the large intestine. J Immunol 174:4365-4372

Lacey DL, Timms E, Tan HL, Kelley MJ, Dunstan CR, Burgess T, Elliott R, Colombero A, Elliott G, Scully S, Hsu H, Sullivan J, Hawkins N, Davy E, Capparelli C, Eli A, Qian YX, Kaufman S, Sarosi I, Shalhoub V, Senaldi G, Guo J, Delaney J, Boyle WJ (1998) Osteoprotegerin ligand is a cytokine that regulates osteoclast differentiation and activation. Cell 93:165-176

Lakkis FG, Arakelov A, Konieczny BT, Inoue Y (2000) Immunologic 'ignorance' of vascularized organ transplants in the absence of secondary lymphoid tissue. Nat Med 6:686-688

Laky K, Lefrancois L, Lingenheld EG, Ishikawa H, Lewis JM, Olson S, Suzuki K, Tigelaar RE, Puddington L (2000) Enterocyte expression of interleukin 7 induces development of γδ T cells and Peyer's patches. J Exp Med 191:1569-1580

Lettice LA, Purdie LA, Carlson GJ, Kilanowski F, Dorin J, Hill RE (1999) The mouse bagpipe gene controls development of axial skeleton, skull, and spleen. Proc Natl Acad Sci U A 96:9695-9700

Lewis FT (1905) The development of the lymphatic system in rabbits. Am J Anat 5:95-111

Liang TS, Hartt JK, Lu S, Martins-Green M, Gao JL, Murphy PM (2001) Cloning, mRNA distribution, and functional expression of an avian counterpart of the chemokine receptor/HIV coreceptor CXCR4. J Leukoc Biol 69:297–305

Liao F, Rabin RL, Smith CS, Sharma G, Nutman TB, Farber JM (1999) CC-chemokine receptor 6 is expressed on diverse memory subsets of T cells and determines responsiveness to macrophage inflammatory protein 3α. J Immunol 162:186–194

Locksley RM, Killeen N, Lenardo MJ (2001) The TNF and TNF receptor superfamilies: integrating mammalian biology. Cell 104:487–501

Lorenz RG, Chaplin DD, McDonald KG, McDonough JS, Newberry RD (2003) Isolated lymphoid follicle formation is inducible and dependent upon lymphotoxin-sufficient B lymphocytes, lymphotoxin β receptor, and TNF receptor I function. J Immunol 170:5475–5482

Lu J, Chang P, Richardson JA, Gan L, Weiler H, Olson EN (2000) The basic helix-loop-helix transcription factor capsulin controls spleen organogenesis. Proc Natl Acad Sci USA 97:9525–9530

Luther SA, Ansel KM, Cyster JG (2003) Overlapping roles of CXCL13, interleukin 7 receptor α, and CCR7 ligands in lymph node development. J Exp Med 197:1191–1198

Luther SA, Bidgol A, Hargreaves DC, Schmidt A, Xu Y, Paniyadi J, Matloubian M, Cyster JG (2002) Differing activities of homeostatic chemokines CCL19, CCL21, and CXCL12 in lymphocyte and dendritic cell recruitment and lymphoid neogenesis. J Immunol 169:424–433

Luther SA, Lesneski MJ, Xu Y, Marquéz G, Cyster JG (2005) Chemokine response profiling of lymphoid tissue inducer cells reveals a role for CXCR4 in Peyer's patch formation. Swiss Med Wkly 135: S3

Luther SA, Lopez T, Bai W, Hanahan D, Cyster JG (2000a) BLC expression in pancreatic islets causes B cell recruitment and lymphotoxin-dependent lymphoid neogenesis. Immunity 12:471–481

Luther SA, Tang HL, Hyman PL, Farr AG, Cyster JG (2000b) Coexpression of the chemokines ELC and SLC by T zone stromal cells and deletion of the ELC gene in the plt/plt mouse. Proc Natl Acad Sci USA 97:12694–12699

Makala LH, Suzuki N, Nagasawa H (2002) Peyer's patches: organized lymphoid structures for the induction of mucosal immune responses in the intestine. Pathobiology 70:55–68

Mangelsdorf DJ, Thummel C, Beato M, Herrlich P, Schutz G, Umesono K, Blumberg B, Kastner P, Mark M, Chambon P, et al. (1995) The nuclear receptor superfamily: the second decade. Cell 83:835–839

Manning MJ, Horton JD (1982) RES structure and function of the Amphibia. In: Cohen, N, Sigel, MM (eds) The Reticuloendothelial System. Plenum Press, New York and London, 423–459

Matsumoto M, Iwamasa K, Rennert PD, Yamada T, Suzuki R, Matsushima A, Okabe M, Fujita S, Yokoyama M (1999) Involvement of distinct cellular compartments in the abnormal lymphoid organogenesis in lymphotoxin-α-deficient mice and alymphoplasia (aly) mice defined by the chimeric analysis. J Immunol 163:1584–1591

Matsushima A, Kaisho T, Rennert PD, Nakano H, Kurosawa K, Uchida D, Takeda K, Akira S, Matsumoto M (2001) Essential role of nuclear factor (NF)-κB-inducing kinase and inhibitor of κB (IκB) kinase α in NF-κB activation through lymphotoxin β receptor, but not through tumor necrosis factor receptor I. J Exp Med 193:631–636

Mebius RE, Miyamoto T, Christensen J, Domen J, Cupedo T, Weissman IL, Akashi K (2001) The fetal liver counterpart of adult common lymphoid progenitors gives rise to all lymphoid lineages, CD45+CD4+CD3– cells, as well as macrophages. J Immunol 166:6593–6601

Mebius RE, Rennert P, Weissman IL (1997) Developing lymph nodes collect CD4+CD3– LTβ+ cells that can differentiate to APC, NK cells, and follicular cells but not T or B cells. Immunity 7:493–504

Mebius RE, Schadee-Eestermans IL, Weissman IL (1998) MAdCAM-1 dependent colonization of developing lymph nodes involves a unique subset of CD4+CD3– hematolymphoid cells. Cell Adhesion Commun 6:97–103

Mebius RE, Streeter PR, Michie S, Butcher EC, Weissman IL (1996) A developmental switch in lymphocyte homing receptor and endothelial vascular addressin expression regulates lymphocyte homing and permits CD4+ CD3–- cells to colonize lymph nodes. Proc Natl Acad Sci USA 93:11019–11024

Miyawaki S, Nakamura Y, Suzuka H, Koba M, Yasumizu R, Ikehara S, Shibata Y (1994) A new mutation, aly, that induces a generalized lack of lymph nodes accompanied by immunodeficiency in mice. Eur J Immunol 24:429–434

Mora JR, Bono MR, Manjunath N, Weninger W, Cavanagh LL, Rosemblatt M, Von Andrian UH (2003) Selective imprinting of gut-homing T cells by Peyer's patch dendritic cells. Nature 424:88–93

Moyron-Quiroz JE, Rangel-Moreno J, Kusser K, Hartson L, Sprague F, Goodrich S, Woodland DL, Lund FE, Randall TD (2004) Role of inducible bronchus associated lymphoid tissue (iBALT) in respiratory immunity. Nat Med 10:927–934

Murray AM, Simm B, Beagley KW (1998) Cytokine gene expression in murine fetal intestine: potential for extrathymic T cell development. Cytokine 10:337–345

Nagasawa T, Hirota S, Tachibana K, Takakura N, Nishikawa S, Kitamura Y, Yoshida N, Kikutani H, Kishimoto T (1996) Defects of B-cell lymphopoiesis and bone-marrow myelopoiesis in mice lacking the CXC chemokine PBSF/SDF-1. Nature 382:635–638

Naito A, Azuma S, Tanaka S, Miyazaki T, Takaki S, Takatsu K, Nakao K, Nakamura K, Katsuki M, Yamamoto T, Inoue J (1999) Severe osteopetrosis, defective interleukin-1 signalling and lymph node organogenesis in TRAF6-deficient mice. Genes Cells 4:353–362

Nakano H, Mori S, Yonekawa H, Nariuchi H, Matsuzawa A, Kakiuchi T (1998) A novel mutant gene involved in T-lymphocyte-specific homing into peripheral lymphoid organs on mouse chromosome 4. Blood 91:2886–2895

Neumann B, Luz A, Pfeffer K, Holzmann B (1996) Defective Peyer's patch organogenesis in mice lacking the 55-kD receptor for tumor necrosis factor. J Exp Med 184:259–264

Ngo VN, Korner H, Gunn MD, Schmidt KN, Riminton DS, Cooper MD, Browning JL, Sedgwick JD, Cyster JG (1999) Lymphotoxin α/β and tumor necrosis factor are required for stromal cell expression of homing chemokines in B and T cell areas of the spleen. J Exp Med 189:403–412

Niess JH, Brand S, Gu X, Landsman L, Jung S, McCormick BA, Vyas JM, Boes M, Ploegh HL, Fox JG, Littman DR, Reinecker HC (2005) CX3CR1-mediated dendritic cell access to the intestinal lumen and bacterial clearance. Science 307:254–258

Nishikawa S, Honda K, Vieira P, Yoshida H (2003) Organogenesis of peripheral lymphoid organs. Immunol Rev 195:72–80

Nishikawa SI, Hashi H, Honda K, Fraser S, Yoshida H (2000) Inflammation, a prototype for organogenesis of the lymphopoietic/hematopoietic system. Curr Opin Immunol 12:342–345

Ohl L, Henning G, Krautwald S, Lipp M, Hardtke S, Bernhardt G, Pabst O, Forster R (2003a) Cooperating mechanisms of CXCR5 and CCR7 in development and organization of secondary lymphoid organs. J Exp Med 197:1199–1204

Ohl L, Henning G, Krautwald S, Lipp M, Hardtke S, Bernhardt G, Pabst O, Förster R (2003b) Cooperative mechanisms of CXCR5 and CCR7 in development and organization of secondary lymphoid organs. J Exp Med 197:1199–1204

Oliver G (2004) Lymphatic vasculature development. Nat Rev Immunol 4:35–45

Owen RL, Piazza AJ, Ermak TH (1991) Ultrastructural and cytoarchitectural features of lymphoreticular organs in the colon and rectum of adult BALB/c mice. Am J Anat 190:10–18

Pabst O, Forster R, Lipp M, Engel H, Arnold HH (2000) NKX2.3 is required for MAdCAM-1 expression and homing of lymphocytes in spleen and mucosa-associated lymphoid tissue. Embo J 19:2015

Pabst O, Herbrand H, Bernhardt G, Förster R (2004) Elucidating the functional anatomy of secondary lymphoid organs. Curr Opin Immunol 16:394–399

Pabst O, Herbrand H, Worbs T, Friedrichsen M, Yan S, Hoffmann MW, Korner H, Bernhardt G, Pabst R, Forster R (2005) Cryptopatches and isolated lymphoid follicles: dynamic lymphoid tissues dispensable for the generation of intraepithelial lymphocytes. Eur J Immunol 35:98–107

Pabst O, Schneider A, Brand T, Arnold HH (1997) The mouse Nkx2-3 homeodomain gene is expressed in gut mesenchyme during pre- and postnatal mouse development. Dev Dyn 209:29–35

Pabst O, Zweigerdt R, Arnold HH (1999) Targeted disruption of the homeobox transcription factor Nkx2-3 in mice results in postnatal lethality and abnormal development of small intestine and spleen. Development 126:2215–2225

Pabst R, Tschernig T (2002) Perivascular capillaries in the lung: an important but neglected vascular bed in immune reactions? J Allergy Clin Immunol 110:209–214

Park SY, Saijo K, Takahashi T, Osawa M, Arase H, Hirayama N, Miyake K, Nakauchi H, Shirasawa T, Saito T (1995) Developmental defects of lymphoid cells in Jak3 kinase-deficient mice. Immunity 3:771–782

Pasparakis M, Alexopoulou L, Episkopou V, Kollias G (1996) Immune and inflammatory responses in TNF α-deficient mice: a critical requirement for TNF α in the formation of primary B cell follicles, follicular dendritic cell networks and germinal centers, and in the maturation of the humoral immune response. J Exp Med 184:1397–1411

Pasparakis M, Alexopoulou L, Grell M, Pfizenmaier K, Bluethmann H, Kollias G (1997) Peyer's patch organogenesis is intact yet formation of B lymphocyte follicles is defective in peripheral lymphoid organs of mice deficient for tumor necrosis factor and its 55-kDa receptor. Proc Natl Acad Sci USA 94:6319–6323

Paxian S, Merkle H, Riemann M, Wilda M, Adler G, Hameister H, Liptay S, Pfeffer K, Schmid RM (2002) Abnormal organogenesis of Peyer's patches in mice deficient for NF-κB1, NF-κB2, and Bcl-3. Gastroenterology 122:1853–1868

Pfeffer K, Matsuyama T, Kundig TM, Wakeham A, Kishihara K, Shahinian A, Wiegmann K, Ohashi PS, Kronke M, Mak TW (1993) Mice deficient for the 55 kd tumor necrosis factor receptor are resistant to endotoxic shock, yet succumb to *L. monocytogenes* infection. Cell 73:457–467

Pihlgren M, Tougne C, Bozzotti P, Fulurija A, Duchosal MA, Lambert PH, Siegrist CA (2003) Unresponsiveness to lymphoid-mediated signals at the neonatal follicular dendritic cell precursor level contributes to delayed germinal center induction and limitations of neonatal antibody responses to T-dependent antigens. J Immunol 170:2824–2832

Rennert PD, Browning JL, Hochman PS (1997) Selective disruption of lymphotoxin ligands reveals a novel set of mucosal lymph nodes and unique effects on lymph node cellular organization. Int Immunol 9:1627–1639

Rennert PD, Browning JL, Mebius R, Mackay F, Hochman PS (1996) Surface lymphotoxin α/α complex is required for the development of peripheral lymphoid organs. J Exp Med 184:1999–2006

Rennert PD, Hochman PS, Flavell RA, Chaplin DD, Jayaraman S, Browning JL, Fu YX (2001) Essential role of lymph nodes in contact hypersensitivity revealed in lymphotoxin-α-deficient mice. J Exp Med 193:1227–1238

Rennert PD, James D, Mackay F, Browning JL, Hochman PS (1998) Lymph node genesis is induced by signaling through the lymphotoxin β receptor. Immunity 9:71–79

Rescigno M, Urbano M, Valzasina B, Francolini M, Rotta G, Bonasio R, Granucci F, Kraehenbuhl JP, Ricciardi-Castagnoli P (2001) Dendritic cells express tight junction proteins and penetrate gut epithelial monolayers to sample bacteria. Nat Immunol 2:361–367

Roberts CW, Shutter JR, Korsmeyer SJ (1994) Hox11 controls the genesis of the spleen. Nature 368:747–749

Rothe J, Lesslauer W, Lotscher H, Lang Y, Koebel P, Kontgen F, Althage A, Zinkernagel R, Steinmetz M, Bluethmann H (1993) Mice lacking the tumour necrosis factor receptor 1 are resistant to TNF-mediated toxicity but highly susceptible to infection by *Listeria monocytogenes*. Nature 364:798–802

Rumbo M, Sierro F, Debard N, Kraehenbuhl JP, Finke D (2004) Lymphotoxin β receptor signaling induces the chemokine CCL20 in intestinal epithelium. Gastroenterology 127:213–223

Sabin FR (1909) The lymphatic system in human embryos, with a consideration of the system as a whole. Am J Anat 9:43–91

Schacht V, Ramirez MI, Hong YK, Hirakawa S, Feng D, Harvey N, Williams M, Dvorak AM, Dvorak HF, Oliver G, Detmar M (2003) T1α/podoplanin deficiency disrupts normal lymphatic vasculature formation and causes lymphedema. EMBO J 22:3546–3556

Scheu S, Alferink J, Potzel T, Barchet W, Kalinke U, Pfeffer K (2002) Targeted disruption of LIGHT causes defects in costimulatory T cell activation and reveals cooperation with lymphotoxin β in mesenteric lymph node genesis. J Exp Med 195:1613–1624

Searle AG (1964) The genetics and morphology of two "luxoid" mutations in the house mouse. Genet Res 5:171–197

Shankey TV, Clem LW (1980) Phylogeny of immunoglobulin structure and function. IX. Intramolecular heterogeneity of shark 19S IgM antibodies to the dinitrophenyl hapten. J Immunol 125:2690–2698

Shikina T, Hiroi T, Iwatani K, Jang MH, Fukuyama S, Tamura M, Kubo T, Ishikawa H, Kiyono H (2004) IgA class switch occurs in the organized nasopharynx- and gut-associated lymphoid tissue, but not in the diffuse lamina propria of airways and gut. J Immunol 172:6259–6264

Shimizu Y, Rose DM, Ginsber MH (1999) Integrins in the immune system. Adv Immunol 72:325–380

Shinkura R, Matsuda F, Sakiyama T, Tsubata T, Hiai H, Paumen M, Miyawaki S, Honjo T (1996) Defects of somatic hypermutation and class switching in alymphoplasia (aly) mutant mice. Int Immunol 8:1067–1075

Sitnicka E, Brakebusch C, Martensson IL, Svensson M, Agace WW, Sigvardsson M, Buza-Vidas N, Bryder D, Cilio CM, Ahlenius H, Maraskovsky E, Peschon JJ, Jacobsen SE (2003) Complementary signaling through flt3 and interleukin-7 receptor α is indispensable for fetal and adult B cell genesis. J Exp Med 198:1495–1506

Sitnicka E, Bryder D, Theilgaard-Monch K, Buza-Vidas N, Adolfsson J, Jacobsen SE (2002) Key role of flt3 ligand in regulation of the common lymphoid progenitor but not in maintenance of the hematopoietic stem cell pool. Immunity 17:463–472

Sock E, Rettig SD, Enderich J, Bosl MR, Tamm ER, Wegner M (2004) Gene targeting reveals a widespread role for the high-mobility-group transcription factor Sox11 in tissue remodeling. Mol Cell Biol 24:6635–6644

Spahn TW, Fontana A, Faria AM, Slavin AJ, Eugster HP, Zhang X, Koni PA, Ruddle NH, Flavell RA, Rennert PD, Weiner HL (2001) Induction of oral tolerance to cellular immune responses in the absence of Peyer's patches. Eur J Immunol 31:1278–1287

Spahn TW, Herbst H, Rennert PD, Lugering N, Maaser C, Kraft M, Fontana A, Weiner HL, Domschke W, Kucharzik T (2002) Induction of colitis in mice deficient of Peyer's patches and mesenteric lymph nodes is associated with increased disease severity and formation of colonic lymphoid patches. Am J Pathol 161:2273–2282

Sun Z, Unutmaz D, Zou YR, Sunshine MJ, Pierani A, Brenner-Morton S, Mebius RE, Littman DR (2000) Requirement for RORγ in thymocyte survival and lymphoid organ development. Science 288:2369–2373

Suto J, Wakayama T, Imamura K, Goto S, Fukuta K (1995) Incomplete development of the spleen and the deformity in the chimeras between asplenic mutant (Dominant hemimelia) and normal mice. Teratology 52:71–77

Tachibana K, Hirota S, Iizasa H, Yoshida H, Kawabata K, Kataoka Y, Kitamura Y, Matsushima K, Yoshida N, Nishikawa S, Kishimoto T, Nagasawa T (1998) The chemokine receptor CXCR4 is essential for vascularization of the gastrointestinal tract. Nature 393:591–594

Taylor RT, Lugering A, Newell KA, Williams IR (2004) Intestinal cryptopatch formation in mice requires lymphotoxin α and the lymphotoxin β receptor. J Immunol 173:7183–7189

Tribioli C, Lufkin T (1999) The murine Bapx1 homeobox gene plays a critical role in embryonic development of the axial skeleton and spleen. Development 126:5699–5711

Tripp RA, Topham DJ, Watson SR, Doherty PC (1997) Bone marrow can function as a lymphoid organ during a primary immune response under conditions of disrupted lymphocyte trafficking. J Immunol 158:3716–3720

Tumanov A, Kuprash D, Lagarkova M, Grivennikov S, Abe K, Shakhov A, Drutskaya L, Stewart C, Chervonsky A, Nedospasov S (2002) Distinct role of surface lymphotoxin expressed by B cells in the organization of secondary lymphoid tissues. Immunity 17:239–250

Wang CC, Biben C, Robb L, Nassir F, Barnett L, Davidson NO, Koentgen F, Tarlinton D, Harvey RP (2000) Homeodomain factor Nkx2-3 controls regional expression of leukocyte homing coreceptor MAdCAM-1 in specialized endothelial cells of the viscera. Dev Biol 224:152–167

Wang J, Foster A, Chin R, Yu P, Sun Y, Wang Y, Pfeffer K, Fu YX (2002) The complementation of lymphotoxin deficiency with LIGHT, a newly discovered TNF family member, for the restoration of secondary lymphoid structure and function. Eur J Immunol 32:1969–1979

Wang JH, Nichogiannopoulou A, Wu L, Sun L, Sharpe AH, Bigby M, Georgopoulos K (1996) Selective defects in the development of the fetal and adult lymphoid system in mice with an Ikaros null mutation. Immunity 5:537–549

Wang Y, Wang J, Sun Y, Wu Q, Fu YX (2001) Complementary effects of TNF and lymphotoxin on the formation of germinal center and follicular dendritic cells. J Immunol 166:330–337

Weih DS, Yilmaz ZB, Weih F (2001) Essential role of RelB in germinal center and marginal zone formation and proper expression of homing chemokines. J Immunol 167:1909–1919

Weih F, Caamano J (2003) Regulation of secondary lymphoid organ development by the nuclear factor-κB signal transduction pathway. Immunol Rev 195:91–105

Weih F, Carrasco D, Durham SK, Barton DS, Rizzo CA, Ryseck RP, Lira SA, Bravo R (1995) Multiorgan inflammation and hematopoietic abnormalities in mice with a targeted disruption of RelB, a member of the NF-κB/Rel family. Cell 80:331–340

Wigle JT, Harvey N, Detmar M, Lagutina I, Grosveld G, Gunn MD, Jackson DG, Oliver G (2002) An essential role for Prox1 in the induction of the lymphatic endothelial cell phenotype. EMBO J 21:1505–1513

Wigle JT, Oliver G (1999) Prox1 function is required for the development of the murine lymphatic system. Cell 98:769–778

Wong BR, Rho J, Arron J, Robinson E, Orlinick J, Chao M, Kalachikov S, Cayani E, Bartlett FS, 3rd, Frankel WN, Lee SY, Choi Y (1997) TRANCE is a novel ligand of the tumor necrosis factor receptor family that activates c-Jun N-terminal kinase in T cells. J Biol Chem 272:25190–25194

Wright DE, Bowman EP, Wagers AJ, Butcher EC, Weissman IL (2002) Hematopoietic stem cells are uniquely selective in their migratory response to chemokines. J Exp Med 195:1145–1154

Wu HY, Nguyen HH, Russell MW (1997a) Nasal lymphoid tissue (NALT) as a mucosal immune inductive site. Scand J Immunol 46:506–513

Wu L, Nichogiannopoulou A, Shortman K, Georgopoulos K (1997b) Cell-autonomous defects in dendritic cell populations of Ikaros mutant mice point to a developmental relationship with the lymphoid lineage. Immunity 7:483–492

Yamamoto M, Kweon MN, Rennert PD, Hiroi T, Fujihashi K, McGhee JR, Kiyono H (2004) Role of gut-associated lymphoreticular tissues in antigen-specific intestinal IgA immunity. J Immunol 173:762–769

Yamamoto M, Rennert P, McGhee JR, Kweon MN, Yamamoto S, Dohi T, Otake S, Bluethmann H, Fujihashi K, Kiyono H (2000) Alternative mucosal immune system: organized Peyer's patches are not required for IgA responses in the gastrointestinal tract. J Immunol 164:5184–5191

Yasumizu R, Miyawaki S, Koba M, Kondoh-Tanaka M, Amoh Y, Nishio N, Yamamoto Y, Watanabe H, Ikehara S (2000) Pathology of ALY mice: congenital immunodeficiency with lymph node and Peyer's patch defects. Immunobiology 202:213–225

Yilmaz ZB, Weih DS, Sivakumar V, Weih F (2003) RelB is required for Peyer's patch development: differential regulation of p52-RelB by lymphotoxin and TNF. Embo J 22:121–130

Yin L, Wu L, Wesche H, Arthur CD, White JM, Goeddel DV, Schreiber RD (2001) Defective lymphotoxin-beta receptor-induced NF-κB transcriptional activity in NIK-deficient mice. Science 291:2162–2165

Yokota Y, Mansouri A, Mori S, Sugawara S, Adachi S, Nishikawa S, Gruss P (1999) Development of peripheral lymphoid organs and natural killer cells depends on the helix-loop-helix inhibitor Id2. Nature 397:702–706

Yoshida H, Honda K, Shinkura R, Adachi S, Nishikawa S, Maki K, Ikuta K, Nishikawa SI (1999) IL-7 receptor α^+ $CD3^-$ cells in the embryonic intestine induces the organizing center of Peyer's patches. Int Immunol 11:643–655

Yoshida H, Kawamoto H, Santee S, Hashi H, Honda K, Nishikawa S, Ware C, Katsura Y, Nishikawa S (2001) Expression of $\alpha_4\beta_7$ integrin defines a distinct pathway of lymphoid progenitors committed to T cells, fetal intestinal lymphotoxin producer, NK, and dendritic cells. J Immunol 167:2511–2521

Yoshida H, Naito A, Inoue J, Satoh M, Santee-Cooper SM, Ware CF, Togawa A, Nishikawa S (2002) Different cytokines induce surface lymphotoxin-$\alpha\beta$ on IL-7 receptor-α cells that differentially engender lymph nodes and Peyer's patches. Immunity 17:823–833

Yuan L, Moyon D, Pardanaud L, Breant C, Karkkainen MJ, Alitalo K, Eichmann A (2002) Abnormal lymphatic vessel development in neuropilin 2 mutant mice. Development 129:4797–4806

Zapata A, Amemiya C (2000) Phylogeny of lower vertebrates and their immunological structures. Curr Top Microbiol Immunol 248:67–110

Zapata AG, Torroba M, Vicente A, Varas A, Sacedon R, Jimenez E (1995) The relevance of cell microenvironments for the appearance of lympho-haemopoietic tissues in primitive vertebrates. Histol Histopathol 10:761–778

Zhao X, Sato A, Dela Cruz CS, Linehan M, Luegering A, Kucharzik T, Shirakawa AK, Marquez G, Farber JM, Williams I, Iwasaki A (2003) CCL9 is secreted by the follicle-associated epithelium and recruits dome region Peyer's patch CD11b+ dendritic cells. J Immunol 171:2797–2803

Lymphoid Tissue Inducer Cells in Intestinal Immunity

I. I. Ivanov · G. E. Diehl · D. R. Littman (✉)

Howard Hughes Medical Institute, Skirball Institute of Biomolecular Medicine,
New York University School of Medicine, New York, NY 10016, USA
littman@saturn.med.nyu.edu

1	Introduction	60
2	Development of Organized GALT Structures	60
2.1	Functions of RORγt in Lymphoid Organogenesis and T Cell Development	61
2.2	Structure and Function of Organized GALT Structures	64
2.2.1	Peyer's Patches	65
2.2.2	Isolated Lymphoid Follicles	67
2.2.3	Cryptopatches	70
2.3	Cryptopatches as Organizing Centers for Localized Mucosal Responses	71
3	Dendritic Cells, a Double-Edged Sword	73
4	LTi Cells and Ectopic Lymphoid Follicles in Autoimmunity	77
5	Conclusions	77
References		78

Abstract During fetal development, lymphoid tissue inducer cells (LTis) seed the developing lymph node and Peyer's patch anlagen and initiate the formation of both types of lymphoid organs. In the adult, a similar population of cells, termed lymphoid tissue inducer-like cells (LTi-like cells), supports the formation of organized gut-associated lymphoid tissue (GALT) in the intestine, including both isolated lymphoid follicles (ILFs) and cryptopatches (CPs). Both LTi and LTi-like cells require expression of the transcription factor RORγt for their differentiation and function, and mice lacking RORγt lack lymph nodes, Peyer's patches, and other organized GALT. In ILFs and cryptopatches, LTi-like cells are in close contact with different populations of intestinal dendritic cells (DCs), including a subpopulation recently shown to extend dendrites and sample luminal microflora. This interaction may allow for communication between the intestinal lumen and the immune cells in the lamina propria, which is necessary for maintaining homeostasis between the commensal microflora and the intestinal immune system. The potential functional implications of the organization of LTi-like cells, DCs, and lymphocytes in the lamina propria are discussed in the context of maintenance of homeostasis and of infectious diseases, particularly HIV infection.

1
Introduction

In the intestine, a balance must be maintained between potentially harmful bacteria and an extensive network of cells that constitute the gut-associated lymphoid tissues (GALT). The mechanisms that govern this homeostasis remain poorly understood. When the homeostasis is compromised, the outcome can range from inflammatory bowel disease to food allergies to inflammation-associated malignancies. In this review, we discuss recent studies that shed light on the organization of immune cells in the intestine and provide clues as to how these interact with luminal microorganisms. We describe the role for an orphan nuclear receptor, RORγt, in the development of lymphoid tissue inducer (LTi) cells during fetal life and of intestinal cryptopatch (CP) cells postnatally, resulting in the genesis of secondary lymphoid organs and tertiary lymphoid follicles, respectively. We also review recent studies showing that dendritic cells (DCs) communicate with the intestinal lumen and transport bacteria from the lumen to the lamina propria (LP). Finally, we propose a model that describes how sensing of microbial content by specialized DCs that extend processes across epithelia can regulate the immune response to the microflora while maintaining the integrity of the intestinal epithelium.

A single layer of intestinal epithelial cells protects the internal organs from more than 700 species of resident gut bacteria totaling approximately 10^{14} cells [1–4]. The mucosal immune system contains and regulates this permanent "infection," but it also supports it, because of the advantages provided by the microorganisms. The immune system must sense changes in the composition of the microflora. These changes may alert the host to the presence of pathogenic bacteria and activate prompt defense mechanisms. It remains unclear, however, how host defenses can discriminate between commensal and pathogenic bacteria, because they share antigens and express identical Toll-like receptor (TLR) ligands. The intestinal immune system must also have the capacity to recognize and become tolerized against food antigens. Thus the mucosal immune system must handle a number of "nonself" antigens differently—some antigens will induce regulatory or tolerogenic responses, others will be sequestered, and yet others will induce different types of protective immune responses.

2
Development of Organized GALT Structures

The GALT consists of secondary lymphoid organs [Peyer's patches (PPs) and the mesenteric lymph nodes (MLNs)], tertiary organized lymphoid tissues

[CPs and isolated lymphoid follicles (ILFs)], dispersed cells [intraepithelial T lymphocytes (IELs) and LP T and B lymphocytes], and an organized network of specialized DCs. In addition, Paneth cells, specialized epithelial cells at the base of the intestinal crypts, secrete antimicrobial peptides that exert their action in the lumen of the intestine. Together, these diverse cells and organized lymphoid structures are thought to regulate the microflora while also defending the host from breaches in epithelial integrity and preventing inflammatory responses against harmless antigens. How these different functions are accomplished remains poorly understood, but it is clear that there must be extensive communication between the immune system components within the intestinal mucosa. In addition, the epithelial cell compartment is also regulated by interactions with components of the mucosal immune system. Recent studies with genetically modified mice have advanced our understanding of the organization and relationship between GALT components. However, the mechanisms and mediators involved in the cross talk between these components have yet to be elucidated.

In general, the PPs, ILFs, and CPs have been ascribed different functions based on their developmental and structural differences. However, several studies, as outlined below, have observed redundant or overlapping functions between PPs and ILFs. CP function remains undetermined, although our recent studies suggest that these cells are similar to the LTi cells that, in the fetus, are required for development of all lymph nodes and PPs. The CP cells, like fetal LTi cells, are characterized by the expression of the orphan nuclear hormone receptor RORγt, which is necessary for the development of all three types of the organized GALT within the LP, as well as for development of lymph nodes [5, 6].

2.1
Functions of RORγt in Lymphoid Organogenesis and T Cell Development

RORγ and the closely related RORγt isoform are retinoic acid receptor-related transcription factors for which no ligand has yet been identified. These proteins are encoded by overlapping transcripts with alternative start sites and differ in sequence at their amino termini. During T cell development, RORγt is expressed in $CD4^+CD8^+$ (double positive, DP) thymocytes, the precursors for $CD4^+$ helper and $CD8^+$ cytotoxic T cells. In our early studies, we found that forced RORγ expression in T cells resulted in inhibition of NFAT-mediated induction of IL-2 transcription. This was due to competition for NFAT binding sites on DNA by RORγ [7]. In a separate study, He et al. isolated RORγt in a screen for cDNA clones that inhibited Fas-mediated activation-induced cell death in a T cell line [8]. This most likely reflects the ability of RORγt to block

NFAT-dependent induction of FasL. In mice lacking expression of RORγ and RORγt, survival of DP thymocytes was dramatically reduced, and fewer T cells differentiated to maturity. This was not related to a defect in FasL expression, but, instead, was due to the requirement for RORγt to direct expression of the antiapoptotic factor Bcl-xL in DP thymocytes. Forced expression of Bcl-xL in the mutant mice rescued development of thymocytes and restored normal T cell numbers in the periphery [9]. We have proposed that the function of RORγt in the thymus is to prolong the life span of DP thymocytes, giving them the opportunity to be selected into the mature T cell pool by interaction of their receptors with MHC molecules and thus avoiding "death by neglect." Because the T cell receptor α locus can undergo sequential V to J segment rearrangements, resulting in expression of new TCRs, a longer life span increases the opportunity for selection by host MHC-peptide complexes. Indeed, in the absence of RORγt, only proximal V_α to J_α rearrangements were observed, resulting in a limited TCR repertoire [10].

A second major function of RORγt, revealed in the analysis of the mutant mice, is to direct the development of lymph nodes and PPs. None of these secondary lymphoid organs developed in the absence of this nuclear receptor, although development of splenic follicles was normal [9]. A similar phenotype was observed in mice lacking the inhibitory HLH transcription factor Id2 [11]. In the absence of either RORγt or Id2, there was a loss of the fetal $CD4^+CD3^-IL$-$7R\alpha^+$ cells proposed by Mebius and Nishikawa to be involved in development of lymphoid tissues [12–15]. These cells, now named lymphoid tissue inducer (LTi) cells, are best defined by the expression of RORγt [5]. LTi cells can be readily visualized in and isolated from mice in which a GFP reporter has been inserted at the start site of the *RORγt* gene [5]. They have been observed in embryos as early as day 12.5 of gestation, in aggregates in regions where lymph nodes and PPs will develop. Many, but not all, LTi cells express high levels of CD4. In addition to IL-7Rα, they also express the lymphotoxin $\alpha_1\beta_2$ heterotrimer (LT), the related TNF family member TRANCE, and the chemokine receptors CXCR5 and CCR7.

Lymph node and PP development in the fetus has been proposed to be initiated by localized production in mesenchymal "organizing" centers of the chemokines CXCL13/BLC, the CXCR5 ligand, and CCL19/ELC or CCL21/SLC, the CCR7 ligands. The LTi cells then migrate toward the organizer, where they induce a cascade of events by LT-mediated triggering of the LTβ receptor and the downstream NF-κB pathway through NIK, a kinase deficient in lymphoid organ-defective *aly/aly* mice. This results in upregulation of the integrin ligands ICAM-1 and VCAM-1 on the stroma as well as expression of chemokines that recruit B and T cells and more LTi cells in a positive feedback loop. Finally, the cells in the newly formed clusters reorganize to form an organized lymph

Table 1 Development of LNs and organized GALT as well as induction of sIgA production in different mouse models

Model	PP	MLN	PLN	ILFs	CPs	LP B cells	sIgA
$LT\alpha^{-/-}$	−	−	−	−	−	−	−
$LT\beta R^{-/-}$	−	−	−	−	−	−	−
aly/aly	−	−	−	−	+	−	−
$LT\beta^{-/-}$	−	+	+/−	−	−	−	−
$TNF^{-/-}$	Less	+	+	+	+	+	+
$TNFR-I^{-/-}$	Less/small	+	+	−	+	++	Low
$TNFR-II^{-/-}$	+	+	+	+	+	+	+
$TRANCE^{-/-}$	+	−	−	NR	NR	NR	NR
$ROR\gamma^{-/-}$	−	−	−	−	−	NR	NR
$IL-7R\alpha^{-/-}$	−	+	+	Atrophied	+ (less)	NR	NR
$\gamma_c^{-/-}$	−	−	−	−	−	Very few	NR
$Id2^{-/-}$	−	−	−	−	−	NR	NR
$IL-7^{-/-}$	−	−	−	NR	NR	NR	NR
μMT	+ (small)	+	+	−	+	+	+ (half)
RAG-KO	+ (small)	+	+	−	+ (large)	−	−
$AID^{-/-}$	+	+	+	++ Hyperplasic	+	+ (IgM+)	−
Germ-free	+ (small)	+	+	−	+	Few	Very low
$TCR\beta X\delta^{-/-}$	+	+	+	+	+	+	+

NR, not reported

node or PP structure with B cell follicles, T cell areas, and specialized vasculature [16]. This series of events is thought to apply in general to development of lymphoid organs, but there are some differences as to which gene products are required for each type of organ, as listed in Table 1. Although the early inductive events are now reasonably well characterized, there remain many details to be worked out. For example, the LT signal, although essential for lymph node development, is not sufficient to induce expression of ICAM-1 and VCAM-1 and the development of the lymph nodes; therefore, the LTi cells are clearly providing other essential signals [5]. It is also not yet known how the mesenchymal cell response to LTi cells results in subsequent organization of lymphoid tissues.

A third function that we can now ascribe to RORγt is its requirement in the development of tertiary lymphoid tissues in the lamina propria in small intestine and colon. We observed RORγt-expressing cells in both CPs and

ILFs, and these structures were absent in the RORγt-deficient mice. Because RORγt⁺ cells in the lamina propria have features similar to those of LTi cells, we believe that they perform inductive functions similar to those that occur during fetal development of secondary lymphoid organs. We will describe studies on the functions and potential relationship between CPs and ILFs and speculate as to the potential role of RORγt⁺ LTi-like cells in the genesis of ectopic lymphoid follicles in autoimmune diseases.

Fetal LTi cells and adult LTi-like cells thus play a central role in the development of secondary lymphoid organs and organized GALT and require the expression of RORγt. RORγt-deficient animals differ significantly from other models that lack organized GALT and/or peripheral lymph nodes (PLNs) (see Table 1), such as $LT\alpha^{-/-}$, $LT\beta^{-/-}$, $LT\beta R^{-/-}$, and *aly/aly* or $NIK^{-/-}$ animals. In the latter models, the defects are at later stages of lymphoid organ development, whereas the RORγt (and Id2) deficiencies result in early abrogation of inducer cell development.

2.2
Structure and Function of Organized GALT Structures

To simplify the discussion of immune responses, mucosal immune sites are customarily divided into inducer (or inductive) and effector sites. The inducer sites are generally identified as secondary lymphoid organs, which in the intestine are the PPs and MLNs. The effector sites are within the LP, where there are populations of B and T lymphocytes as well as multiple populations of DCs and other myeloid cells, and the epithelium, where the IELs reside. It is thought that antigens come in contact with the immune system in the inductive sites, where they are delivered either actively by DCs or passively through M cells. Upon antigen presentation in the inductive site, lymphocytes differentiate into effector cells and migrate to effector sites. This separation of inducer and effector sites rests on the assumption that induction of immune responses occurs only in organized lymphoid follicles of secondary lymphoid organs (PPs and MLNs in the intestine), whereas effectors (plasma cells and activated T cells) accumulate and act in the LP.

Recent findings suggest that this conceptual separation of inductive and effector sites is not so clear-cut in vivo. For example, PPs and intact MLN architecture have been reported to be dispensable for antigen-specific B cell responses and IgA production [17, 18]. However, other types of lymphoid aggregates in the intestine, such as ILFs, may also serve as inductive sites, and these have different developmental requirements than PPs. The appearance of functional ILFs may be dependent on signals received by other GALT structures, such as CPs, or DCs in the LP. In addition, the LP, which was considered an exclusive effector site, may have an additional role in B cell activation and class switching [19]. The primary argument for the exclusive inductive capacity of PPs and MLNs was that these were thought to be the only sites where antigen gained access to the mucosal immune system, which is required for the inductive phase of an immune response. PPs contain follicular-associated epithelium (FAE) with specialized intestinal epithelial cells, the M cells, which sieve antigen from the lumen and deliver it to subpopulations of DCs. These DCs can then present the antigen in the context of a germinal center (GC) reaction in the PP or migrate to the MLN and induce immune responses there. However, recent studies have described at least four alternative means of antigen uptake directly into the LP, thus circumventing the PP. M cells were also found in ILFs [20] as well as dispersed in the villus intestinal epithelium [21]. Thus antigen can potentially gain access to the mucosa through both ILFs and villus M cells. Other studies have demonstrated that LP DCs can extend dendrites through the epithelial tight junctions and sample luminal antigens directly [22, 23]. Although it is thought that migration of DCs to the MLN is required to induce an immune response [24], it remains possible that antigen presentation or induction of immune functions can occur directly within the LP. Finally, epithelial cells can directly transfer IgG-bound antigen by using the intestinal neonatal Fc receptor (FcRn) as a shuttle [25], thus delivering the antigen into the LP, where it will most likely be taken up by phagocytic immune cells.

Despite the lack of a clear functional delineation between inducer and effector sites, the existence of distinct immune structures within the intestines is well established. We discuss recent advances in our understanding of their structure and function during immune responses below.

2.2.1
Peyer's Patches

The Peyer's patch (PP) is the largest organized lymphoid tissue of the small intestine. The central structures are B cell follicles, which are usually multiple and large. The number of B cell follicles defines the size of the PP. In mice PPs contain fewer than 10 follicles, usually 3–4, whereas human PPs may be several centimeters long and contain many tens of follicles [26]. T cells are also present in the PP. The T cell areas are around high endothelial venules (HEVs), between the B cell follicles. The luminal side of the PP is lined with a specialized epithelium, called follicle-associated epithelium (FAE). FAE lacks crypts or villi and, in contrast to the columnar villous epithelium, is cuboid, has few goblet cells, and does not contain secretory cells such as Paneth cells. The major feature of FAE is the presence of specialized epithelial cells called M cells. M cells are derived from adjacent crypts and have specialized microfolds instead of microvilli on their luminal surface, which allow for transcytosis of luminal antigens [27]. On the PP side M cells possess large pockets that are tightly associated with PP immune cells, represented by clusters of DCs, CD4$^+$ T cells, and B cells [28, 29]. M cells participate in the formation of a regional environment bellow the FAE that differs in composition of immune cells from the rest of the PP and the villous epithelium. This region is also known as the subepithelial dome (SED). M cells are the major portals of antigen entry into the mucosa and thus direct and deliver the antigen to immune cells in the SED [30–32]. Pathogenic microorganisms, such as virulent *Salmonella* species, *Yersinia* species, *Shigella flexneri*, Poliovirus, and reoviruses may take advantage of the M cells to gain access to the intestinal mucosa.

As in other immune inductive sites, PP DCs are probably responsible for initiating and directing the subsequent immune response. In the PP, several populations of DCs have been described [33]. The first is found directly below the SED. These cells are CD11c$^+$, DEC205$^-$, and M342$^-$ and are also found in the B cell follicle outside of GCs. These cells are mainly immature myeloid DCs (CD11b$^+$ CD8α^-) [34] and appear to take up antigens transported by M cells. The second population is found in the intrafollicular region and is seen in close proximity with T cells. These cells are mainly lymphoid DCs (CD11b$^-$ CD8α^+) [34] and also express DEC205 and M342, which correlate with DC maturation. "Double negative" DCs (CD11b$^-$ CD8α^-) are found in both locations.

DCs in the PP induce intestine-specific immune responses. Surface phenotypic analysis of CD11c$^+$ DC populations revealed that PP DCs express higher levels of MHC class II molecules, but similar levels of costimulatory and adhesion molecules, compared with splenic DCs [35]. DCs isolated from the spleen induce a Th1-biased response characterized by high levels of IFNγ production. In contrast, DCs isolated from PPs, especially those of the myeloid lineage, induce a Th2 response that includes elevated IL-4 and IL-10 and reduced IFNγ production by T cells [34, 35]. In addition, stimulation with CD40L or RANKL leads to IL-10 production by DCs from PPs, but IL-12 production by DCs from lymph nodes [34–36]. Thus, there exist significant functional differences between DCs from different tissues.

One of the most prominent roles of the PP is the formation of GCs after antigenic stimulation, with subsequent production of IgA. Class switching to IgA occurs in the GCs, and the resulting plasmablasts migrate out of the PP to the LP to form plasma cells and produce sIgA [37, 38]. B cells play a major role in the organization of the PP in general and the FAE in particular, because B cell-deficient mice have very small PPs, FAE and M cell numbers [39].

PPs also play a major role in the activation of T cells and their homing to the LP. Because PPs are on the major route of lymphocyte recirculation, small naïve T cells enter the T cell areas of the PP using L-selectin and CCR7 [40]. After antigen stimulation, secretion of retinoic acid by intestinal DCs causes the upregulation on T cells of the gut homing receptors α4β7 and CCR9 and downregulation of E selectin ligands [41], allowing the T cells to preferentially migrate to the LP.

2.2.2
Isolated Lymphoid Follicles

ILFs are relatively large lymphoid aggregates found throughout the LP, in both small intestine and colon, with the highest density in the antimesenteric wall of the small intestine [20, 42]. They are most abundant in the distal ileum [42], which may be related to their developmental requirement for intestinal flora. ILFs are composed of a single B cell follicle and thus resemble a small PP. Their similarity to PPs is further underlined by the presence of a GC and M cells. A recent study implied that ILFs can serve as inductive sites for mucosal immune responses, especially following signals from pathogenic bacteria [43]. ILFs are composed of a large central cluster of B cells surrounded by a ring of RORγt$^+$c-kit$^+$IL-7Rα$^+$ cells (see below and Fig. 1F). In addition, a large number of DCs are present in the ILF [20] (Fig. 2). Besides size and general morphology, ILFs appear postnatally [44], whereas PPs develop during late fetal life. Although both ILFs and PPs require LTβR signaling for development, ILFs, but not PPs, require LTβR signaling for maintenance through adulthood: Treatment of adult mice with LTβR-Ig eliminates ILFs, but not PPs or MLNs [44]. In addition, ILF development requires stimulation by commensal intestinal microflora [42]. Thus ILFs were absent in germ-free mice, which have small PPs [20], but ILF development was induced by recolonization with normal flora [42]. Furthermore, ILF hyperplasia correlated with the increased commensal bacterial load in activation induced cytidine-deaminase (AID)-deficient mice that cannot class switch and therefore lack IgA. The ILF hyperplasia was abolished when bacterial load was decreased by antibiotic treatment [45]. Together, these studies suggest that ILFs form continuously throughout adult life, in response to the commensal microflora, and that RORγt$^+$ cells are essential for their induction.

ILFs may be functionally redundant or complementary to PPs. They may contribute to the production of antigen-specific sIgA [17] or may serve as inductive sites of pathogen-specific immune responses in vivo [43]. One possibility is that ILFs form in the absence of PPs, when IgA levels are low, or in response to the microflora to supplement levels of sIgA, thus serving as a second line of defense and aiding the PP. Another possible role for ILFs is that they are responsible for the induction of sIgA against bacterial stimuli, whereas

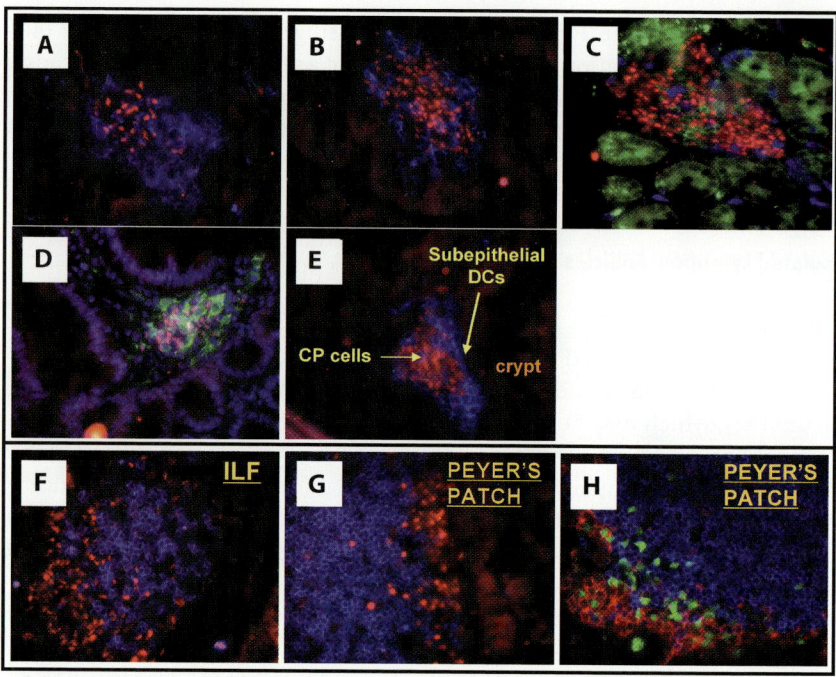

Fig. 1A–H RORγt⁺ cells act as inducers of all organized GALT in small intestinal LP. Different sized cryptopatches (CPs) (**A–C**) are present at the bottom of villi near the crypt areas (**D, E**). Cryptopatches contain large clusters of RORγt⁺ cells (*red*) surrounded by CD11c⁺ DCs (*blue* in **A, B**, and **E** and *green* in **D**). Very few B and T cells are present in CPs (**C**). RORγt⁺ cells are also present in ILFs (**F**) and around B cell follicles in the PP (**G, H**). All sections are at ×40 magnification. *Colors*: **A, B, E** *Red* (RORγ), *blue* (CD11c); **C** *red* (RORγ), *blue* (CD3), *green* (B220); **D** *red* (RORγ), *blue* (DAPI), *green* (CD11c); **F, G** *red* (RORγ), *blue* (B220); **H** *green* (RORγt), *blue* (B220), *red* (CD11c)

PPs and MLNs are more important in the production of antigen-specific sIgA after oral immunization [17, 18, 43].

Most studies point to a function of ILFs as sensors of intestinal microflora, receiving signals from the lumen and probably transmitting these signals to the mucosal immune system. Thus the close association of ILFs with DCs and RORγt⁺c-kit⁺ cells would allow ILFs to receive signals from the DCs that sample the lumen of the intestine. The presence of hundreds of organized lymphoid structures throughout the LP, as opposed to the limited number of PPs, would allow for faster and more efficient sampling and activation of local immune responses. Keeping the immune response localized would also

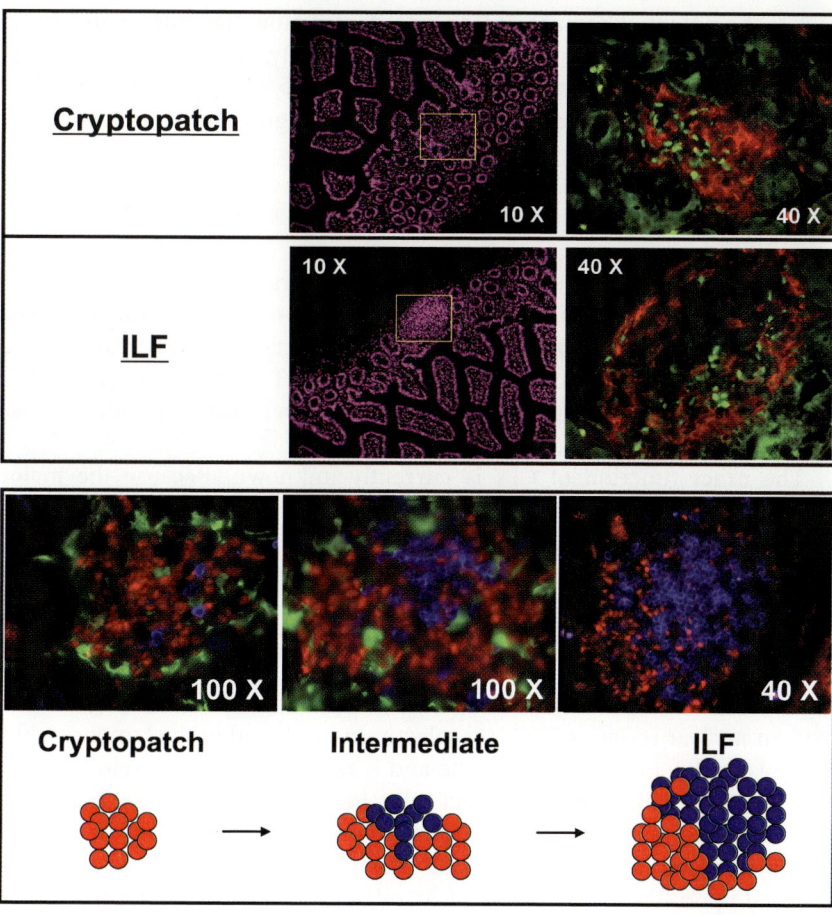

Fig. 2 Cryptopatches and ILFs. *Top and middle panels*: Cryptopatches are small lymphoid aggregates consisting mainly of RORγt⁺ lymphoid tissue inducer-like cells and dendritic cells (DCs). ILFs are large aggregates that are readily detectable with DAPI staining and consist of a large B cell follicle surrounded by RORγt⁺ inducer-like cells and DCs. Sections were obtained from the small intestine of an adult RORγt-GFP-KI mouse. RORγt⁺ cells (*green*) and DCs (*red*) were stained with antibodies against GFP (Alexa 488) and CD11c (PE). *Left panels*: DAPI staining only. *Bottom panel*: Different stages of ILF development. In this model RORγ⁺ cells in the cryptopatch receive signals from DCs and induce stromal cell production of chemokines, such as CXCL13, to recruit B cells and form ILFs. Structures intermediate between CPs and ILFs, containing small clusters of B cells, are often seen in the LP. Sections were obtained from the small intestine of a heterozygous CX_3CR1-GFP-KI mouse. Staining is with anti-RORγ⁺ Cy3 (*red*) and B220-APC for B cells (*blue*). In the first two panels CX_3CR1^+ DCs (*green*) were stained with an antibody against GFP (Alexa 488)

reduce the potential damage caused by inflammation, therefore maintaining the integrity of the intestinal barrier. Additionally, ILF-based immune responses may precede those in PPs and MLNs, which would require more time to develop because of the requirement for cell migration to and from these sites.

2.2.3
Cryptopatches

Cryptopatches (CPs) were first described as clusters of c-kit$^+$Lin$^-$ lymphoid-like cells and DCs in the LP of the small intestine [46]. Their name is derived from their location in proximity to the bottom of crypt villous areas. CPs are distinguished from ILFs by the lack of both B and T lymphocytes [20]. It has been estimated that about 1,500 CPs accumulate over time in the adult mouse intestine [46, 47].

The exact function of CPs is currently unknown. Because the major lymphoid-like cells in CPs express the lymphoid precursor markers c-kit and IL-7Rα, CPs were postulated to be involved in the extrathymic pathway of IEL differentiation. Initial reconstitution experiments, as well as transfer of Lin$^-$c-kit$^+$IL-7Rα$^+$ CP cells from nude mice into *scid* mice, supported this hypothesis, as IELs were generated in the immunodeficient host [48]. However, we have recently shown that, in immune-competent mice, CP cells do not give rise to IELs. This conclusion was made possible by the finding that the orphan nuclear receptor RORγt is selectively expressed in the lymphoid-like CP cells in the adult small intestine and is required for the development of CPs. RORγt$^{-/-}$ mice completely lack CPs ([6], Fig. 3), but there is no reduction in the number of TCRγδ IELs. The reduced TCRαβ IEL numbers were due to compromised thymic output in the mutant mice, and these cells were restored upon forced expression of Bcl-xL, despite continued absence of CP cells. To determine which cells are precursors of the IEL, we performed fate-mapping experiments. When RORγt-Cre transgenic mice were crossed with ROSA26-GFP reporter mice that express GFP only after Cre-mediated excision of a transcriptional stop signal, all DP-derived T cells, including TCRαβ IELs, and all CP cells expressed GFP. In contrast, when the ROSA26-GFP mice were crossed to CD4-Cre mice (in which Cre expression is present in DP cells and CD4 lineage T cells but not CP cells), GFP could only be seen in the TCRαβ IELs, but not in CP cells. These experiments supported the finding that most, if not all, of the TCRαβ IEL are derived from CD4$^+$CD8$^+$ DP thymocytes rather than from CP cells [6].

In addition, the fate-mapping studies indicated that the RORγt$^+$ fetal LTi cells and adult CP cells have no apparent lineage progeny. This finding suggests that RORγt$^+$ LTi cells and CP cells are terminally differentiated cells

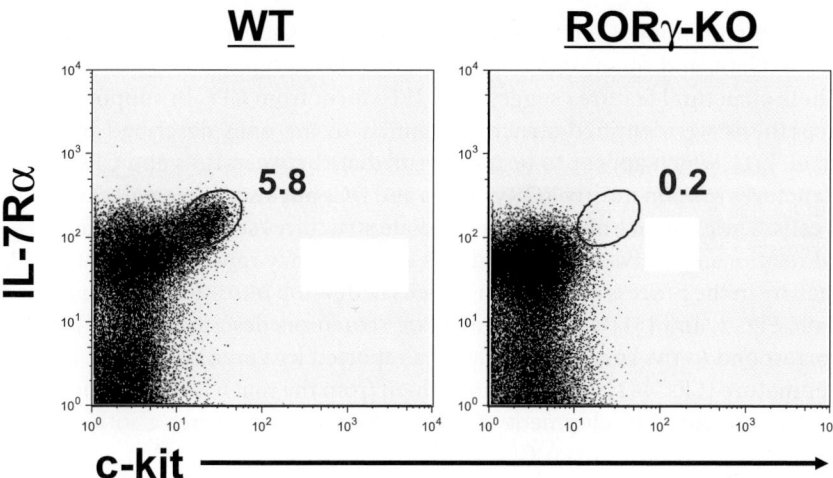

Fig. 3 RORγ-KO mice lack CP cells. No c-kit^{hi}IL-7Rα^{hi} CP cells are detected in RORγ-KO and RORγt-KO (not shown) mice. Representative staining of total LP lymphocytes is shown. The plots were gated on CD45$^+$ lymphocytes. The numbers indicate percentage of CD45$^+$ lymphocytes

whose function is to induce lymphoid structures in the appropriate microenvironment. Once secondary lymphoid organs are induced during fetal development, LTi cells appear to no longer be necessary. In contrast, the RORγt$^+$ CP cells are thought to be continuously replenished in adult animals. Reconstitution experiments have shown that CPs and ILFs in LTα and common γ chain ($γ_c$)-deficient mice can be reconstituted by the transfer of wild-type bone marrow (BM), indicating that adult BM can be a source of precursors for LTi-like cells [49, 50].

2.3
Cryptopatches as Organizing Centers for Localized Mucosal Responses

In adult mice heterozygous for the *RORγt*^{GFP} allele, expression of the GFP reporter was limited to DP thymocytes and to cells in the lamina propria of the small and large intestine. In the LP, all Lin$^-$c-kit$^+$IL-7Rα$^+$ CP cells [48] were GFP$^+$. We also utilized a monoclonal antibody against RORγ/RORγt to assess its expression in wild-type mice. Combining these two approaches revealed that CPs consist almost exclusively of RORγt$^+$ cells tightly clustered and surrounded by DCs (Fig. 1A–E). ILFs contain a peripheral layer of RORγt$^+$ cells in addition to the major B cell follicle (Fig. 1F) and may thus represent a later stage in GALT development than the CP. Interestingly, RORγt$^+$ cells were also found surrounding B cell follicles in the PP (Fig. 1G,H), providing a potential mechanistic and functional link between all three types of organized GALT. These structural features suggest that ILFs form from CPs. In support of this hypothesis we identified structures similar to the ones described by Pabst et. al. [51], which appear to be an intermediate between ILFs and CPs. These structures contain mostly RORγt$^+$ cells and DCs but also have small clusters of B cells. The existence of these intermediate structures suggests a developmental relationship between ILFs and CPs and they may represent activated CPs that are in the process of recruiting B cells to develop into an ILF (unpublished data, Fig. 2, and [51]). The intermediate structures described here may also correspond to the small B220$^+$ clusters reported by Lorenz et al. and labeled "immature ILFs" [42], to distinguish them from the much larger mature ILFs.

The temporal development of the two types of structures also hints that ILFs may be derived from CPs. In the mouse, CPs first develop around 1–2 weeks of age and ILFs are not observed until the colonization of the intestine by microflora around weaning time (3–4 weeks) [20, 46].

In addition, as can be seen from Table 1, mice deficient in organized GALT lack either both ILFs and CPs or only ILFs. For example *aly/aly*, IL-7Rα, and RAG-KO mice have CPs but lack ILFs, but there is no mouse model that specifically lacks CPs while still preserving ILFs. The ILF-like aggregates in RAG-KO mice [20] are most likely enlarged CPs and not ILFs because they do not contain any B cells. It is possible that the CPs are hyperactivated in the RAG-KO LP and recruit, through a positive feedback loop, the only available lymphoid-like cells in this environment. As a result, these RORγt$^+$ cells form large CPs instead of ILFs.

CPs may thus activate the intestinal stroma to recruit B cells and form ILFs and in this way participate in an integrated mucosal immune network. In the case of fetal LTi cells, developmentally timed signals are likely to activate the inducer function of these cells (such as lymphotoxin $\alpha_1\beta_2$ and other still undefined mediators) and subsequent development of lymph nodes and PPs. If RORγt$^+$ CP cells have a similar inducer function, it is likely that this is regulated by environmental signals rather than by developmental timing. Environmental signals emanating in the lumen may be transmitted to the RORγt$^+$ cells through the surrounding layer of DCs. This may induce the recruitment of B cells and generation of ILFs. In support of the hypothesis that RORγt$^+$ cells help recruit naïve B cells to LP, RORγt-KO mice lack CPs and have very few B cells in the LP (I.I. Ivanov and D.R. Littman, unpublished data). Correspondingly B cells accumulate in the spleen and peritoneal cavity (our unpublished data and [52]). Additionally, naïve B cells require intact LTβR-signaling on stromal cells for their recruitment to the LP [53, 54]. Together, these data suggest that LTβR-signaling on cryptopatch stroma, most likely induced by RORγt⁺ CP cells, is necessary for the recruitment of naïve B cells to the LP. Formation of ILFs would then allow for production of sIgA.

DCs probably have an essential role in CP function. Large clusters of DCs are present at the periphery of the CP, surrounding the RORγt⁺ cells as shown in Fig. 1. These DCs are located directly in the subepithelial space of the crypts and may be the first to receive signals from penetrating bacteria or bacteria present in the crypts, which would be a signal for a failure in immune protection. Alternatively, DCs may transmit signals from the lumen by direct sampling of its content. The latter was suggested by the presence at the periphery of the CP of a population of DCs that express the fractalkine receptor CX_3CR1, as can be seen in Fig. 2. These DCs were recently demonstrated to form a dense network under the basal lamina and to project dendrites into the lumen of the intestine, especially in the terminal ileum [22]. The CX_3CR1-expressing DCs can transport bacteria into the LP with these transepithelial dendrites [22]. DCs that transport bacteria into the lumen may then transmit the information to the CP as well as to the MLN. In our model, this transport may induce the differentiation of CP to ILFs. Interestingly, mature ILFs, are mostly present in the terminal ileum [42], which is colonized by microflora and is the only region of the small intestine that contains these transepithelial dendrites. Figure 4 represents schematically a model of the possible function of CPs and ILFs.

The strategic location of CPs at the base of crypts may indicate that these structures have functions in addition to inducing differentiation of B cell follicles. For example, in response to luminal signals, possibly mediated by the epithelium-associated network of DCs, CPs may induce innate immune responses in the nearby crypt epithelium. Following signals from the lumen, RORγt⁺ CP cells or associated DCs may thus modify the function of Paneth cells by inducing secretion of bioactive molecules (e.g., defensins), or they may participate in the regeneration of epithelium from epithelial stem cells in the crypt. The latter is an especially attractive possibility in light of the finding of Medzhitov and colleagues that TLR-mediated signaling supplied by the intestinal microflora is required for regeneration of the intestinal epithelium after chemical or radiation-induced damage [55].

3
Dendritic Cells, a Double-Edged Sword

In the model that we propose (Fig. 4), DCs continuously survey the intestinal lumen for commensal and pathogenic microorganisms and communicate with other cells in the lamina propria and the epithelium to activate innate

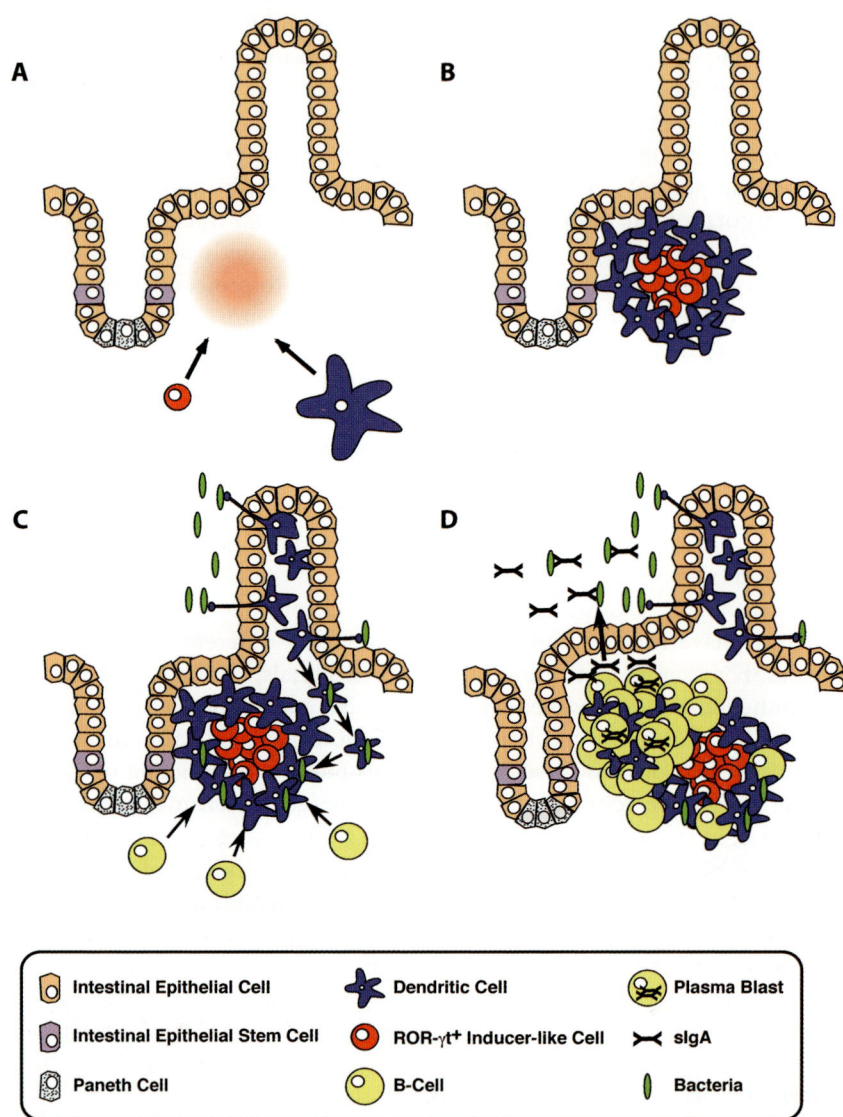

Fig. 4A–D Model of cryptopatch (*CP*) function in sIgA production **A** The initial stages and order of cell recruitment in CP and ILF formation are unclear. RORγt$^+$ LTi-like cells and DCs are recruited to the base of villi. The signals for this recruitment may initiate from the DCs, the RORγt$^+$ LTi-like cells, or the stroma. However, RORγt$^+$ cells were shown to be the major inducer population in fetal lymph node and PP anlagen and may also play a similar role in the adult. **B** A CP, consisting of RORγt-expressing LTi-like cells as well as dendritic cells, is formed. **C** CPs may receive signals from the lumen through the sampling action of subepithelial DCs. DCs may deliver bacterial antigens to the CP in addition to migrating to mesenteric lymph nodes. Activation of CP cells may lead to induction of B cell recruitment signals from the stroma. **D** The recruited B cells form clusters, resulting in ILF formation. B cells are then activated and class-switch to IgA. IgA-producing cells may differentiate into plasmablasts/plasma cells in the lamina propria to secrete sIgA into the lumen

host defense mechanisms. In this model, activation of the DCs by microbial products induces recruitment of B cells as well as some LP T cells into the CP, resulting in formation of ILFs. This could be due to direct action of CP-associated DCs on B and T cells, to activation of CP stromal cells by the DC, or to DC-mediated activation of the RORγt$^+$ CP cells, which, in turn, would activate the stromal cells, resulting in lymphocyte recruitment. An important outcome would be the production of sIgA, which limits the concentration of bacteria in the intestinal crypts. The introduction of antigen would cause the maturation of a CP into an ILF and allow for a rapid and localized immune response. Additionally, DCs will migrate to the MLN to induce both mucosal and systemic immune responses.

The direct detection of antigens by DCs allows for rapid recognition of pathogens. The DCs form a complex network throughout the intestine and can rapidly transmit danger signals and recruit immune effector cells. However, in some pathogenic settings, such as HIV infection, this network and direct recruitment may lead to an enhancement of infection. DCs can bind HIV through the cell surface C-type lectin DC-SIGN, which results in virus uptake and enhanced infection of cocultivated T cells [56, 57]. This interaction may also allow intact virus to exploit the trafficking properties of DC to disseminate from the mucosa to secondary lymphoid organs [56, 57]. In addition, the interaction of intestinal DC with effector memory T cells could explain the sustained loss of these cells that has been reported in HIV and SIV infections.

Activated memory T cells express the chemokine receptor CCR5. This is a major coreceptor for both HIV and SIV, making memory T cells a primary target for both viruses. Mattapallil et al. used quantitative PCR to show that at the peak of SIV infection 30%–60% of CD4$^+$ memory T cells throughout the body are infected with the virus. Most of these infected cells disappear within

4 days [58]. As a consequence, over one-half of all memory CD4$^+$ T cells in SIV-infected macaques are destroyed directly by the virus during the acute phase of infection.

Because of the constant activation by oral antigens and the surveillance necessary in the GI tract, a much higher percentage of T cells in the gut are memory T cells and an easy target for HIV infection. In 1995, the massive depletion of CD4$^+$ T cells in the gut was first reported [59]. It wasn't until 1998 that studies in macaques demonstrated how quickly this depletion occurred. Veazey et al. reported that 14–21 days after infection with SIV there was a dramatic decrease in CD4$^+$ T cells in the gut [60]. Strikingly, at this point in infection there was no decrease in blood or lymph node CD4$^+$ T cells. In addition, the decrease of T cells seems to be a direct effect of the virus, as peak virus production in the GI tract in SIV infection coincides with peak number of infected CD4$^+$ T cells [61]. There is a corresponding depletion of CD4$^+$ cells in other mucosal areas, as similar depletion has been observed in the vaginal and lung mucosa [62, 63]. It was further demonstrated that most infected cells were not recently activated T cells but were resting memory cells [61].

The findings with SIV were recently correlated with two studies of HIV-infected patients. In HIV$^+$ patients, there is a significant and preferential depletion of mucosal CD4$^+$ T cells compared with peripheral blood CD4$^+$. This depletion occurs mainly in the LP instead of in the PP in all stages of disease [64, 65]. As in macaques infected with SIV, this depletion occurs preferentially within CCR5$^+$ CD4$^+$ T cells [65].

Cross-sectional analysis of a cohort of primary HIV-1 infection subjects showed that although chronic suppression of HIV-1 permits near-complete immune recovery of the peripheral blood CD4$^+$ T cell population, a significantly greater CD4$^+$ T cell loss persists in the GI mucosa, despite up to 5 years of fully suppressive therapy [64].

It is formally possible that DC-SIGN-mediated uptake of HIV represents a mechanism for long-term retention of infectious HIV particles within DCs. Intestinal DCs therefore represent a potentially sizable reservoir for HIV and may be important in the transport and dissemination of the virus. Local dissemination in the lamina propria could involve not only T helper cells but also the lymphoid-like CP cells. In mouse, about one-third to one-half of these RORγt$^+$ cells express CD4, and these cells also express a variety of chemokine receptors that can function as coreceptors for HIV entry. The equivalent cell population in humans has not yet been described, but it is highly likely to be present, because ILFs have been identified in human lamina propria. If these cells also express CD4, they are highly likely to be targets of HIV within the intestine, and this may contribute to pathogenesis of viral infection. Understanding the contribution of intestinal DCs and the RORγt$^+$

CP cells to initiation of immune responses in the LP may therefore lead to important insights for designing strategies to eliminate HIV from the body.

4
LTi Cells and Ectopic Lymphoid Follicles in Autoimmunity

Several autoimmune diseases, including Crohn's disease, rheumatoid arthritis, and type I diabetes, are marked by formation of ectopic lymphoid organ-like structures within the affected tissues. The contribution of such ectopic follicles to disease pathogenesis remains unexplored. The role of LTi cells or related inducer cells (such as those found in CPs) in these lesions has yet to be explored. Forced expression of CXCL13/BLC in pancreatic islet cells resulted in the local formation of lymphoid follicles, but this was independent of LTi cells, because follicles were also observed in ROR$\gamma^{-/-}$ mice ([66] and unpublished collaborative result). However, CXCL13 expression by stromal cells is induced by LTβR signaling. As LTi-like cells are the producers of LT$\alpha\beta$, this system may bypass the requirement for the cells. In autoimmune diseases, inflammatory stimuli may result in activation of LTi or CP-like cells, particularly in the intestine, and this could induce excessive follicle formation. Consistent with this notion, the number of ILFs is increased in dextran sulfate-induced colitis in mice [67] and also in Crohn's disease [68] and ulcerative colitis [69] in humans . Such tertiary lymphoid tissue could have a central role in autoimmune disease. Because nuclear receptors are readily amenable to pharmacological manipulation, inhibition of RORγt function in vivo may be achievable and may provide a means to control inflammatory bowel disease.

5
Conclusions

The intestinal immune system is a dynamic environment. By necessity, many types of detection and inductive sites must exist throughout the intestine. The intestinal immune system is constantly bombarded with different types of antigens, which it must rapidly identify and respond to accordingly. If the antigen is a food antigen, the immune system must become tolerant; if the antigen is a non-pathogenic commensal bacteria, the immune system must work to contain it in the lumen of the intestine; if the antigen is a pathogenic bacteria or virus, the immune system must initiate a protective immune response. The DC-CP-ILF axis may play a major role in integrating signals from the lumen or the crypt, thus allowing for the rapid detection of and response to a variety of antigens while limiting the response to a local region. This would allow for control of pathogenic microbes while stronger responses in either the PP or MLN are being generated. Consequently, this will result in faster containment as well as limit the potential damage to the delicate balance of the intestine.

The mechanisms that are involved in sampling microorganisms and mounting appropriate responses can potentially also be turned against the host, resulting in autoimmune inflammatory bowel disease or in persistent infections. A better understanding of the role of the intestinal DC-CP-ILF axis in immune responses will be necessary to determine its importance in human disease.

References

1. Sonnenburg JL, Xu J, Leip DD, Chen CH, Westover BP, Weatherford J, Buhler JD, Gordon JI: Glycan foraging in vivo by an intestine-adapted bacterial symbiont. *Science* 2005, 307:1955–1959.
2. Macpherson AJ, Uhr T: Compartmentalization of the mucosal immune responses to commensal intestinal bacteria. *Ann NY Acad Sci* 2004, 1029:36–43.
3. Macpherson AJ, Harris NL: Interactions between commensal intestinal bacteria and the immune system. *Nat Rev Immunol* 2004, 4:478–485.
4. Macpherson AJ, Geuking MB, McCoy KD: Immune responses that adapt the intestinal mucosa to commensal intestinal bacteria. *Immunology* 2005, 115:153–162.
5. Eberl G, Marmon S, Sunshine MJ, Rennert PD, Choi Y, Littman DR: An essential function for the nuclear receptor RORγ_t in the generation of fetal lymphoid tissue inducer cells. *Nat Immunol* 2004, 5:64–73.
6. Eberl G, Littman DR: Thymic origin of intestinal $\alpha\beta$ T cells revealed by fate mapping of RORγt+ Cells. *Science* 2004, 305:248–251.
7. Littman DR, Sun Z, Unutmaz D, Sunshine MJ, Petrie HT, Zou YR: Role of the nuclear hormone receptor ROR γ in transcriptional regulation, thymocyte survival, and lymphoid organogenesis. *Cold Spring Harb Symp Quant Biol* 1999, 64:373–381.
8. He YW, Deftos ML, Ojala EW, Bevan MJ: RORγ t, a novel isoform of an orphan receptor, negatively regulates Fas ligand expression and IL-2 production in T cells. *Immunity* 1998, 9:797–806.
9. Sun Z, Unutmaz D, Zou YR, Sunshine MJ, Pierani A, Brenner-Morton S, Mebius RE, Littman DR: Requirement for RORγ in thymocyte survival and lymphoid organ development. *Science* 2000, 288:2369–2373.
10. Guo J, Hawwari A, Li H, Sun Z, Mahanta SK, Littman DR, Krangel MS, He YW: Regulation of the TCRα repertoire by the survival window of CD4$^+$CD8$^+$ thymocytes. *Nat Immunol* 2002, 3:469–476.

11. Yokota Y, Mansouri A, Mori S, Sugawara S, Adachi S, Nishikawa S, Gruss P: Development of peripheral lymphoid organs and natural killer cells depends on the helix-loop-helix inhibitor Id2. *Nature* 1999, 397:702-706.
12. Mebius RE, Miyamoto T, Christensen J, Domen J, Cupedo T, Weissman IL, Akashi K: The fetal liver counterpart of adult common lymphoid progenitors gives rise to all lymphoid lineages, CD45+CD4+CD3− cells, as well as macrophages. *J Immunol* 2001, 166:6593-6601.
13. Mebius RE, Rennert P, Weissman IL: Developing lymph nodes collect CD4+CD3− LTβ+ cells that can differentiate to APC, NK cells, and follicular cells but not T or B cells. *Immunity* 1997, 7:493-504.
14. Yoshida H, Honda K, Shinkura R, Adachi S, Nishikawa S, Maki K, Ikuta K, Nishikawa SI: IL-7 receptor α^+ $CD3^-$ cells in the embryonic intestine induces the organizing center of Peyer's patches. *Int Immunol* 1999, 11:643-655.
15. Adachi S, Yoshida H, Kataoka H, Nishikawa S: Three distinctive steps in Peyer's patch formation of murine embryo. *Int Immunol* 1997, 9:507-514.
16. Eberl G, Littman DR: The role of the nuclear hormone receptor RORγt in the development of lymph nodes and Peyer's patches. *Immunol Rev* 2003, 195:81-90.
17. Yamamoto M, Kweon MN, Rennert PD, Hiroi T, Fujihashi K, McGhee JR, Kiyono H: Role of gut-associated lymphoreticular tissues in antigen-specific intestinal IgA immunity. *J Immunol* 2004, 173:762-769.
18. Yamamoto M, Rennert P, McGhee JR, Kweon MN, Yamamoto S, Dohi T, Otake S, Bluethmann H, Fujihashi K, Kiyono H: Alternate mucosal immune system: organized Peyer's patches are not required for IgA responses in the gastrointestinal tract. *J Immunol* 2000, 164:5184-5191.
19. Fagarasan S, Kinoshita K, Muramatsu M, Ikuta K, Honjo T: In situ class switching and differentiation to IgA-producing cells in the gut lamina propria. *Nature* 2001, 413:639-643.
20. Hamada H, Hiroi T, Nishiyama Y, Takahashi H, Masunaga Y, Hachimura S, Kaminogawa S, Takahashi-Iwanaga H, Iwanaga T, Kiyono H, et al.: Identification of multiple isolated lymphoid follicles on the antimesenteric wall of the mouse small intestine. *J Immunol* 2002, 168:57-64.
21. Jang MH, Kweon MN, Iwatani K, Yamamoto M, Terahara K, Sasakawa C, Suzuki T, Nochi T, Yokota Y, Rennert PD, et al.: Intestinal villous M cells: an antigen entry site in the mucosal epithelium. *Proc Natl Acad Sci USA* 2004, 101:6110-6115.
22. Niess JH, Brand S, Gu X, Landsman L, Jung S, McCormick BA, Vyas JM, Boes M, Ploegh HL, Fox JG, et al.: CX3CR1-mediated dendritic cell access to the intestinal lumen and bacterial clearance. *Science* 2005, 307:254-258.
23. Rescigno M, Urbano M, Valzasina B, Francolini M, Rotta G, Bonasio R, Granucci F, Kraehenbuhl JP, Ricciardi-Castagnoli P: Dendritic cells express tight junction proteins and penetrate gut epithelial monolayers to sample bacteria. *Nat Immunol* 2001, 2:361-367.
24. Macpherson AJ, Uhr T: Induction of protective IgA by intestinal dendritic cells carrying commensal bacteria. *Science* 2004, 303:1662-1665.
25. Spiekermann GM, Finn PW, Ward ES, Dumont J, Dickinson BL, Blumberg RS, Lencer WI: Receptor-mediated immunoglobulin G transport across mucosal barriers in adult life: functional expression of FcRn in the mammalian lung. *J Exp Med* 2002, 196:303-310.

26. Cornes JS: Peyer's patches in the human gut. *Proc R Soc Med* 1965, 58:716.
27. Owen RL, Jones AL: Epithelial cell specialization within human Peyer's patches: an ultrastructural study of intestinal lymphoid follicles. *Gastroenterology* 1974, 66:189–203.
28. Bjerke K, Brandtzaeg P, Fausa O: T cell distribution is different in follicle-associated epithelium of human Peyer's patches and villous epithelium. *Clin Exp Immunol* 1988, 74:270–275.
29. Yamanaka T, Straumfors A, Morton H, Fausa O, Brandtzaeg P, Farstad I: M cell pockets of human Peyer's patches are specialized extensions of germinal centers. *Eur J Immunol* 2001, 31:107–117.
30. Owen RL: Sequential uptake of horseradish peroxidase by lymphoid follicle epithelium of Peyer's patches in the normal unobstructed mouse intestine: an ultrastructural study. *Gastroenterology* 1977, 72:440–451.
31. Sicinski P, Rowinski J, Warchol JB, Jarzabek Z, Gut W, Szczygiel B, Bielecki K, Koch G: Poliovirus type 1 enters the human host through intestinal M cells. *Gastroenterology* 1990, 98:56-58.
32. Wolf JL, Rubin DH, Finberg R, Kauffman RS, Sharpe AH, Trier JS, Fields BN: Intestinal M cells: a pathway for entry of reovirus into the host. *Science* 1981, 212:471–472.
33. Kelsall BL, Strober W: Distinct populations of dendritic cells are present in the subepithelial dome and T cell regions of the murine Peyer's patch. *J Exp Med* 1996, 183:237–247.
34. Iwasaki A, Kelsall BL: Unique functions of CD11b+, CD8 α+, and double-negative Peyer's patch dendritic cells. *J Immunol* 2001, 166:4884–4890.
35. Iwasaki A, Kelsall BL: Freshly isolated Peyer's patch, but not spleen, dendritic cells produce interleukin 10 and induce the differentiation of T helper type 2 cells. *J Exp Med* 1999, 190:229–239.
36. Williamson E, Bilsborough JM, Viney JL: Regulation of mucosal dendritic cell function by receptor activator of NF-κ B (RANK)/RANK ligand interactions: impact on tolerance induction. *J Immunol* 2002, 169:3606–3612.
37. Craig SW, Cebra JJ: Peyer's patches: an enriched source of precursors for IgA-producing immunocytes in the rabbit. *J Exp Med* 1971, 134:188–200.
38. Guy-Grand D, Griscelli C, Vassalli P: The gut-associated lymphoid system: nature and properties of the large dividing cells. *Eur J Immunol* 1974, 4:435–443.
39. Golovkina TV, Shlomchik M, Hannum L, Chervonsky A: Organogenic role of B lymphocytes in mucosal immunity. *Science* 1999, 286:1965–1968.
40. Mora JR, Bono MR, Manjunath N, Weninger W, Cavanagh LL, Rosemblatt M, Von Andrian UH: Selective imprinting of gut-homing T cells by Peyer's patch dendritic cells. *Nature* 2003, 424:88–93.
41. Iwata M, Hirakiyama A, Eshima Y, Kagechika H, Kato C, Song SY: Retinoic acid imprints gut-homing specificity on T cells. *Immunity* 2004, 21:527–538.
42. Lorenz RG, Chaplin DD, McDonald KG, McDonough JS, Newberry RD: Isolated lymphoid follicle formation is inducible and dependent upon lymphotoxin-sufficient B lymphocytes, lymphotoxin β receptor, and TNF receptor I function. *J Immunol* 2003, 170:5475–5482.

43. Lorenz RG, Newberry RD: Isolated lymphoid follicles can function as sites for induction of mucosal immune responses. *Ann NY Acad Sci* 2004, 1029:44–57.
44. Newberry RD, McDonough JS, McDonald KG, Lorenz RG: Postgestational lymphotoxin/lymphotoxin β receptor interactions are essential for the presence of intestinal B lymphocytes. *J Immunol* 2002, 168:4988–4997.
45. Fagarasan S, Muramatsu M, Suzuki K, Nagaoka H, Hiai H, Honjo T: Critical roles of activation-induced cytidine deaminase in the homeostasis of gut flora. *Science* 2002, 298:1424–1427.
46. Kanamori Y, Ishimaru K, Nanno M, Maki K, Ikuta K, Nariuchi H, Ishikawa H: Identification of novel lymphoid tissues in murine intestinal mucosa where clusters of c-kit+ IL-7R+ Thy1+ lympho-hemopoietic progenitors develop. *J Exp Med* 1996, 184:1449–1459.
47. Oida T, Suzuki K, Nanno M, Kanamori Y, Saito H, Kubota E, Kato S, Itoh M, Kaminogawa S, Ishikawa H: Role of gut cryptopatches in early extrathymic maturation of intestinal intraepithelial T cells. *J Immunol* 2000, 164:3616–3626.
48. Saito H, Kanamori Y, Takemori T, Nariuchi H, Kubota E, Takahashi-Iwanaga H, Iwanaga T, Ishikawa H: Generation of intestinal T cells from progenitors residing in gut cryptopatches. *Science* 1998, 280:275–278.
49. Suzuki K, Oida T, Hamada H, Hitotsumatsu O, Watanabe M, Hibi T, Yamamoto H, Kubota E, Kaminogawa S, Ishikawa H: Gut cryptopatches: direct evidence of extrathymic anatomical sites for intestinal T lymphopoiesis. *Immunity* 2000, 13:691–702.
50. Taylor RT, Lugering A, Newell KA, Williams IR: Intestinal cryptopatch formation in mice requires lymphotoxin α and the lymphotoxin β receptor. *J Immunol* 2004, 173:7183–7189.
51. Pabst O, Herbrand H, Worbs T, Friedrichsen M, Yan S, Hoffmann MW, Korner H, Bernhardt G, Pabst R, Forster R: Cryptopatches and isolated lymphoid follicles: dynamic lymphoid tissues dispensable for the generation of intraepithelial lymphocytes. *Eur J Immunol* 2005, 35:98–107.
52. Zhang N, Guo J, He YW: Lymphocyte accumulation in the spleen of retinoic acid receptor-related orphan receptor γ-deficient mice. *J Immunol* 2003, 171:1667–1675.
53. Kang HS, Chin RK, Wang Y, Yu P, Wang J, Newell KA, Fu YX: Signaling via LTβR on the lamina propria stromal cells of the gut is required for IgA production. *Nat Immunol* 2002, 3:576–582.
54. Suzuki K, Meek B, Doi Y, Honjo T, Fagarasan S: Two distinctive pathways for recruitment of naïve and primed IgM+ B cells to the gut lamina propria. *Proc Natl Acad Sci U S A* 2005, 102:2482–2486.
55. Rakoff-Nahoum S, Paglino J, Eslami-Varzaneh F, Edberg S, Medzhitov R: Recognition of commensal microflora by toll-like receptors is required for intestinal homeostasis. *Cell* 2004, 118:229–241.
56. Geijtenbeek TB, Kwon DS, Torensma R, van Vliet SJ, van Duijnhoven GC, Middel J, Cornelissen IL, Nottet HS, KewalRamani VN, Littman DR, et al.: DC-SIGN, a dendritic cell-specific HIV-1-binding protein that enhances trans-infection of T cells. *Cell* 2000, 100:587–597.

57. Kwon DS, Gregorio G, Bitton N, Hendrickson WA, Littman DR: DC-SIGN-mediated internalization of HIV is required for trans-enhancement of T cell infection. *Immunity* 2002, 16:135–144.
58. Mattapallil JJ, Douek DC, Hill B, Nishimura Y, Martin M, Roederer M: Massive infection and loss of memory CD4+ T cells in multiple tissues during acute SIV infection. *Nature* 2005, 434:1093–1097.
59. Schneider T, Jahn HU, Schmidt W, Riecken EO, Zeitz M, Ullrich R: Loss of CD4 T lymphocytes in patients infected with human immunodeficiency virus type 1 is more pronounced in the duodenal mucosa than in the peripheral blood. Berlin Diarrhea/Wasting Syndrome Study Group. *Gut* 1995, 37:524–529.
60. Veazey RS, DeMaria M, Chalifoux LV, Shvetz DE, Pauley DR, Knight HL, Rosenzweig M, Johnson RP, Desrosiers RC, Lackner AA: Gastrointestinal tract as a major site of CD4+ T cell depletion and viral replication in SIV infection. *Science* 1998, 280:427–431.
61. Li Q, Duan L, Estes JD, Ma ZM, Rourke T, Wang Y, Reilly C, Carlis J, Miller CJ, Haase AT: Peak SIV replication in resting memory CD4+ T cells depletes gut lamina propria CD4+ T cells. *Nature* 2005, 434:1148–1152.
62. Veazey RS, Marx PA, Lackner AA: Vaginal CD4+ T cells express high levels of CCR5 and are rapidly depleted in simian immunodeficiency virus infection. *J Infect Dis* 2003, 187:769–776.
63. Vajdy M, Veazey R, Tham I, deBakker C, Westmoreland S, Neutra M, Lackner A: Early immunologic events in mucosal and systemic lymphoid tissues after intrarectal inoculation with simian immunodeficiency virus. *J Infect Dis* 2001, 184:1007–1014.
64. Mehandru S, Poles MA, Tenner-Racz K, Horowitz A, Hurley A, Hogan C, Boden D, Racz P, Markowitz M: Primary HIV-1 infection is associated with preferential depletion of CD4+ T lymphocytes from effector sites in the gastrointestinal tract. *J Exp Med* 2004, 200:761–770.
65. Brenchley JM, Schacker TW, Ruff LE, Price DA, Taylor JH, Beilman GJ, Nguyen PL, Khoruts A, Larson M, Haase AT, et al.: CD4+ T cell depletion during all stages of HIV disease occurs predominantly in the gastrointestinal tract. *J Exp Med* 2004, 200:749–759.
66. Luther SA, Lopez T, Bai W, Hanahan D, Cyster JG: BLC expression in pancreatic islets causes B cell recruitment and lymphotoxin-dependent lymphoid neogenesis. *Immunity* 2000, 12:471–481.
67. Spahn TW, Herbst H, Rennert PD, Lugering N, Maaser C, Kraft M, Fontana A, Weiner HL, Domschke W, Kucharzik T: Induction of colitis in mice deficient of Peyer's patches and mesenteric lymph nodes is associated with increased disease severity and formation of colonic lymphoid patches. *Am J Pathol* 2002, 161:2273–2282.
68. Kaiserling E: Newly-formed lymph nodes in the submucosa in chronic inflammatory bowel disease. *Lymphology* 2001, 34:22–29.
69. Yeung MM, Melgar S, Baranov V, Oberg A, Danielsson A, Hammarstrom S, Hammarstrom ML: Characterisation of mucosal lymphoid aggregates in ulcerative colitis: immune cell phenotype and TcR-γδ expression. *Gut* 2000, 47:215–227.

Specificity and Plasticity of Memory Lymphocyte Migration

J. Rodrigo Mora · U. H. von Andrian (✉)

CBR Institute for Biomedical Research and Department of Pathology,
Harvard Medical School, 200 Longwood Ave, Boston, MA 02115, USA
uva@cbr.med.harvard.edu

1	Introduction	84
2	Homing of Naive T and B Cells	85
3	Migration of Antigen-Experienced Lymphocytes	92
3.1	Homing of Effector/Memory T Cells	92
3.2	Tissue-Specific Homing Receptors: "Zip Codes" Shape Immune Responses	93
3.3	Homing of Antibody-Secreting Cells (ASC)	97
4	Teaching Lymphocytes Where to Go: Mechanisms Driving "Gut" Versus "Peripheral" Homing	99
5	Modulation of Lymphocyte Homing for Therapeutic Purposes	103
6	Re-educating Tissue-Specific T Cells— A New Platform for Immunomodulation?	105
7	Future Directions	107
References		109

Abstract To exert immunological activity, T and B cells must leave the blood and enter different extravascular compartments in the body. An essential step in this process is their adhesion to microvascular endothelium and subsequent diapedesis into a target tissue. Naive and effector/memory T and B cells possess distinct repertoires of traffic molecules that restrict their ability to interact with specialized microvessels in different anatomic compartments and thus exhibit distinct patterns of migration. In addition, antigen-experienced lymphocytes are subdivided into different subsets based on their expression of characteristic sets of adhesion receptors that favor their accumulation in certain target organs, such as the skin and the gut. This article focuses on recent discoveries that have broadened our understanding of the "imprinting" mechanisms responsible for the generation of tissue-specific effector/memory lymphocytes, especially in the intestine. We discuss how gut-specific homing is acquired, maintained, and modulated and how these mechanisms might be harnessed to develop improved vaccine protocols and treatments for intestinal autoimmune diseases.

1
Introduction

Lymphocyte responses to pathogens are triggered by engagement of antigen receptors with cognate pathogen-derived antigens presented by other cells. The initial priming encounter and the transmission of additional prerequisite costimulatory signals for lymphocyte activation occur in the specialized environment of lymphoid organs. Subsequently, the antigen-primed cells relocate to peripheral sites of infection and exert effector activities on renewed antigen challenge. To achieve this, the rare antigen-specific lymphocytes must travel between lymphoid and nonlymphoid organs via the blood and then exit the circulation to enter antigen-containing tissues. An essential step in this migration process is the adhesion of circulating lymphocytes to the endothelium of postcapillary venules, a complex, multistep cascade of events mediated by specialized adhesion receptors and chemoattractant pathways (Butcher 1991; von Andrian and Mackay 2000). In the first step, lymphocytes are captured ("tethering") and interact loosely with the endothelial cells ("rolling"). Tethering and rolling are mediated by members of the selectin family (L-, P-, and E-selectin) and their glycoprotein ligands (Ley and Kansas 2004); the two α4-integrins, α4β1 (VLA-4) and α4β7, can also mediate these initial adhesion steps in some cases (Alon et al. 1995; Berlin et al. 1995). Once T cells have begun to roll, they can undergo an "activation" step, which is usually (although not exclusively) mediated by chemokines, secreted polypeptides that are presented on the endothelial surface (Rot and von Andrian 2004). Chemokines bind to specific G protein-coupled receptors on rolling lymphocytes and trigger intracellular signals that lead to firm arrest ("sticking") of T cells on the endothelial surface. The sticking step is mediated by lymphocyte-expressed integrins (e.g., LFA-1, α4β7, and α4β1), which undergo rapid, chemoattractant-induced conformational changes to assume an extended configuration. This transient structural shift greatly enhances the affinity of integrins for their endothelial ligands (e.g., ICAM-1, ICAM-2, VCAM-1, MAdCAM-1), most of which belong to the immunoglobulin superfamily (Carman and Springer 2003; von Andrian and Mackay 2000). Only when all steps are successfully taken can a T cell transmigrate ("diapedese") into a tissue.

Although the multistep adhesion paradigm applies to all leukocytes, the molecules involved in the different steps vary depending on the leukocyte population, tissue, and inflammatory context (Butcher and Picker 1996; Cyster 2003; Springer 1994; von Andrian and Mackay 2000). Recent advances in the field have unveiled several examples for this exquisite degree of specialization, in particular for T cell migration. At the same time, new observations highlight a previously unexpected degree of dynamic plasticity and malleability in the trafficking behavior of effector/memory T cells. These findings open the possibility that the expression of tissue-specific traffic molecules on lymphocytes can be custom-modified, which might allow us to tailor cellular immune responses for therapeutic purposes.

In this review, we discuss the migratory pathways of naive as well as effector/memory T and B cells, including antibody-secreting cells (ASC, i.e., plasmablasts and plasma cells), with special emphasis on the mechanisms responsible for generating gut-tropic lymphocytes.

2
Homing of Naive T and B Cells

Naive lymphocytes preferentially migrate to secondary lymphoid organs, such as lymph nodes, Peyer's patches (PP), appendix, tonsils, and the spleen, tissues where they can meet their cognate antigen in the proper cellular milieu to become activated (Mackay et al. 1990; von Andrian and Mackay 2000).

Naive T cells express L-selectin, which allows them to interact and roll in specialized postcapillary microvessels known as high endothelial venules (HEV) in peripheral (PLN) and mesenteric (MLN) lymph nodes and Peyer's patches (PP) (Bargatze et al. 1995; von Andrian 1996) (Fig. 1A and Table 1). HEV in PLN and MLN express L-selectin ligands collectively known as PNAd (peripheral node addressin), which are sialylated, sulfated, and fucosylated glycoproteins (Ley and Kansas 2004; Streeter et al. 1988). In addition, the chemokines CCL21/SLC and probably also CCL19/ELC are presented in HEV of LN and PP. These chemokines activate CCR7 expressed on naive T and B cells as well as central memory T cells (Okada et al. 2002; Stein et al. 2000; Warnock et al. 2000; Weninger et al. 2001), which triggers the activation of LFA-1 (and/or $\alpha 4\beta 7$) and lymphocyte arrest in HEV (Bargatze et al. 1995; Warnock et al. 1998). Recent findings indicate that T cell responsiveness to these chemokine signals in HEV is enhanced by the presence of blood-borne sphingosine-1-phosphate, which acts through a T cell-expressed receptor, $S1P_1$ (Halin et al. 2005).

Naive B cells and central memory T cells use the same traffic molecules as naive T cells to home to PLN. However, unlike naive T cells, they can additionally use CXCR4 for integrin activation; the CXCR4 ligand CXCL12/SDF1α is presented in PLN HEV (Okada et al. 2002; Scimone et al. 2004) (Fig. 1B and Table 2). In addition, the CXCR5-CXCL13 pathway can also support B cell homing (Ebisuno et al. 2003; Okada et al. 2002). Thus B cells and central memory T cells are less dependent on CCR7 signals for homing to PLN than naive T cells. On the other hand, naive B cells express ~50% less L-selectin than naive

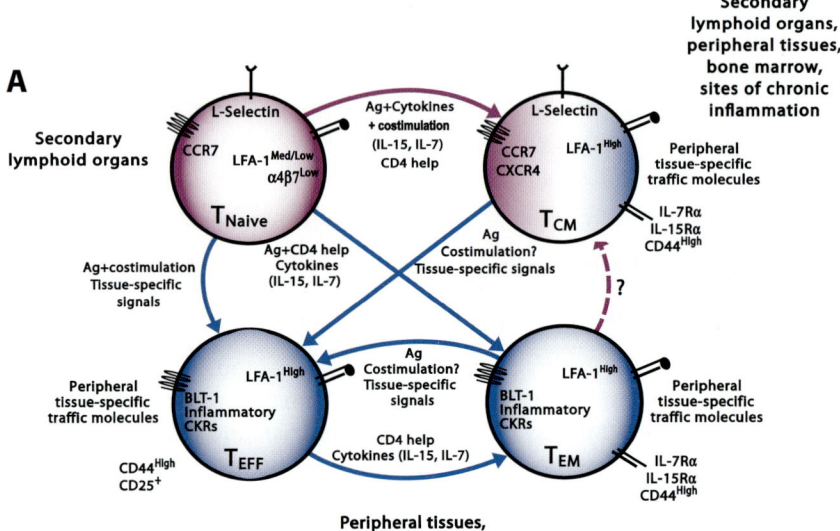
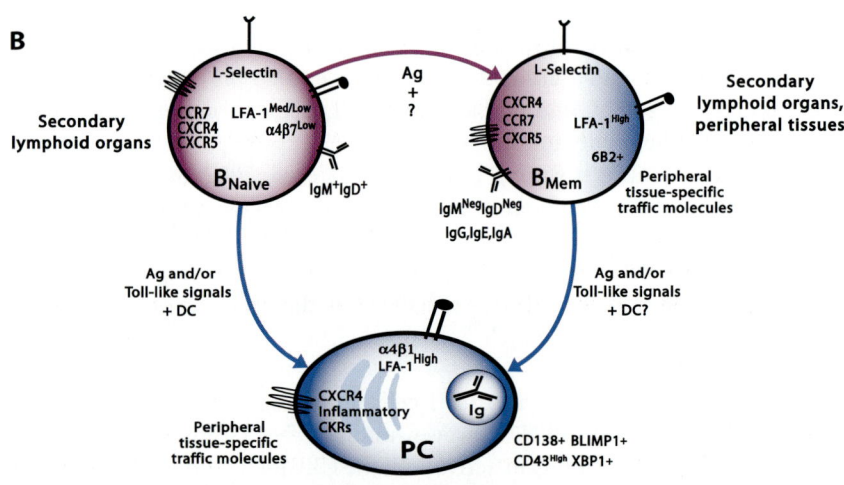

Fig. 1A, B Differentiation and migratory pathways of naive and antigen experienced T and B cells. **A** Naive T cells (T_{Naive}) express L-selectin, CCR7, intermediate levels of LFA-1, and low levels of $\alpha 4\beta 7$, which allow them to migrate into SLO, such as LN, PP, and the spleen. Once they are activated by their cognate antigen, they proliferate and can differentiate into T_{EM}, T_{CM}, or T_{EFF}. The latter two are long-lived because they express receptors for IL-7 and IL-15, which provide essential signals for survival and homeostatic proliferation. T_{CM} remain L-selectin$^+$ and CCR7$^+$ and continue to recirculate through SLO, analogous to T_{Naive}. However, T_{CM} can also migrate to peripheral inflamed tissues and the bone marrow, and they respond more vigorously to antigen than T_{Naive}. The mostly short-lived T_{EFF} and the long-lived T_{EM} (which can arise from T_{EFF}) also respond quickly and very efficiently to recall antigen and, unlike T_{CM} (at least in some settings), they exert more rapid effector activity, such as cytokine secretion and cytotoxicity. T_{CM}, T_{EFF}, and T_{EM} express inflammation-seeking traffic receptors as well as peripheral tissue-specific homing receptors for the small bowel or the skin. T_{CM} and T_{EM} give rise to T_{EFF} on reactivation. T_{EM} can also give rise to T_{CM} over longer time intervals, although the mechanisms and the extent to which this occurs at physiological precursor levels are unclear. **B** Naive B cells (B_{Naive}, IgM$^+$/IgD$^+$) express L-selectin, CCR7, CXCR4, CXCR5, and low levels of $\alpha 4\beta 7$, which target them to SLO. When activated, B cells give rise to ASC, either plasmablasts or plasma cells (*PC*), which do not divide. These cells are mostly short-lived, except for a subset of bone marrow-resident plasma cells that persist for very long times. PC express CD138 (syndecan-1), CD43, and the transcription factors Blimp-1 and XBP-1. Some activated B cells become memory B cells (B_{Mem}, 6B2$^+$), which are long-lived and can proliferate and give rise to PC (and more B_{Mem}) on re-encounter with the antigen and/or TLR agonists. ASC (and probably also B_{Mem}) can exhibit specific tropism for mucosal tissues, bone marrow, and probably other peripheral tissues. B_{Mem} can also express receptors for SLO. *IL-7Rα/IL-15Rα*, α-subunit of the IL-7 and IL-15 receptors; *BLT-1*, leukotriene B4 receptor. *Colors* indicate preferential migratory specificity: *purple*, recirculating through SLO; *blue*, tropism for nonlymphoid organs and inflammation

T cells, which reduces their ability to engage in productive rolling interactions in HEV and results in an approximately fivefold lower homing efficiency in PLN (Gauguet et al. 2004; Tang et al. 1998). This example highlights a regulatory mechanism of leukocyte traffic that is often overlooked: The recruitment efficiency of any given cell population is not merely decided by the presence or absence of relevant receptor-ligand pairs, but can be greatly influenced by relatively subtle shifts in the expression level of critical homing receptors.

In PP, HEV do not express PNAd in the lumen (Streeter et al. 1988). Instead, they express high levels of mucosal addressin cell adhesion molecule-1 (MAdCAM-1) (Nakache et al., 1989). MAdCAM-1 can interact with both L-selectin and $\alpha 4\beta 7$ (Berg et al., 1993; Berlin et al., 1993). Although the $\alpha 4\beta 7$ integrin is expressed at low levels on naive T cells it plays an important role for lymphocyte migration into PP and MLN (Bargatze et al. 1995; Berlin et al.

Table 1 Multistep adhesion cascade for T cell subpopulations in lymphoid and peripheral tissues[a]

Tissue	Lymph nodes	Peyer's patches	Bone marrow	Skin	Small bowel lamina propria	Colon lamina propria	Central nervous system	Sites of acute inflammation
Lymphocyte subset	Naïve and T_{CM}[b]	Naïve and T_{CM}	T_{CM}	T_{EFF}/T_{EM}[d]	T_{EFF}/T_{EM}	T_{EFF}/T_{EM}	T_{EFF}/T_{EM}	T_{EFF}/T_{EM}
Microvascular bed	HEV[c]	HEV	sinusoids, venules	Venules	Venules	Venules	Venules	Venules
Tethering and rolling	L-selectin– PNAd	L-selectin– PNAd $\alpha 4\beta 7^{Low}$– MAdCAM-1	L-selectin– PSGL-1 P-/E-selectin ligands– $\alpha 4\beta 1$– P-/E-selectin VCAM-1?	P-/E-selectin ligands– P-/E-selectin* $\alpha 4\beta 1$– VCAM-1?** *Steady-state, increased in inflammation **Inflammation only?	$\alpha 4\beta 7^{High}$– MAdCAM-1* P-selectin ligands– $\alpha 4\beta 1$– VCAM-1** *Steady-state, increased in inflammation **Inflammation only?	$\alpha 4\beta 7^{High}$– MAdCAM-1* $\alpha 4\beta 1$– VCAM-1* P-selectin ligands– P-selectin?** *Steady-state, increased in inflammation **Inflammation only?	$\alpha 4\beta 1$– VCAM-1* P-selectin ligands– P-selectin** *Steady-state, increased in inflammation **Inflammation only?	P-/E-selectin ligands– P-/E-selectin CD44– Hyaluromate
Integrin activation	CCR7– CCL19/ CCL21 CXCR4– CXCL12* *T_{CM} only	CCR7– CCL19/ CCL21	CXCR4– CXCL12 Non PTx-sensitive[e]	CCR4–CCL17* CCR10–CCL27* CCR8–CCL1** *Steady-state, increased in inflammation **Non-inflamed skin only?	CCR9–CCL25 Other chemokine receptors in inflammation?	CCR6 - CCL20* *Inflammation only?	CXCR3– CXCL9/ CXCL10/ CXCL11?* CCR5– CCL3/4/5?* *Inflammation only?	CCR5– CCL3/4/5 CCR2–CCL2 CXCR3– CXCL9/10/11 BLT-1–BLT[f]

Table 1 (continued)

Tissue	Lymph nodes	Peyer's patches	Bone marrow	Skin	Small bowel lamina propria	Colon lamina propria	Central nervous system	Sites of acute inflammation
Firm adhesion	LFA-1–ICAM-1/-2	LFA-1–ICAM-1/-2 $\alpha 4\beta 7^{Low}$–MAdCAM-1	$\alpha 4\beta 1$–VCAM-1	LFA-1–ICAM-1* $\alpha 4\beta 1$–VCAM-1?** *Steady-state, increased in inflammation **Inflammation only?	$\alpha 4\beta 7^{High}$–MAdCAM-1* $\alpha 4\beta 1$–VCAM-1** LFA-1–ICAM-1? *Steady-state, increased in inflammation **Inflammation only	$\alpha 4\beta 7^{High}$–MAdCAM-1 $\alpha 4\beta 1$–VCAM-1* *Steady-state, increased in inflammation	$\alpha 4\beta 1$–VCAM-1* *Steady-state, increased in inflammation	LFA-1–ICAM-1 $\alpha 1\beta 1/\alpha 2\beta 1$–collagen $\alpha 4\beta 1$–VCAM-1/fibronectin
Diapedesis	CCR7–CCL19/CCL21?	CCR7–CCL19/CCL21?	Unknown PTx-sensitive	CCR10–CCL27? CCR8–CCL1?	CCR9–CCL25?	Unknown	Unknown CXCR3–CXCL9/CXCL10/CXCL11?	CCR5–CCL3/4/5? CCR2–CCL2? CXCR3–CXCL9/10/11? BLT1–LTB4

[a] This table illustrates the adhesion mechanisms operating under steady-state (non-inflammatory) conditions, unless otherwise specified; [b] T_{CM}: central memory T cells; [c] HEV: high endothelial venules; [d] T_{EFF}/T_{EM}: effector and effector memory T cells; [e] PTx: Pertussis toxin; [f] BLT1/LTB4: leukotriene B4 (LTB4) receptor and its ligand

Table 2 Multistep adhesion cascade for B cells and antibody secreting cells (ASC) in lymphoid and peripheral tissues[a]

Tissue	Lymph nodes	Peyer's patches	Bone marrow	Skin[c]	Small bowel lamina propria	Colon lamina propria	Central nervous system	Sites of acute inflammation
Lymphocyte subset	Naïve, B_{MEM}[b]	Naïve, B_{MEM}	ASC, B_{MEM}?	ASC, B_{MEM}?	ASC, B_{MEM}?	ASC, B_{MEM}?	ASC, B_{MEM}?	ASC
Microvascular bed	HEV[d]	HEV	sinusoids, venules	Venules	Venules	Venules	Venules	Venules
Tethering and rolling	L-selectin–PNAd	L-selectin–PNAd $\alpha 4\beta 7^{Low}$–MAdCAM-1	P-/E-selectin ligands–P-/E-selectin? $\alpha 4\beta 1$–VCAM-1?	P-/E-selectin ligands–P-/E-selectin?* $\alpha 4\beta 1$–VCAM-1?** *Steady-state, increased in inflammation **Inflammation	$\alpha 4\beta 7^{High}$–MAdCAM-1* $\alpha 4\beta 1$–VCAM-1? P-selectin ligands–P-selectin?** *Steady-state, increased in inflammation **Inflammation	$\alpha 4\beta 7^{High}$–MAdCAM-1* $\alpha 4\beta 1$–VCAM-1* P-selectin ligands–P-selectin?** *Steady-state, increased in inflammation **Inflammation only?	$\alpha 4\beta 1$–VCAM-1?* P-selectin ligands–P-selectin?** *Steady-state, increased in inflammation **Inflammation only?	P-/E-selectin ligands–P-/E-selectin
Integrin activation	CCR7–CCL19/CCL21 CXCR4–CXCL12 (CXCR5–CXCL13)	CCR7–CCL19/CCL21 CXCR4–CXCL12 CXCR5–CXCL13	CXCR4–CXCL12?	CCR4–CCL17?* CCR10–CCL27?* CXCR3–CXCL10/CXCL11?** *Steady-state, increased in inflammation **Inflammation only?	CCR9–CCL25 CCR10–CCL28? Other chemokine receptors in inflammation?	CCR10–CCL28?	CXCR3–CXCL9/CXCL10/CXCL11?* *Inflammation only?	CCR5–CCL3/4/5 CCR2–CCL2 CXCR3–CXCL9/10/11

Table 2 (continued)

Tissue	Lymph nodes	Peyer's patches	Bone marrow	Skin[c]	Small bowel lamina propria	Colon lamina propria	Central nervous system	Sites of acute inflammation
Firm adhesion	LFA-1–ICAM-1 α4β1–VCAM-1?	LFA-1–ICAM-1 α4β7^{Low}–MAdCAM-1	α4β1–VCAM-1?	LFA-1–ICAM-1?* α4β1–VCAM-1?** *Steady-state, increased in inflammation **Inflammation only?	α4β7^{High}–MAdCAM-1* α4β1–VCAM-1?** LFA-1–ICAM-1? *Steady-state, increased in inflammation **Inflammation only	α4β7^{High}–MAdCAM-1* α4β1–VCAM-1?* *Steady-state, increased in inflammation	α4β1–VCAM-1?* *Steady-state, increased in inflammation	LFA-1–ICAM-1 α1β1/α2β1–collagen? α4β1–VCAM-1/fibronectin?
Diapedesis	Unknown	Unknown	CXCR4–CXCL12?	CCR10–CCL27?	CCR9–CCL25?	CCR10–CCL28?	CXCR3–CXCL9/CXCL10/CXCL11? *Inflammation only?	CCR5–CCL3/4/5? CCR2–CCL2? CXCR3–CXCL9/10/11?

[a] This table illustrates the adhesion mechanisms operating under steady-state (non-inflammatory) conditions, unless otherwise specified; [b] Most of the evidence on B cell homing has been obtained for naïve B cells and ASC. Due to the difficulties identifying and isolating them, the evidence for B$_{MEM}$ homing is scarce; [c] There is very limited evidence showing skin homing potential for ASC; [d] HEV: high endothelial venules

1993; Berlin-Rufenach et al. 1999; Wagner et al. 1996) (Table 1). MAdCAM-1 on PP HEV contributes to both rolling and sticking in these organs (Bargatze et al. 1995; Berg et al. 1993; Berlin et al. 1993). Firm arrest of naive T cells in PP HEV is mediated by LFA-1 and α4β7, which are activated by CCL21-CCR7 (Bargatze et al. 1995; Warnock et al. 1998). Naive B cells also use L-selectin and α4β7 to interact with PP HEV, and, as in PLN, they can make use of CXCR4, CXCR5, and CCR7 for integrin activation (Okada et al. 2002) (Table 2). Interestingly, there seems to be a spatial distinction between T and B cell firm arrest in PP, with T cells sticking preferentially within interfollicular HEV segments, whereas B cells were found to arrest preferentially in follicle-associated HEV (Warnock et al. 2000).

A special case are MLN whose HEV express a mosaic of both PNAd (Streeter et al. 1988) and MAdCAM-1 (Nakache et al. 1989), thus supporting both the PLN-like and PP-like adhesion cascades for lymphocyte homing (Streeter et al. 1988; Wagner et al. 1996).

3
Migration of Antigen-Experienced Lymphocytes

3.1
Homing of Effector/Memory T Cells

When naive T cells find their cognate antigen in the context of appropriate costimulatory signals, usually provided by dendritic cells (DC), they are activated, proliferate, and differentiate into effector or memory T cells. Antigen-experienced T cells differ significantly from naive T cells in their migratory properties. In particular, the former migrate much better to nonlymphoid tissues and sites of inflammation (Mackay et al. 1990; Masopust et al. 2001; Reinhardt et al. 2001; Weninger et al. 2001). In addition, memory cells can be further divided into two main categories, based on distinct migratory and functional characteristics (Sallusto et al. 1999) (Fig. 1A and Table 1). The central-memory T cells (T_{CM}) maintain the expression of L-selectin and CCR7 and, like naive T cells, can migrate into secondary lymphoid organs (Weninger et al. 2001). In addition, T_{CM} upregulate inflammation-seeking traffic molecules and also express high levels of CXCR4, which allows them to migrate efficiently to sites where the CXCR4 ligand CXCL12 is highly expressed, such as the bone marrow (Mazo et al. 2005) and also PLN (Scimone et al. 2004). Consistent with their memory status, T_{CM} express IL-7Rα (Kaech et al. 2003) and can respond faster and more vigorously than naive T cells when reencountering cognate antigen (Manjunath et al. 2001; Sallusto et al. 1999; Wherry et al. 2003).

In contrast to CCR7$^+$ T$_{CM}$, effector T cells (T$_{EFF}$, short-lived) and effector memory T cells (T$_{EM}$, long-lived IL-7Rα^+) do not express CCR7, and most are also L-selectin$^-$. Therefore, T$_{EM}$ and T$_{EFF}$ cannot recirculate efficiently through LN or PP (Sallusto et al. 1999; Weninger et al. 2001). However, they migrate efficiently to peripheral/nonlymphoid tissues, like liver, lungs, skin, gut lamina propria, and sites of inflammation (Masopust et al. 2001; Reinhardt et al. 2001; Sallusto et al. 1999; Weninger et al. 2001). In addition, in some assays, only T$_{EFF}$ and T$_{EM}$, but not T$_{CM}$, have immediate effector/cytotoxic activity (Manjunath et al. 2001; Sallusto et al., 1999). However, it should be cautioned that, in some studies, in vivo differentiated T cells with a T$_{CM}$ phenotype have been observed to exert effector functions as rapidly and efficiently as T$_{EM}$ (Debes et al. 2002; Unsoeld et al. 2002), and T$_{CM}$ that arise after viral infections are superior to T$_{EM}$ at conferring long-lived antiviral protection (Wherry et al., 2003). It should also be pointed out that in vivo generated T$_{CM}$ can be CCR7$^+$ and simultaneously express homing receptors for peripheral tissues, such as the skin and the gut. Indeed, although a CCR7$^+$ and L-selectin^{High} phenotype is predictive of a memory cell's capacity to home to LN, this does not preclude that such cells can also infiltrate peripheral tissues (Campbell et al. 2001). Given these observations, the distinctions between T$_{CM}$ and T$_{EM}$ can be rather subtle. In the absence of a broad consensus on defining functional subset characteristics, we will refer to T$_{CM}$ as antigen-experienced T cells with PLN homing capacity (i.e., memory marker-expressing T cells that are L-selectin^{High} and CCR7$^+$), whereas T$_{EM}$ and T$_{EFF}$ are memory cells that lack either one or both of these homing receptors.

We recently described a method to differentiate and expand CD8 T cells with a T$_{CM}$ or T$_{EFF}$ phenotype by activating naive T cells with antigen for 48 h followed by culture for at least 5 days in IL-15 or IL-2, respectively (Manjunath et al. 2001). This strategy has allowed us to characterize the in vivo migratory properties of each T cell subset and to perform intravital microscopy (IVM) to dissect the molecular mechanisms involved in the interaction of these cells with PLN HEV and microvessels in bone marrow and inflamed tissues (Goodarzi et al. 2003; Mazo et al. 2005; Scimone et al. 2004; Weninger et al. 2001) (Table 1).

3.2
Tissue-Specific Homing Receptors: "Zip Codes" Shape Immune Responses

Although T$_{EFF}$ and T$_{EM}$ share the propensity to migrate through nonlymphoid tissues, some subsets have been shown to possess remarkable migratory selectivity for certain nonlymphoid tissues, such as the gut and the skin (Guy-Grand et al. 1978; Kantele et al. 1999b) (Fig. 2A and Table 1). For ex-

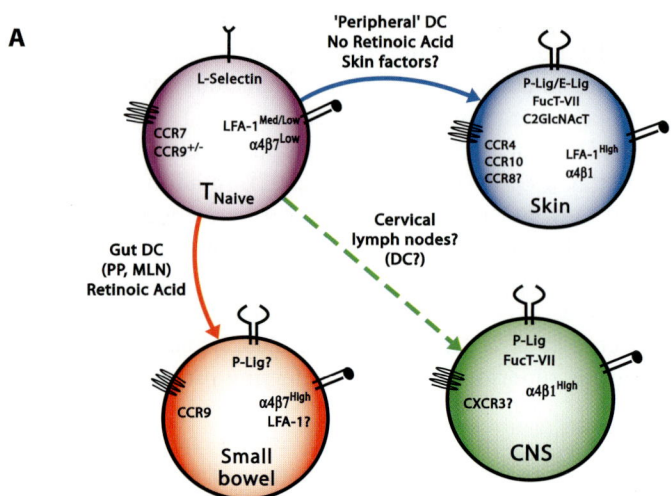

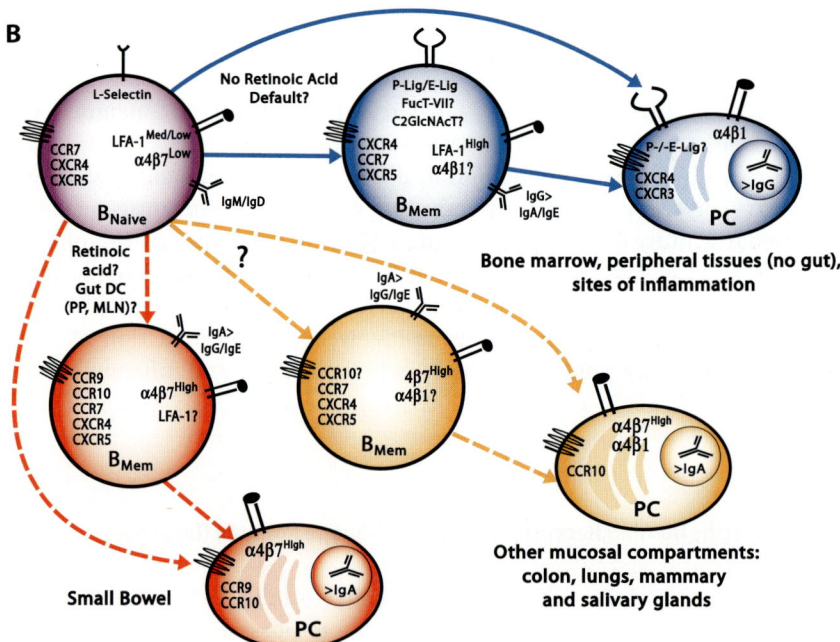

Fig. 2A, B Tissue specificity of antigen-experienced T and B cells. **A** When naive T cells are activated by dendritic cells from PP or MLN or in the presence of RA, the resulting T_{EFF}/T_{EM} become $\alpha 4\beta 7^{High}$ and CCR9$^+$. By contrast, when T cells are activated in the absence of RA or by DC from PLN, they upregulate skin-homing molecules, i.e., ligands for P-selectin (*P-Lig*) and E-selectin (*E-Lig*) and CCR4. T cells activated in cervical LN were recently shown to exhibit tropism for the CNS; it is still unknown how this homing preference is imprinted on T cells. **B** Similarly, naive B cell activation in gut-associated lymphoid tissues generates ASC and B$_{Mem}$ that upregulate $\alpha 4\beta 7$ and probably CCR9, which target them to the small bowel. It is not known whether gut-DC and/or RA are important to induce gut-homing ASC or B$_{Mem}$. ASC in mucosal tissues also express CCR10, which is probably important for their homing into all mucosal compartments. It is unknown where and how CCR10 is upregulated on mucosal ASC and whether ASC and B$_{Mem}$ with tropism for "peripheral" tissues or the bone marrow (*BM*) require specific imprinting signals. *PP*, Peyer's patches; *MLN*, mesenteric lymph nodes; *P-/E-Lig*, P- and/or E-selectin ligands; *FucT-VII*, fucosyltransferase-VII; *C2GlcNAcT*, core 2 1,6-*N*-acetylglucosaminyltransferase. *Colors* indicate preferential migratory specificity: *purple*, recirculating through SLO; *blue*, tropism for nonlymphoid organs and inflammation; *red*, small intestine; green, CNS; *orange*, mucosal sites

ample, skin-tropic T_{EFF}/T_{EM} express E- and P-selectin ligands (Fuhlbrigge et al. 1997; Picker et al. 1991) and the chemokine receptors CCR4 (Campbell et al. 1999) and/or CCR10 (Morales et al. 1999), which are critical for efficient T cell homing into the skin (Biedermann et al. 2002; Homey et al. 2002; Reiss et al. 2001; Rossiter et al. 1993, 1994; Silber et al. 1994; Tietz et al. 1998; Yan et al. 1994). E- and P-selectin are upregulated on endothelial cells exposed to inflammatory mediators in most tissues, including the skin. However, unlike most other microvascular beds, noninflamed skin venules express functional E- and P-selectin constitutively, as evidenced by the high frequency of rolling leukocytes in intact skin (Janssen et al. 1994; Nolte et al. 1994; Weninger et al. 2000). Both CCR4 and/or CCR10 play a role in skin T cell homing under steady-state and inflammatory conditions (Homey et al. 2002; Reiss et al. 2001; Soler et al. 2003), although other chemokine receptors, like CXCR3, contribute in acute inflammatory states (Flier et al. 2001). The ligands for CCR4 and CCR10 (CCL17/TARC and CCL27/CTACK, respectively) have been found on inflamed and noninflamed skin endothelium (Campbell et al. 1999; Chong et al. 2004; Homey et al. 2002). In normal human skin, CCR8 is expressed by most resident T cells (Schaerli et al. 2004), but the function of CCR8 and its skin-expressed ligand CCL1 remains to be determined.

Conversely, T cells that migrate to the small intestine lamina propria mostly do not express skin-homing receptors listed above but express the integrin $\alpha 4\beta 7$ (Berlin et al. 1993; Wagner et al. 1996) and the chemokine receptor

CCR9 (Zabel et al. 1999). These traffic molecules are essential for efficient T cell migration into the small bowel, at least in the absence of inflammation (Hamann et al. 1994; Hosoe et al. 2004; Johansson-Lindbom et al. 2003; Svensson et al. 2002; Wagner et al. 1996). Indeed, the principal α4β7 ligand, MAdCAM-1, is expressed in gut lamina propria venules (Nakache et al. 1989), and the CCR9 ligand CCL25/TECK is strongly expressed by epithelial cells in the small intestine (Kunkel et al. 2000), and in lamina propria venules (Hosoe et al. 2004; Papadakis et al. 2000). However, genetic ablation of CCR9 caused only a mild reduction in the number of (mostly TCRγδ$^+$) small bowel intraepithelial lymphocytes (IEL) (Uehara et al. 2002; Wurbel et al. 2001). Nevertheless, CCL25 blockade or CCR9 deficiency significantly reduced the number of antigen-specific CD8 T cells in the small intestine after intraperitoneal immunization (Johansson-Lindbom et al. 2003; Svensson et al. 2002). It is not clear whether these seemingly contradictory observations are due to compensatory mechanisms developed in mice with inborn CCR9 deficiency. Alternatively, CCR9 might be more important for the migration of recently generated CD8 T$_{EFF}$ to the small bowel, rather than for steady-state traffic under unstimulated conditions, which has a very slow turnover (Klonowski et al. 2004). In addition, a substantial proportion of CD4 effector T cells can migrate to the small bowel independently of CCR9 (Stensted et al. 2006).

Interestingly, T cell homing into the large intestine seems to be controlled, at least in part, by distinct mechanisms. Although α4β7 is also important for T cell migration into this gut compartment, even under inflammatory conditions (Hesterberg et al. 1996; Picarella et al. 1993), α4β1 has also been implicated (Soriano et al. 2000). Notably, the colon lamina propria is mostly devoid of CCR9-expressing cells, and CCL25 is not expressed in this tissue (Kunkel et al. 2000; Papadakis et al. 2000; Zabel et al. 1999). Accordingly, CCR9 desensitization (or CCL25 blockade) significantly blocked the firm adhesion of T cells in small bowel venules but had no effect on T cell adhesion in the colon (Hosoe et al. 2004). These results suggest that there may be other chemoattractant pathway(s) that direct T cell migration to the colon mucosa (Kunkel and Butcher 2002). For example, the chemokine CCL28/MEC is highly expressed by colonic epithelial cells (Pan et al. 2000), although its receptor CCR10 is only found on mucosal antibody-secreting cells (ASC), but not intestinal T cells (Kunkel et al. 2003).

Another β7 integrin, αEβ7, has also been associated to gut homing. In fact, αE knockout mice have a slight reduction in the number of IEL and lamina propria T cells (Schon et al. 1999). However, some studies have shown that αEβ7 is neither necessary (Lefrancois et al. 1999) nor sufficient (Austrup et al. 1995) to target circulating T cells to the gut. Moreover, no ligand for αEβ7 has been detected so far on intestinal venules. E-cadherin, the only known ligand for αEβ7, is only expressed on epithelial cells. Nevertheless, it has recently been shown that αEβ7 is necessary for the induction of intestinal graft-versus-host disease (GVHD) (El-Asady et al. 2005), suggesting that this integrin may play a role in lymphocyte retention/survival or function in the gut mucosa (Cepek et al. 1994; Higgins et al. 1998). Indeed, recent evidence suggests that αEβ7 is induced on T cells after they have gained entrance into the gut (Ericsson et al. 2004).

Of note, $CD4^+$ $CD25^+$ ($Foxp3^+$) regulatory T cells (T_{REG}) also exhibit tissue specificity, particularly T_{CM}- and T_{EM}-like phenotypes (Huehn et al. 2004), and gut- and skin-homing molecules (Colantonio et al. 2002; Iellem et al. 2003; Nagatani et al. 2004). This homing receptor versatility may allow T_{REG} to exert their suppressor function in secondary lymphoid organs during initial priming events or in peripheral tissues during the effector phase. In fact, recent evidence suggests that T_{CM}-like and T_{EFF}-like T_{REG} fulfill different roles in the regulation of immune responses, with T_{CM}-like T_{REG} exerting their regulatory activity in secondary lymphoid tissues and T_{EFF}-like T_{REG} acting in inflamed tissues (Huehn et al. 2004). It will be interesting to explore whether tissue-specificity (e.g., gut- versus skin-specific T_{REG}) is also induced during T_{REG} activation. In this line, a recent report suggests that T_{EFF}-like T_{REG} need fucosyltransferase-VII (FucT-VII), an enzyme that is essential to synthesize P-/E-selection ligands (skin-homing receptors) to exert their regulatory activity in the skin (Siegmund et al. 2005).

3.3
Homing of Antibody-Secreting Cells (ASC)

After encountering an antigen in secondary lymphoid organs, conventional B cells (B-2 cells) become either ASC with no proliferative capacity or memory B cells (Bmem), which can proliferate and give rise to ASC upon reactivation (McHeyzer-Williams and McHeyzer-Williams 2005) (Fig. 1B). B cells responding to T cell-independent antigens mainly differentiate into short-lived IgM-secreting ASC. However, if B cells receive T cell help shortly after activation, they can form germinal centers where they undergo affinity maturation and class switching (McHeyzer-Williams and McHeyzer-Williams 2005). ASC that secrete IgG (and, to a lesser extent, IgE and IgA) leave lymphoid tissues and travel primarily to the bone marrow, where a small fraction become long-lived plasma cells (Cyster 2003; Kunkel and Butcher 2003). CXCR4 and probably α4β1, LFA-1, P-selectin ligands, and CD22 are important for ASC lodging in the bone marrow (Hargreaves et al. 2001; Nitschke et al. 1999; Sawada et al. 1998; Underhill et al. 2002). However, it is not clear to what extent each of these pathways contributes to homing, survival, or retention of plasma cells in this compartment. Some ASC also home into sites of inflammation; this migration event is probably mediated by CXCR3 (Cyster 2003).

Early studies have shown that IgA-secreting plasma cells (IgA-ASC) migrate preferentially into the gut (McDermott and Bienenstock 1979; Rudzik et al. 1975; Tseng 1981). Indeed, human intestinal plasma cells express α4β7 (Farstad et al. 1995), and studies in β7 knockout mice have established that this integrin is also critical for murine ASC accumulation in the gut (Wagner et al. 1996) (Fig. 2B and Table 2). Recent observations indicate that plasma cells in mucosal compartments, including the small intestine, colon, rectum, mammary gland, salivary gland, and trachea, express CCR10 (Kunkel and Butcher 2003; Kunkel et al. 2003; Pan et al. 2000; Wilson and Butcher 2004). This is relevant because the CCR10 ligand CCL28 is expressed by most mucosal epithelial cells (Pan et al. 2000; Wang et al. 2000) and selectively attracts IgA-ASC (Kunkel et al. 2003; Lazarus et al. 2003). In fact, IgA-ASC require CCL28 to home efficiently to the colon lamina propria (Hieshima et al., 2004). Moreover, a subset of IgA-ASC also respond to the CCR9-ligand CCL25 (Bowman et al. 2002), and recent evidence shows that ASC, analogously to T cells, require CCR9 to home to the small intestine (Hieshima et al. 2004; Kunkel et al. 2003; Pabst et al. 2004) (Fig. 2B and Table 2). In addition, CCL28 supports IgA-ASC homing to the small bowel mucosa (Hieshima et al. 2004). It is not clear how and why ASC apparently require both chemokine pathways for optimal migration into this tissue.

As mentioned before, CCR10 is also expressed on skin-homing T cells (Homey et al. 2002; Reiss et al. 2001). However, CCR10$^+$ T cells do not express α4β7, and therefore they cannot home efficiently to the gut. Conversely, CCR10$^+$ mucosal ASC do not express E- and P-selectin ligands and are therefore excluded from the skin. This is a particularly illustrative example of how the combination of multiple receptors, and not the expression of a particular one, determines the overall homing potential of lymphocytes (Butcher 1991).

T cell-dependent B cell responses also generate long-lived memory B cells (B_{Mem}), which can give rise to ASC (and more B_{Mem}) when they become stimulated (Bernasconi et al. 2002; McHeyzer-Williams and McHeyzer-Williams 2005). It is thought that B_{Mem} recirculate through both lymphoid and peripheral tissues, but their migratory behavior has been difficult to study because of their physiologically low abundance. However, B_{Mem} conferring protection against intestinal pathogens express α4β7, indicating that these cells, like their T cell counterparts, respond to tissue-specific imprinting signals (Weitkamp et al. 2005; Williams et al. 1998). In addition, it has been estimated that B-1 cells from the peritoneal cavity comprise uo to 50% of the gut-associated IgA-ASC (Kroese et al. 1989a, 1989b). However, it is unclear whether these cells rely on the same homing mechanisms as B-2 cell-derived IgA-ASC to reach the gut mucosa.

4
Teaching Lymphocytes Where to Go: Mechanisms Driving "Gut" Versus "Peripheral" Homing

Naive T cells have the capacity to acquire any set of homing receptors on activation. However, the site of antigen entry exerts a strong influence on the traffic pattern that lymphocytes acquire. For example, pathogens entering through the skin, such as herpes simplex virus, preferentially generate lymphocytes with skin-homing receptors (Gonzalez et al. 2005; Kantele et al. 2003; Koelle et al. 2002, 2005). On the other hand, oral vaccination induces higher levels of $\alpha 4\beta 7$ on effector/memory T cells (Kantele et al. 1999b; Lundin et al. 2002; Rojas et al. 2003; Rott et al. 1997) and B cells (Gonzalez et al. 2003; Kantele et al. 1997, 1999a, 2005; Quiding-Jarbrink et al. 1997; Youngman et al. 2002) than parenteral administration of the same antigen. Importantly, among memory B and CD8 T cells, only $\alpha 4\beta 7^+$ (but not $\alpha 4\beta 7^{Neg}$) cells carried protection against intestinal rotavirus infection on adoptive transfer (Rose et al. 1998; Williams et al. 1998). In agreement with these observations, it has been shown that the homing potential of activated lymphocytes depends on the lymphoid tissue environment; T cells activated in MLN express higher levels of $\alpha 4\beta 7$ and CCR9 as compared to those activated in skin-draining PLN (Campbell and Butcher 2002; Svensson et al. 2002). Conversely, skin-homing receptors (selectin ligands) are preferentially induced when T cells are activated in skin-draining PLN (Campbell and Butcher 2002).

In lymphoid tissues, DC are essential for efficient T cell activation (Jung et al. 2002; Probst and van den Broek 2005). DC modulate a number of T- and B cell properties in a tissue-specific fashion, such as Th1/Th2 bias (Everson et al. 1998; Iwasaki and Kelsall 1999; Rissoan et al. 1999) and antibody isotype switching (Sato et al. 2003; Spalding and Griffin 1986; Spalding et al. 1984). Recent work by several groups, including ours, has shown that DC are also responsible for the imprinting of tissue-specific homing potential. Intestinal DC from PP and MLN are sufficient to imprint activated T cells with the gut homing receptors $\alpha 4\beta 7$ and CCR9 (Dudda et al., 2004, 2005; Johansson-Lindbom et al. 2003; Mora et al. 2003, 2005; Stagg et al. 2002), and a pronounced capacity to home to the small bowel mucosa (Mora et al. 2003) (Fig. 3A). On the other hand, DC from peripheral lymph nodes (PLN-DC) induce higher levels of E- and P-selectin ligands on T cells compared with intestinal DC (Dudda et al. 2004, 2005; Mora et al., 2005). Fucosyltransferase-VII (FucT-

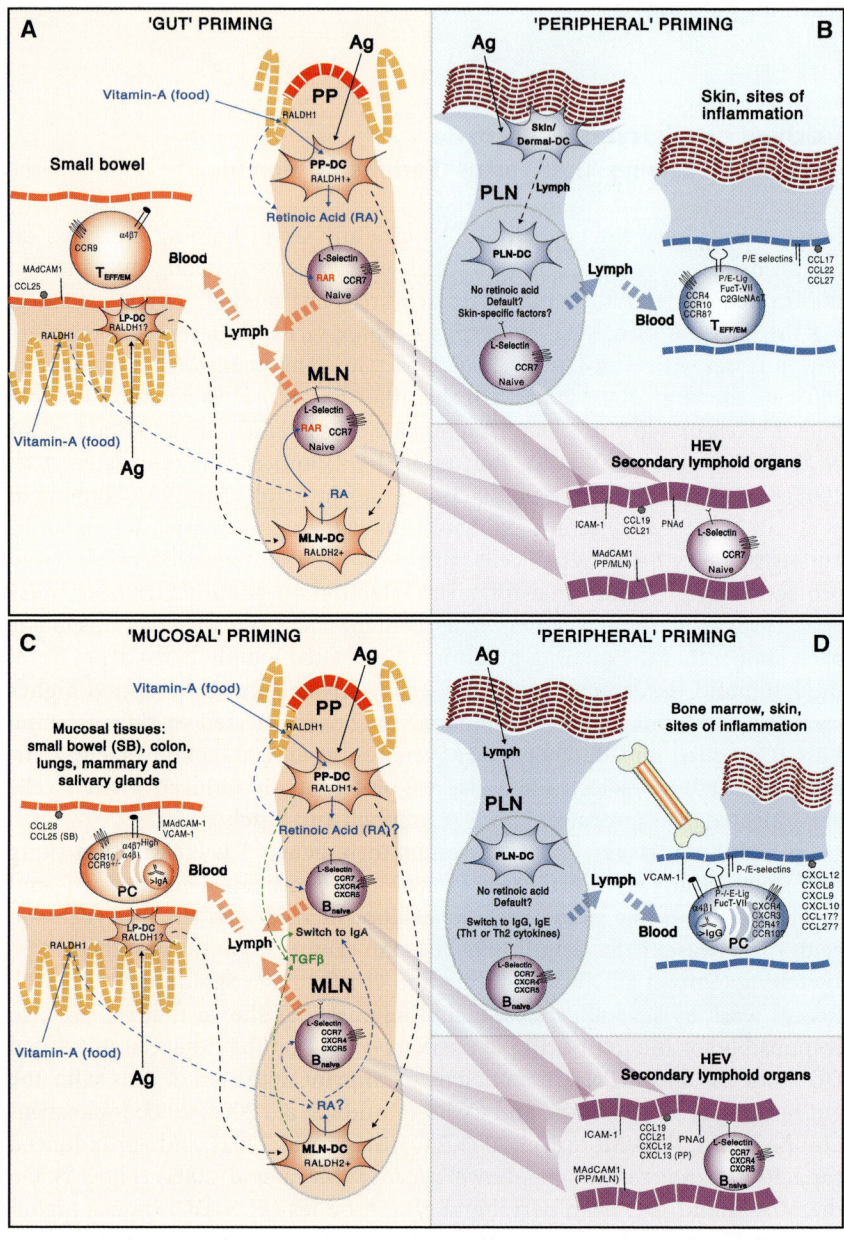

Fig. 3A–D Imprinting mechanisms for gut- and skin-specific lymphocytes. Naive T and B cells access PLN, MLN, and PP through high endothelial venules (*HEV*) and become activated when they encounter a cognate antigen in the local T cell area or follicles, respectively. Once a lymphocyte has become activated in the lymphoid organs, it gives rise to tissue-seeking T_{EFF} that leave the SLO via lymphatics or (from the spleen), enter directly into the blood, and home to peripheral organs through specialized postcapillary venules that express tissue-specific traffic molecules (*vascular addressins*). **A** PP-DC and MLN-DC express critical enzymes to metabolize vitamin-A (retinol) into RA, particularly retinaldehyde dehydrogenases (RALDH-1 and -2). T cell encounter of antigen in the presence of DC-derived RA induces gut-homing receptors and suppresses skin-homing molecules. This requires RA signaling through the RAR family of RA-receptors. It is likely that DC from lamina propria (*LP-DC*) can also make RA, but RA can be synthesized by other cells in the intestinal mucosa, such as enterocytes, which express RALDH-1. **B** When T cells are activated in skin-draining PLN, they are exposed to DC that cannot synthesize RA. The T cells then upregulate skin-homing molecules. The induction of this migratory preference appears to reflect the default differentiation pathway that T cells take on stimulation without gut-specific signals. However, it is still possible that skin-associated DC or other environmental factors are needed to upregulate CCR8 or CCR10 on cutaneous T cells. **C** B cells that become activated by oral antigens upregulate gut-homing molecules. Similar to the situation with T cells, we propose that PP-DC and MLN-DC, possibly by virtue of their ability to produce RA, may also trigger the acquisition of gut homing molecules by antigen-experienced B cells. In addition, B cells are exposed to other factors in the intestinal microenvironment, including TGFβ and RA, which promote isotype switching to IgA. **D** Conversely, when B cells are activated in PLN or the spleen, they are not exposed to RA or other mucosal signals. It is not known whether there are specific imprinting signals for ASC or B_{Mem} targeting to the BM or other peripheral tissues

VII) is an essential enzyme for the generation of selectin ligands (Maly et al. 1996). Accordingly, PLN-DC induce higher levels of FucT-VII in CD8 T cells compared with DC from PP (PP-DC) (Mora et al. 2005). Interestingly, DC from spleen, glutaraldehyde-fixed DC (from any lymphoid tissue), or stimulation by anti-CD3 and anti-CD28 (without DC) also induced high levels of E- and P-selectin ligands on CD8 T cells (Mora et al. 2005). These results suggest that the acquisition of skin-homing molecules (at least E-/P-selectin ligands and probably also CCR4) may be a default pathway whenever T cells are activated in the absence of gut-derived signals (Mora et al. 2005) (Fig. 3A). However, it must be cautioned that CCR10 and CCR8 (which can also be expressed on skin-homing T cells) are not induced by these in vitro conditions, suggesting that they might be controlled by skin-specific environmental cues.

A recent report has shown that mice depleted of vitamin A have dramatically reduced numbers of effector/memory T cells in the gut mucosa, but not elsewhere (Iwata et al. 2004). Concomitant in vitro experiments showed that the presence of the vitamin A metabolite retinoic acid (RA) during T cell activation induces α4β7 and CCR9 on T cells, even in the absence of DC (Iwata et al. 2004). RA also blocked the activation-induced default upregulation of E- and P-selectin ligands on T cells (Iwata et al. 2004), a phenomenon that was also observed when T cells were activated in the presence of PP-DC, even when the PP-DC did not present the activating antigen (Mora et al. 2005). Importantly, gut DC (from PP and MLN) express higher levels of retinaldehyde dehydrogenases (RALDHs), which are essential enzymes for RA biosynthesis (Iwata et al. 2004). These enzymes were not detected in DC from PLN or spleen. Blocking RALDHs in DCs or RA receptors in T cells significantly decreased the induction of α4β7 by PP-DC and MLN-DC (Iwata et al. 2004). Therefore, the ability to produce RA is an important mechanism by which gut DC induce gut-homing molecules and suppress skin-homing molecules on T cells (Fig. 3A).

It should be mentioned that even though intestinal DC are sufficient to induce gut homing molecules in vitro, it is formally possible that other sources of RA may contribute in vivo. For example, enterocytes in the small intestine express high levels of RALDH-1 (Iwata et al. 2004), and it has been shown that RA can be produced by a small intestinal epithelial cell line in vitro (Lampen et al., 2000) (Fig. 3A). On the other hand, intraperitoneal immunization efficiently generates gut-homing T cells (Campbell and Butcher 2002; Johansson-Lindbom et al. 2003; Svensson et al. 2002), and some nonintestinal viral infections also induce the generation of α4β7$^+$ T cells (Masopust et al. 2004). Thus it is possible that gut-homing T cells can be imprinted in regions other than gut-associated lymphoid tissues. It will be interesting to determine whether RA synthesis can be induced in nonintestinal DC under inflammatory or infectious conditions and whether there are additional, RA-independent mechanisms of intestinal imprinting (Mora and von Andrian 2004). Moreover, the expression of α4β7 and CCR9 is not always linked. For example, naive CD8 T cells express high levels of CCR9 (Carramolino et al. 2001) but low levels of α4β7 (Mora et al. 2003), and T cells infiltrating the colon mucosa are α4β7^{High}, but CCR9$^-$ (Zabel et al. 1999). Because RA induces both gut-homing molecules simultaneously (Iwata et al. 2004), these findings suggest that there are additional mechanisms that may regulate the expression of α4β7 and/or CCR9 (Mora and von Andrian 2004).

It should also be emphasized that although PP-DC generate T cells that potently migrate to the small intestine, PP-DC-induced effector T cells do not migrate efficiently to the colon (Mora et al. 2003). Moreover, T cells activated with appendix-derived DC did not migrate better to the colon mucosa than those activated with PP-DC (Mora and von Andrian, unpublished observations), suggesting that there additional, still unknown factors involved in the imprinting of colon-homing T cells (assuming that specific colon-tropic T cells exist).

As discussed above, many IgA-ASC express $\alpha 4\beta 7$ and CCR10, and some also express CCR9 (Cyster 2003; Kunkel and Butcher 2003). PP-DC can affect B cell function in a tissue-specific fashion by promoting class-switching to IgA (Sato et al. 2003; Spalding and Griffin 1986; Spalding et al. 1984). Similarly, B cell exposure to RA induces class-switching to IgA (Tokuyama and Tokuyama 1999). Therefore, it will be interesting to determine whether gut DC and/or RA can also imprint gut tropism in ASC and to understand how is this linked to IgA switching (Fig. 3B).

5
Modulation of Lymphocyte Homing for Therapeutic Purposes

Some genetic defects in adhesion mechanisms result in variable degrees of immunodeficiency, for example, leukocyte adhesion deficiency (LAD)-1 (lack of functional $\beta 2$ integrins) (Kishimoto et al. 1987), LAD-2 (deficiency in selectin ligands) (Etzioni et al. 1992), or LAD-3 (defects in integrin activation) (Kinashi et al. 2004). These paradigmatic "experiments of nature" imply that the manipulation of leukocyte adhesion/homing could be a useful immunotherapeutic tool. In fact, a mAb against the integrin LFA-1 (efalizumab) is being used in the clinic for the treatment of psoriasis (Lebwohl et al. 2003). Anti-LFA may also be effective in the treatment of refractive cutaneous GVHD (Stoppa et al. 1991) and possibly other inflammatory/immune-mediated diseases. However, blocking either LFA-1 or one of its ligand ICAM-1 has not been successful in stroke, myocardial infarction, and traumatic shock (Schreiber et al. 2001; Yacyshyn et al. 2002; Yonekawa and Harlan 2005). On the other hand, because LFA-1 and ICAM-1 are required for lymphocyte adhesion in a multitude of tissues, interfering with these molecules could cause undesired immunosuppression. It has been postulated that modulating lymphocyte adhesion in a tissue-specific fashion could be an effective and less immunosuppressive alternative in this regard.

Recent events have prompted intense discussion on the validity of this argument. Clinical trials with Natalizumab (Tysabri), a mAb that blocks the binding of both $\alpha 4\beta 1$ (VLA-4) to VCAM-1 and $\alpha 4\beta 7$ to MAdCAM-1 on Th1 cells that infiltrate the brain and gut, respectively (von Andrian and Engelhardt 2003), have shown that the mAb is efficacious in the treatment of both Crohn disease (Ghosh et al. 2003) and, especially, multiple sclerosis (Miller et al. 2003). These exciting clinical results were initially hailed as validation of the approach of blocking traffic molecules to treat autoimmune inflammatory diseases. However, Natalizumab was subsequently withdrawn from the market when it was learned that a small percentage of patients treated with this drug developed progressive multifocal leukoencephalopathy (PML), a deadly opportunistic CNS infection caused by JC polyomavirus. The occurrence of PML in this setting was unanticipated because this condition is normally only seen in patients with severely impaired cell-mediated immunity, such as in AIDS, leukemia, or organ transplantation. The majority of humans have detectable antibody titers against JC virus, and many individuals test positive for viral DNA but never experience viral disease. Therefore, although Natalizumab blocked the entry of encephalitogenic $CD4^+$ T cells and the subsequent CNS demyelination, the drug apparently also inhibited the prerequisite immunosurveillance by (presumably) a subset of T cells that normally protect the brain against JC virus infection.

Another tissue with defined homing specificity is the skin. Consistent with the role of E- and P-selectin in skin homing, mice lacking these receptors have a compromised delayed-type contact hypersensitivity response and suffer from spontaneous skin infections (Hirata et al. 2002; Staite et al. 1996). In nonhuman primates, recruitment of lymphocytes into DTH skin depended on VCAM-1 and E-selectin (Silber et al. 1994), and blocking of the E-selectin ligand CLA prevented migration of human T cells into human skin transplanted into SCID mice (Biedermann et al. 2002). However, blocking E-selectin alone was ineffective in clinical trials for psoriasis (Bhushan et al. 2002). This failure could have been due to the redundancy of P- and E-selectin expression and function in the skin (Schon et al. 2004; Staite et al. 1996; Weninger et al. 2000). Similarly, although blocking the CCR10-ligand CCL27 effectively decreased skin inflammation in DTH and atopic dermatitis in mice (Homey et al. 2002), there is likely redundancy among the skin-associated chemokine receptors CCR10 and CCR4, at least in some settings of skin inflammation (Reiss et al. 2001). Moreover, it is possible that other inflammation-induced receptors play a role in inflamed skin. In fact, clinical trials are currently underway targeting CCR1 and CXCR3 in psoriasis (Johnson et al. 2005).

The gut mucosa is arguably the most paradigmatic example of tissue-specific homing. Blockade of $\alpha 4\beta 7$ in a spontaneous model of colitis in nonhuman primates rapidly reverts the disease (Hesterberg et al. 1996). Similarly, in a chronic colitis model caused by transfer of $CD45RB^{Hi}$ CD4 T cells into SCID mice, blocking $\beta 7$ integrins and/or MAdCAM-1 inhibited the development of colitis (Picarella et al. 1997). Consistent with these data, Natalizumab has been efficacious in clinical trials of Crohn disease (Ghosh et al. 2003). However, as discussed above, there are important safety concerns associated with global inhibition of $\alpha 4$ integrins (Steinman 2005). Nevertheless, a recent trial in ulcerative colitis selectively targeting the gut-homing receptor α4β7 has successfully reached its therapeutic end point (Feagan et al. 2005). Because this approach does not interfere with α4β1 pathway in the CNS, it seems less likely to elicit susceptibility to PML or other opportunistic infections.

Another pathology involving the gut is GVHD, and interfering with the function of α4 or α4β7 has been effective in preventing gut and liver (but not cutaneous) GVDH in mice (Murai et al. 2003; Petrovic et al. 2004; Tanaka et al. 1995). However, it is possible that other molecules induced on inflammation are also involved in this pathology, for example, the chemokine receptors CXCR3 (Duffner et al. 2003) and CCR5 (Murai et al. 2003).

Interestingly, in some studies of acute experimental colitis, blocking tissue-specific homing receptors has been only partially or not at all effective. For instance, blocking VCAM-1, but not the α4β7 ligand MAdCAM-1, was shown to attenuate DSS colitis (Soriano et al. 2000). This could be due in part to the fact that DSS-induced colitis does not depend on T and B lymphocytes (Axelsson et al. 1996). In addition, it is possible that other non-tissue-specific adhesion molecules induced under inflammatory conditions could (at least in part) override the role of some tissue-specific homing receptors and addressins. Consistent with this possibility, blocking the CCR6-ligand CCL20 (in addition to MAdCAM-1) was necessary to decrease the accumulation of T and B cells in DSS-induced colitis (Teramoto et al. 2005). Additionally, blocking α1β1, a collagen-binding integrin upregulated in many inflammatory settings, decreases TNBS-induced acute colitis in mice (Fiorucci et al. 2002). Moreover, it has been found in humans that CCR2 is expressed by most CD4 T cells infiltrating the lamina propria in Crohn's ileitis (Connor et al. 2004), suggesting that this receptor (with or without CCR9) might play a role in this intestinal pathology. Furthermore, in SAMP-1/Yit mice, a strain that develops spontaneous chronic enteritis similar to Crohn's disease, blocking ICAM-1 plus VCAM-1 reduced inflammation (Burns et al. 2001). Interestingly, blocking β7, α4β7, or MAdCAM-1 alone did not prevent ileitis, but blocking L-selectin in combination with MAdCAM-1 or α4 ameliorated the disease, suggesting that under chronic intestinal inflammation, non-gut-specific molecules such as α4β1 and L-selectin might play important roles in the pathogenesis of these diseases (Rivera-Nieves et al. 2005). However, using the same mouse model, another group has reported recently that blocking MAdCAM-1 alone was not only effective but even better than VCAM-1 blockade (Matsuzaki et al. 2005). Whether the discrepancies among these reports could have been due to differences in experimental treatment schedules or some other factors remains to be determined.

6
Re-educating Tissue-Specific T Cells—
A New Platform for Immunomodulation?

An important question is whether effector/memory lymphocytes, after having been imprinted to express a set of tissue-specific homing molecules, can change or modulate their homing potential. There is mounting evidence that the answer to this question is affirmative in most if not all cases. For example, CD4 T cells can sequentially up- or downregulate the skin-homing receptor CLA when they are reactivated under Th1 or Th2 conditions, respectively (Teraki and Picker 1997). T_{EM} cells can spontaneously reacquire L-selectin and CCR7 expression and thus revert to a T_{CM} phenotype in vivo (Wherry et al. 2003). In addition, most TCRαβ/CD8αβ T cells in the intestinal lamina propria are $\alpha 4\beta 7^{Low/neg}$ (Mora et al. 2003). Indeed, recent findings suggest that α4β7 is downregulated whereas αEβ7 is upregulated after T cells have entered the intestinal mucosa (Ericsson et al. 2004). Even skin and gut homing commitment are not immutable properties but apparently reflect rather dynamic functional states. T cells that have been imprinted with gut- or skin-homing potential by intestinal DC or PLN-DC, respectively, become "reprogrammed" when they are restimulated by the "opposite" DC (Dudda et al. 2005; Mora et al. 2005) (Fig. 4A). Consistent with a pivotal role of RA during intestinal imprinting (Iwata et al. 2004), memory T cells that were restimulated in the presence of exogenous RA acquired a marked gut-homing phenotype irrespective of their prior tissue commitment or the nature of the stimulus (i.e., antibodies or DC from different tissues) used for reactivation (Mora and von Andrian, unpublished observations). Re-education of memory lymphocytes may also be possible in humans. When volunteers were immunized orally or parenterally and then reimmunized with *Salmonella* through the same or the opposite pathway with respect to the first immunization, the last immunization was dominant over the first one regarding the expression of the gut-homing receptor α4β7 on antigen-specific ASC (Kantele et al. 2005). Thus memory B cells may also possess plasticity in their homing commitment (Fig. 3B). The new concept that has emerged from the above observations is that tissue selectivity is a dynamic and pliable property of lymphocytes. This plasticity could be an attractive target for therapeutic intervention. On one hand, the pharmacological provision of homing instructions may allow for improved targeting of effector/memory lymphocytes to improve vaccination protocols in infectious diseases or cancer. On the other hand, it might be possible to divert pathogenic lymphocytes away from a site of autoimmune attack to other tissues where the redirected cells remain harmless.

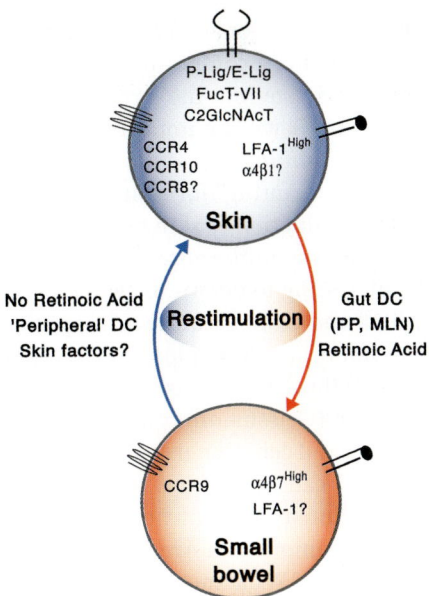

Fig. 4 Plasticity in lymphocyte homing potential. Effector/memory T cells with gut-homing potential are rapidly converted to skin-homing T cells if they are reactivated with peripheral DC (i.e., in the absence of RA). Reciprocally, cutaneous effector/memory T cells readily acquire a gut-homing phenotype when they are restimulated by intestinal DC (i.e., in the presence of RA)

7
Future Directions

A growing body of evidence indicates that the division between T_{CM} and T_{EFF}/T_{EM} can be complex and fluid. For example, some human cells with a T_{CM} phenotype express not only LN homing receptors but also traffic molecules for peripheral tissues, and such cells have been detected in extralymphoid organs (Campbell et al. 2001). In addition, at least in certain mouse models, some T_{CM}-like cells exhibit immediate effector activity comparable to that of T_{EFF} (Debes et al. 2002; Unsoeld et al. 2002; Wherry et al. 2003). Given these observations, there are no universally accepted criteria for unambiguous distinction between these memory T cell subsets, other than their differential capacity to migrate to PLN.

The molecular mechanisms driving the homing of effector/memory lymphocytes to the small intestine and the skin have been partially elucidated. Although gut DC and RA seem to be necessary and sufficient to imprint T cell with small bowel tropism under steady-state conditions, it will be interesting to explore whether there are additional mechanisms to generate gut-homing lymphocytes under inflammatory conditions. Moreover, T cells seem to require different signals to migrate into the large bowel (Kunkel and Butcher 2002; Mora et al. 2003), and it will be important to determine the specific multistep cascade for colon homing.

Is there truly "homing imprinting" for tissues other than the gut? Recent evidence suggests that the induction of skin homing (at least selectin ligands and CCR4) is a default pathway in the absence of gut-derived signals (Mora et al. 2005). It will be interesting to determine whether other skin-associated receptors, such as CCR10 and CCR8, require skin-specific molecular signals. In addition, it will be important to explore other proposed tissue-specific lymphocyte imprinting pathways, such as those for the lung (Ainslie et al. 2002; Xu et al. 2003), liver (Geissmann et al. 2005; Sato et al. 2005), bone marrow (Mazo et al. 2005), and central nervous system (Calzascia et al. 2005).

Similarly, although ASC can exhibit gut tropism, which depends on the site of antigen encounter (Kunkel and Butcher 2003), it is presently unknown whether and how B cells get imprinted. Are tissue-specific DC and/or RA involved in this process (Fig. 3B)? What mechanisms coordinate the expression of $\alpha 4\beta 7$ and CCR10 and/or CCR9 in ASC? How is B cell imprinting correlated with switching to IgA versus IgG production?

Most studies on lymphocyte migration to the gut have focused on steady-state, noninflamed conditions. However, recent evidence suggests that other adhesion molecules, different from the canonical gut-specific homing receptors, may be invoked under inflammatory conditions (Rivera-Nieves et al. 2005). To devise optimal therapeutic strategies, it will be important to dissect the relative contribution of tissue-specific versus non-tissue-specific traffic molecules in different inflammatory settings.

Because gut-associated DC play an active role in programming T cells to express gut-homing molecules (Iwata et al. 2004; Mora and von Andrian 2004), it will be important to understand how DC themselves are "educated" to acquire this tissue-specific imprinting potential. It is likely that "DC education" happens in the periphery after bone marrow-derived DC precursors have established a tissue residence, but the alternative, a priori specialization of precursors in the bone marrow, has not been ruled out. Wherever DC imprinting specialization may have its origin, the signals involved in this process are unknown. Possible candidates include the gut microflora, signals through toll-like receptors, the influence of epithelial and/or other stromal cells, intrinsic differentiation programs triggered during hematopoiesis, or a mixture of these diverse factors. The elucidation of this mechanism(s) may have implications for the design or improvement of DC-based vaccines targeting mucosal immune responses, such as in HIV and cancer.

Acknowledgements Supported by NIH Grants HL-62524, HL-54936, HL-56949, and AI-061663.

References

Ainslie MP, McNulty CA, Huynh T, Symon FA, and Wardlaw AJ (2002). *Thorax* 57, 1054-9.
Alon R, Kassner PD, Carr MW, Finger EB, Hemler ME, and Springer TA (1995). *J Cell Biol* 128, 1243–1253.
Austrup F, Rebstock S, Kilshaw PJ, and Hamann A (1995). *Eur J Immunol* 25, 1487–91.
Axelsson LG, Landstrom E, Goldschmidt TJ, Gronberg A, and Bylund-Fellenius AC (1996). *Inflamm Res* 45, 181–91.
Bargatze RF, Jutila MA, and Butcher EC (1995). *Immunity* 3, 99–108.
Berg EL, McEvoy LM, Berlin C, Bargatze RF, and Butcher EC (1993). *Nature* 366, 695–698.
Berlin C, Bargatze RF, von Andrian UH, Szabo MC, Hasslen SR, Nelson RD, Berg EL, Erlandsen SL, and Butcher EC (1995). *Cell* 80, 413–422.
Berlin C, Berg EL, Briskin MJ, Andrew DP, Kilshaw PJ, Holzmann B, Weissman IL, Hamann A, and Butcher EC (1993). *Cell* 74, 185–195.
Berlin-Rufenach C, Otto F, Mathies M, Westermann J, Owen MJ, Hamann A, and Hogg N (1999). *J Exp Med* 189, 1467–1478.
Bernasconi NL, Traggiai E, and Lanzavecchia A (2002). *Science* 298, 2199–202.
Bhushan M, Bleiker TO, Ballsdon AE, Allen MH, Sopwith M, Robinson MK, Clarke C, Weller RP, Graham-Brown RA, Keefe M, Barker JN, and Griffiths CE (2002). *Br J Dermatol* 146, 824–31.
Biedermann T, Schwarzler C, Lametschwandtner G, Thoma G, Carballido-Perrig N, Kund J, de Vries JE, Rot A, and Carballido JM (2002). *Eur J Immunol* 32, 3171–3180.
Bowman EP, Kuklin NA, Youngman KR, Lazarus NH, Kunkel EJ, Pan J, Greenberg HB, and Butcher EC (2002). *J Exp Med* 195, 269–75.
Burns RC, Rivera-Nieves J, Moskaluk CA, Matsumoto S, Cominelli F, and Ley K (2001). *Gastroenterology* 121, 1428–36.
Butcher EC (1991). *Cell* 67, 1033–1036.
Butcher EC, and Picker LJ (1996). *Science* 272, 60–66.
Calzascia T, Masson F, Di Berardino-Besson W, Contassot E, Wilmotte R, Aurrand-Lions M, Ruegg C, Dietrich PY, and Walker PR (2005). *Immunity* 22, 175–84.
Campbell DJ, and Butcher EC (2002). *J Exp Med* 195, 135–141.
Campbell J, Haraldsen G, Pan J, Rottman J, Qin S, Ponath P, Andrew DP, Warnke R, Ruffing N, Kassam N, Wu L, and Butcher EC (1999). *Nature* 400, 776–780.
Campbell JJ, Murphy KE, Kunkel EJ, Brightling CE, Soler D, Shen Z, Boisvert J, Greenberg HB, Vierra MA, Goodman SB, Genovese MC, Wardlaw AJ, Butcher EC, and Wu L (2001). *J Immunol* 166, 877–884.
Carman CV, and Springer TA (2003). *Curr Opin Cell Biol* 15, 547–56.
Carramolino L, Zaballos A, Kremer L, Villares R, Martin P, Ardavin C, Martinez AC, and Marquez G (2001). *Blood* 97, 850–7.
Cepek KL, Shaw SK, Parker CM, Russell GJ, Morrow JS, Rimm DL, and Brenner MB (1994). *Nature* 10, 190–193.

Chong BF, Murphy JE, Kupper TS, and Fuhlbrigge RC (2004). *J Immunol* 172, 1575–1581.
Colantonio L, Iellem A, Sinigaglia F, and D'Ambrosio D (2002). *Eur J Immunol* 32, 3506–14.
Connor SJ, Paraskevopoulos N, Newman R, Cuan N, Hampartzoumian T, Lloyd AR, and Grimm MC (2004). *Gut* 53, 1287–94.
Cyster JG (2003). *Immunol Rev* 194, 48–60.
Debes GF, Hopken UE, and Hamann A (2002). *J Immunol* 168, 5441–7.
Dudda JC, Lembo A, Bachtanian E, Huehn J, Siewert C, Hamann A, Kremmer E, Forster R, and Martin SF (2005). *Eur J Immunol* 35, 1056–1065.
Dudda JC, Simon JC, and Martin S (2004). *J Immunol* 172, 857–863.
Duffner U, Lu B, Hildebrandt GC, Teshima T, Williams DL, Reddy P, Ordemann R, Clouthier SG, Lowler K, Liu C, Gerard C, Cooke KR, and Ferrara JL (2003). *Exp Hematol* 31, 897–902.
Ebisuno Y, Tanaka T, Kanemitsu N, Kanda H, Yamaguchi K, Kaisho T, Akira S, and Miyasaka M (2003). *J Immunol* 171, 1642–6.
El-Asady R, Yuan R, Liu K, Wang D, Gress RE, Lucas PJ, Drachenberg CB, and Hadley GA (2005). *J Exp Med* 201, 1647–57.
Ericsson A, Svensson M, Arya A, and Agace WW (2004). *Eur J Immunol* 34, 2720–9.
Etzioni A, Frydman M, Pollack S, Avidor I, Phillips ML, Paulson JC, and Gershoni-Baruch R (1992). *N Engl J Med* 327, 1789.
Everson MP, Lemak DG, McDuffie DS, Koopman WJ, McGhee JR, and Beagley KW (1998). *J Interferon Cytokine Res* 18, 103–15.
Farstad IN, Halstensen TS, Lazarovits AI, Norstein J, Fausa O, and Brandtzaeg P (1995). *Scand J Immunol* 42, 662–72.
Feagan BG, Greenberg GR, Wild G, Fedorak RN, Pare P, McDonald JW, Dube R, Cohen A, Steinhart AH, Landau S, Aguzzi RA, Fox IH, and Vandervoort MK (2005). *N Engl J Med* 352, 2499–507.
Fiorucci S, Mencarelli A, Palazzetti B, Sprague AG, Distrutti E, Morelli A, Novobrantseva TI, Cirino G, Koteliansky VE, and de Fougerolles AR (2002). *Immunity* 17, 769–80.
Flier J, Boorsma DM, van Beek PJ, Nieboer C, Stoof TJ, Willemze R, and Tensen CP (2001). *J Pathol* 194, 398–405.
Fuhlbrigge RC, Kieffer JD, Armerding D, and Kupper TS (1997). *Nature* 389, 978–981.
Gauguet JM, Rosen SD, Marth JD, and von Andrian UH (2004). *Blood* 104, 4104–12.
Geissmann F, Cameron TO, Sidobre S, Manlongat N, Kronenberg M, Briskin MJ, Dustin ML, and Littman DR (2005). *PLoS Biol* 3, e113.
Ghosh S, Goldin E, Gordon FH, Malchow HA, Rask-Madsen J, Rutgeerts P, Vyhnalek P, Zadorova Z, Palmer T, and Donoghue S (2003). *N Engl J Med* 348, 24–32.
Gonzalez AM, Jaimes MC, Cajiao I, Rojas OL, Cohen J, Pothier P, Kohli E, Butcher EC, Greenberg HB, Angel J, and Franco MA (2003). *Virology* 305, 93–105.
Gonzalez JC, Kwok WW, Wald A, McClurkan CL, Huang J, and Koelle DM (2005). *J Infect Dis* 191, 243–54.
Goodarzi K, Goodarzi M, Tager AM, Luster AD, and von Andrian UH (2003). *Nat Immunol* 4, 965–973.
Guy-Grand D, Griscelli C, and Vassalli P (1978). *J Exp Med* 148, 1661–1677.

Halin C, Scimone ML, Bonasio R, Gauguet JM, Mempel TR, Quackenbush E, Proia RL, Mandala S, and von Andrian UH (2005). *Blood* 106, 1314–1322.
Hamann A, Andrew DP, Jablonski-Westrich D, Holzmann B, and Butcher EC (1994). *J Immunol* 152, 3282–3293.
Hargreaves DC, Hyman PL, Lu TT, Ngo VN, Bidgol A, Suzuki G, Zou YR, Littman DR, and Cyster JG (2001). *J Exp Med* 194, 45–56.
Hesterberg PE, Winsor-Hines D, Briskin MJ, Soler-Ferran D, Merrill C, Mackay CR, Newman W, and Ringler DJ (1996). *Gastroenterology* 111, 1373–80.
Hieshima K, Kawasaki Y, Hanamoto H, Nakayama T, Nagakubo D, Kanamaru A, and Yoshie O (2004). *J Immunol* 173, 3668–75.
Higgins, J. M. G., Mandlebrot DA, Shaw SK, Russell GJ, Murphy EA, Chen, Y.-T., Nelson WJ, Parker CM, and Brenner MB (1998). *J Cell Biol* 140, 197–210.
Hirata T, Furie BC, and Furie B (2002). *J Immunol* 169, 4307–4313.
Homey B, Alenius H, Muller A, Soto H, Bowman EP, Yuan W, McEvoy L, Lauerma AI, Assmann T, Bunemann E, Lehto M, Wolff H, Yen D, Marxhausen H, To W, Sedgwick J, Ruzicka T, Lehmann P, and Zlotnik A (2002). *Nat Med* 8, 157-165.
Hosoe N, Miura S, Watanabe C, Tsuzuki Y, Hokari R, Oyama T, Fujiyama Y, Nagata H, and Ishii H (2004). *Am J Physiol Gastrointest Liver Physiol* 286, G458-G466.
Huehn J, Siegmund K, Lehmann JC, Siewert C, Haubold U, Feuerer M, Debes GF, Lauber J, Frey O, Przybylski GK, Niesner U, de la Rosa M, Schmidt CA, Brauer R, Buer J, Scheffold A, and Hamann A (2004). *J Exp Med* 199, 303–13.
Iellem A, Colantonio L, and D'Ambrosio D (2003). *Eur J Immunol* 33, 1488–96.
Iwasaki A, and Kelsall BL (1999). *J Exp Med* 190, 229–39.
Iwata M, Hirakiyama A, Eshima Y, Kagechika H, Kato C, and Song SY (2004). *Immunity* 21, 527–38.
Janssen GH, Tangelder GJ, Oude Egbrink MG, and Reneman RS (1994). *Am J Physiol Heart Circ Physiol* 267, H1199–204.
Johansson-Lindbom B, Svensson M, Wurbel MA, Malissen B, Marquez G, and Agace W (2003). *J Exp Med* 198, 963–969.
Johnson Z, Schwarz M, Power CA, Wells, T. N. C., and Proudfoot, A. E. I. (2005). *Trends Immunol*, 26, 268–274.
Jung S, Unutmaz D, Wong P, Sano G, De los Santos K, Sparwasser T, Wu S, Vuthoori S, Ko K, Zavala F, Pamer EG, Littman DR, and Lang RA (2002). *Immunity* 17, 211–20.
Kaech SM, Tan JT, Wherry EJ, Konieczny BT, Surh CD, and Ahmed R (2003). *Nat Immunol* 4, 1191–1198.
Kantele A, Arvilommi H, Iikkanen K, Savilahti E, Makela HP, Herzog C, Furer E, and Kantele JM (2005). *J Infect Dis* 191, 312–7.
Kantele A, Kantele JM, Savilahti E, Westerholm M, Arvilommi H, Lazarovits A, Butcher EC, and Makela PH (1997). *J Immunol* 158, 574–9.
Kantele A, Savilahti E, Tiimonen H, Iikkanen K, Autio S, and Kantele JM (2003). *Eur J Immunol* 33, 3275–83.
Kantele A, Westerholm M, Kantele JM, Makela PH, and Savilahti E (1999a). *Vaccine* 17, 229–36.
Kantele A, Zivny J, Hakkinen M, Elson CO, and Mestecky J (1999b). *J Immunol* 162, 5173–7.
Kinashi T, Aker M, Sokolovsky-Eisenberg M, Grabovsky V, Tanaka C, Shamri R, Feigelson S, Etzioni A, and Alon R (2004). *Blood* 103, 1033–6.

Kishimoto TK, Hollander N, Roberts TM, Anderson DC, and Springer TA (1987). *Cell* 50, 193–202.
Klonowski KD, Williams KJ, Marzo AL, Blair DA, Lingenheld EG, and Lefrancois L (2004). *Immunity* 20, 551–562.
Koelle DM, Gonzalez JC, and Johnson AS (2005). *Am J Reprod Immunol* 53, 172–81.
Koelle DM, Liu Z, McClurkan CM, Topp MS, Riddell SR, Pamer EG, Johnson AS, Wald A, and Corey L (2002). *J Clin Invest* 110, 537–48.
Kroese FG, Butcher EC, Stall AM, and Herzenberg LA (1989a). *Immunol Invest* 18, 47–58.
Kroese FG, Butcher EC, Stall AM, Lalor PA, Adams S, and Herzenberg LA (1989b). *Int Immunol* 1, 75–84.
Kunkel EJ, and Butcher EC (2002). *Immunity* 16, 1–4.
Kunkel EJ, and Butcher EC (2003). *Nat Rev Immunol* 3, 822–9.
Kunkel EJ, Campbell JJ, Haraldsen G, Pan J, Boisvert J, Roberts AI, Ebert EC, Vierra MA, Goodman SB, Genovese MC, Wardlaw AJ, Greenberg HB, Parker CM, Butcher EC, Andrew DP, and Agace WW (2000). *J Exp Med* 192, 761–8.
Kunkel EJ, Kim CH, Lazarus NH, Vierra MA, Soler D, Bowman EP, and Butcher EC (2003). *J Clin Invest* 111, 1001–1010.
Lampen A, Meyer S, Arnhold T, and Nau H (2000). *J Pharmacol Exp Ther* 295, 979–85.
Lazarus NH, Kunkel EJ, Johnston B, Wilson E, Youngman KR, and Butcher EC (2003). *J Immunol* 170, 3799–805.
Lebwohl M, Tyring SK, Hamilton TK, Toth D, Glazer S, Tawfik NH, Walicke P, Dummer W, Wang X, Garovoy MR, and Pariser D (2003). *N Engl J Med* 349, 2004–13.
Lefrancois L, Parker CM, Olson S, Muller W, Wagner N, Schon MP, and Puddington L (1999). *J Exp Med* 189, 1631–8.
Ley K, and Kansas GS (2004). *Nat Rev Immunol* 4, 325–335.
Lundin BS, Johansson C, and Svennerholm AM (2002). *Infect Immun* 70, 5622–7.
Mackay CR, Marston WL, and Dudler L (1990). *J Exp Med* 171, 801–817.
Maly P, Thall AD, Petryniak B, Rogers CE, Smith PL, Marks RM, Kelly RJ, Gersten KM, Cheng G, Saunders TL, Camper SA, Camphausen RT, Sullivan FX, Isogai Y, Hindsgaul O, von Andrian UH, and Lowe JB (1996). *Cell* 86, 643–653.
Manjunath N, Shankar P, Wan J, Weninger W, Crowley MA, Hieshima K, Springer TA, Fan X, Shen H, Lieberman J, and von Andrian UH (2001). *J Clin Invest* 108, 871–878.
Masopust D, Vezys V, Marzo AL, and Lefrancois L (2001). *Science* 291, 2413–7.
Masopust D, Vezys V, Usherwood EJ, Cauley LS, Olson S, Marzo AL, Ward RL, Woodland DL, and Lefrancois L (2004). *J Immunol* 172, 4875–4882.
Matsuzaki K, Tsuzuki Y, Matsunaga H, Inoue T, Miyazaki J, Hokari R, Okada Y, Kawaguchi A, Nagao S, Itoh K, Matsumoto S, and Miura S (2005). *Clin Exp Immunol* 140, 22–31.
Mazo IB, Honczarenko M, Leung H, Cavanagh LL, Bonasio R, Weninger W, Engelke K, Xia L, McEver RP, Koni PA, Silberstein LE, and von Andrian UH (2005). *Immunity* 22, 259–70.
McDermott MR, and Bienenstock J (1979). *J. Immunol.* 122, 1892–1898.
McHeyzer-Williams LJ, and McHeyzer-Williams MG (2005). *Annu Rev Immunol* 23, 487–513.

Miller DH, Khan OA, Sheremata WA, Blumhardt LD, Rice GP, Libonati MA, Willmer-Hulme AJ, Dalton CM, Miszkiel KA, and O'Connor PW (2003). *N Engl J Med* 348, 15–23.

Mora JR, Bono MR, Manjunath N, Weninger W, Cavanagh LL, Rosemblatt M, and von Andrian UH (2003). *Nature* 424, 88–93.

Mora JR, Cheng G, Picarella D, Briskin M, Buchanan N, and von Andrian UH (2005). *J Exp Med* 201, 303–16.

Mora JR, and von Andrian UH (2004). *Immunity* 21, 458–60.

Morales J, Homey B, Vicari AP, Hudak S, Oldham E, Hedrick J, Orozco R, Copeland NG, Jenkins NA, McEvoy LM, and Zlotnik A (1999). *Proc Natl Acad Sci USA* 96, 14470–14475.

Murai M, Yoneyama H, Ezaki T, Suematsu M, Terashima Y, Harada A, Hamada H, Asakura H, Ishikawa H, and Matsushima K (2003). *Nat Immunol* 4, 154–60.

Nagatani K, Sagawa K, Komagata Y, and Yamamoto K (2004). *Ann NY Acad Sci* 1029, 366–70.

Nakache M, Berg EL, Streeter PR, and Butcher EC (1989). *Nature* 337, 179–181.

Nitschke L, Floyd H, Ferguson DJ, and Crocker PR (1999). *J Exp Med* 189, 1513–8.

Nolte D, Schmid P, Jäger U, Botzlar A, Roesken F, Hecht R, Uhl E, Messmer K, and Vestweber D (1994). *Am J Physiol Heart Circ Physiol* 36, H1637-H1642.

Okada T, Ngo VN, Ekland EH, Forster R, Lipp M, Littman DR, and Cyster JG (2002). *J Exp Med* 196, 65–75.

Pabst O, Ohl L, Wendland M, Wurbel MA, Kremmer E, Malissen B, and Forster R (2004). *J Exp Med* 199, 411–6.

Pan J, Kunkel EJ, Gosslar U, Lazarus N, Langdon P, Broadwell K, Vierra MA, Genovese MC, Butcher EC, and Soler D (2000). *J Immunol* 165, 2943–2949.

Papadakis KA, Prehn J, Nelson V, Cheng L, Binder SW, Ponath PD, Andrew DP, and Targan SR (2000). *J Immunol* 165, 5069–5076.

Petrovic A, Alpdogan O, Willis LM, Eng JM, Greenberg AS, Kappel BJ, Liu C, Murphy GJ, Heller G, and van den Brink MR (2004). *Blood* 103, 1542–7.

Picarella D, Hurlbut P, Rottman J, Shi X, Butcher E, and Ringler DJ (1997). *J Immunol* 158, 2099–106.

Picarella DE, Kratz A, Li, C.-b., Ruddle NH, and Flavell RA (1993). *J Immunol* 150, 4136–4150.

Picker LJ, Kishimoto TK, Smith CW, Warnock RA, and Butcher EC (1991). *Nature* 349, 796–798.

Probst HC, and van den Broek M (2005). *J Immunol* 174, 3920–4.

Quiding-Jarbrink M, Nordstrom I, Granstrom G, Kilander A, Jertborn M, Butcher EC, Lazarovits AI, Holmgren J, and Czerkinsky C (1997). *J Clin Invest* 99, 1281–6.

Reinhardt RL, Khoruts A, Merica R, Zell T, and Jenkins MK (2001). *Nature* 410, 101–105.

Reiss Y, Proudfoot AE, Power CA, Campbell JJ, and Butcher EC (2001). *J Exp Med* 194, 1541–1547.

Rissoan MC, Soumelis V, Kadowaki N, Grouard G, Briere F, de Waal Malefyt R, and Liu YJ (1999). *Science* 283, 1183–1186.

Rivera-Nieves J, Olson T, Bamias G, Bruce A, Solga M, Knight RF, Hoang S, Cominelli F, and Ley K (2005). *J Immunol* 174, 2343–52.

Rojas OL, Gonzalez AM, Gonzalez R, Perez-Schael I, Greenberg HB, Franco MA, and Angel J (2003). *Virology* 314, 671–9.
Rose JR, Williams MB, Rott LS, Butcher EC, and Greenberg HB (1998). *J Virol* 72, 726–30.
Rossiter H, Mudde G, van Reijsen F, Kalthoff F, Bruijnzeel-Koomen C, Picker LJ, and Kupper TS (1993). *manuscript*.
Rossiter H, van Reijsen F, Mudde GC, Kalthoff F, Bruijnzeel-Koomen, C. A. E. M., Picker LJ, and Kupper TS (1994). *Eur J Immunol* 24, 205–210.
Rot A, and von Andrian UH (2004). *Annu Rev Immunol* 22, 891–928.
Rott LS, Rose JR, Bass D, Williams MB, Greenberg HB, and Butcher EC (1997). *J Clin Invest* 100, 1204–8.
Rudzik O, Perey DY, and Bienenstock J (1975). *J Immunol* 114, 40–4.
Sallusto F, Lenig D, Forster R, Lipp M, and Lanzavecchia A (1999). *Nature* 401, 708–12.
Sato A, Hashiguchi M, Toda E, Iwasaki A, Hachimura S, and Kaminogawa S (2003). *J Immunol* 171, 3684–90.
Sato T, Thorlacius H, Johnston B, Staton TL, Xiang W, Littman DR, and Butcher EC (2005). *J Immunol* 174, 277–83.
Sawada S, Gowrishankar K, Kitamura R, Suzuki M, Suzuki G, Tahara S, and Koito A (1998). *J Exp Med* 187, 1439–49.
Schaerli P, Ebert L, Willimann K, Blaser A, Roos RS, Loetscher P, and Moser B (2004). *J Exp Med* 199, 1265–1275.
Schon MP, Arya A, Murphy EA, Adams CM, Strauch UG, Agace WW, Marsal J, Donohue JP, Her H, Beier DR, Olson S, Lefrancois L, Brenner MB, Grusby MJ, and Parker CM (1999). *J Immunol* 162, 6641–6649.
Schon MP, Drewniok C, and Boehncke WH (2004). *Curr Drug Targets Inflamm Allergy* 3, 163–8.
Schreiber S, Nikolaus S, Malchow H, Kruis W, Lochs H, Raedler A, Hahn EG, Krummenerl T, and Steinmann G (2001). *Gastroenterology* 120, 1339–46.
Scimone ML, Felbinger TW, Mazo IB, Stein JV, von Andrian UH, and Weninger W (2004). *J Exp Med* 199, 1113–1120.
Siegmund K, Feuerer M, Siewert C, Ghani S, Haubold U, Dankof A, Krenn V, Schon MP, Scheffold A, Lowe JB, Hamann A, Syrbe U, and Huehn J (2005). *Blood*, 106, 3097–3104.
Silber A, Newman W, Sasseville VG, Pauley D, Beall D, Walsh DG, and Ringler DJ (1994). *J Clin Invest* 93, 1554–1563.
Soler D, Humphreys TL, Spinola SM, and Campbell JJ (2003). *Blood* 101, 1677–1682.
Soriano A, Salas A, Sans M, Gironella M, Elena M, Anderson DC, Pique JM, and Panes J (2000). *Lab Invest* 80, 1541–51.
Spalding DM, and Griffin JA (1986). *Cell* 44, 507–15.
Spalding DM, Williamson SI, Koopman WJ, and McGhee JR (1984). *J Exp Med* 160, 941–6.
Springer TA (1994). *Cell* 76, 301–314.
Stagg AJ, Kamm MA, and Knight SC (2002). *Eur J Immunol* 32, 1445–54.
Staite ND, Justen JM, Sly LM, Beaudet AL, and Bullard DC (1996). *Blood* 88, 2973–9.
Stein JV, Rot A, Luo Y, Narasimhaswamy M, Nakano H, Gunn MD, Matsuzawa A, Quackenbush EJ, Dorf ME, and von Andrian UH (2000). *J Exp Med* 191, 61–76.
Steinman L (2005). *Nat Rev Drug Discov* 4, 510–8.

Stensted H, Ericson A, Johansson-Lindbom B, Svensson M, Marsal J, Mack M, Picarella D, Soler D, Marquez G, Briskin M, Agace WW (2006). *Blood*, prepublished January 3, 2006; DOI:10.1182/blood-2005-07-2860

Stoppa AM, Maraninchi D, Blaise D, Viens P, Hirn M, Olive D, Reiffers J, Milpied N, Gaspard MH, and Mawas C (1991). *Transpl Int* 4, 3–7.

Streeter PR, Rouse, B. T. N., and Butcher EC (1988). *J Cell Biol* 107, 1853–1862.

Svensson M, Marsal J, Ericsson A, Carramolino L, Broden T, Marquez G, and Agace WW (2002). *J Clin Invest* 110, 1113–21.

Tanaka T, Ohtsuka Y, Yagita H, Shiratori Y, Omata M, and Okumura K (1995). *Int Immunol* 7, 1183–9.

Tang ML, Steeber DA, Zhang XQ, and Tedder TF (1998). *J Immunol* 160, 5113–21.

Teraki Y, and Picker LJ (1997). *J Immunol* 159, 6018–6029.

Teramoto K, Miura S, Tsuzuki Y, Hokari R, Watanabe C, Inamura T, Ogawa T, Hosoe N, Nagata H, Ishii H, and Hibi T (2005). *Clin Exp Immunol* 139, 421–8.

Tietz W, Allemand Y, Borges E, von Laer D, Hallmann R, Vestweber D, and Hamann A (1998). *J Immunol* 161, 963–970.

Tokuyama H, and Tokuyama Y (1999). *Cell Immunol* 192, 41–7.

Tseng J (1981). *J Immunol* 127, 2039–43.

Uehara S, Grinberg A, Farber JM, and Love PE (2002). *J Immunol* 168, 2811–2819.

Underhill GH, Minges Wols HA, Fornek JL, Witte PL, and Kansas GS (2002). *Blood* 99, 2905–12.

Unsoeld H, Krautwald S, Voehringer D, Kunzendorf U, and Pircher H (2002). *J Immunol* 169, 638–641.

von Andrian UH (1996). *Microcirc* 3, 287–300.

von Andrian UH, and Engelhardt B (2003). *N Engl J Med* 348, 68–72.

von Andrian UH, and Mackay CR (2000). *N Engl J Med* 343, 1020–1034.

Wagner N, Lohler J, Kunkel EJ, Ley K, Leung E, Krissansen G, Rajewsky K, and Muller W (1996). *Nature* 382, 366–370.

Wang W, Soto H, Oldham ER, Buchanan ME, Homey B, Catron D, Jenkins N, Copeland NG, Gilbert DJ, Nguyen N, Abrams J, Kershenovich D, Smith K, McClanahan T, Vicari AP, and Zlotnik A (2000). *J Biol Chem* 275, 22313–22323.

Warnock RA, Askari S, Butcher EC, and von Andrian UH (1998). *J Exp Med* 187, 205–216.

Warnock RA, Campbell JJ, Dorf ME, Matsuzawa A, McEvoy LM, and Butcher EC (2000). *J Exp Med* 191, 77–88.

Weitkamp JH, Kallewaard NL, Bowen AL, Lafleur BJ, Greenberg HB, and Crowe JE, Jr. (2005). *J Immunol* 174, 3454–60.

Weninger W, Crowley MA, Manjunath N, and von Andrian UH (2001). *J Exp Med* 194, 953–966.

Weninger W, Ulfman LH, Cheng G, Souchkova N, Quackenbush EJ, Lowe JB, and von Andrian UH (2000). *Immunity* 12, 665–676.

Wherry EJ, Teichgraber V, Becker TC, Masopust D, Kaech SM, Antia R, von Andrian UH, and Ahmed R (2003). *Nat Immunol* 4, 225–34.

Williams MB, Rose JR, Rott LS, Franco MA, Greenberg HB, and Butcher EC (1998). *J Immunol* 161, 4227–35.

Wilson E, and Butcher EC (2004). *J Exp Med* 200, 805–9.

Wurbel MA, Malissen M, Guy-Grand D, Meffre E, Nussenzweig MC, Richelme M, Carrier A, and Malissen B (2001). *Blood* 98, 2626–32.

Xu B, Wagner N, Pham LN, Magno V, Shan Z, Butcher EC, and Michie SA (2003). *J Exp Med* 197, 1255–67.

Yacyshyn BR, Chey WY, Goff J, Salzberg B, Baerg R, Buchman AL, Tami J, Yu R, Gibiansky E, and Shanahan WR (2002). *Gut* 51, 30–6.

Yan, H.-C., DeLisser HM, Pilewski JM, Barone KM, Szklut PJ, Chang, X.-J., Ahern TJ, Langer-Safer P, and Albelda SM (1994). *J Immunol* 152, 3053–3063.

Yonekawa K, and Harlan JM (2005). *J Leukoc Biol* 77, 129–40.

Youngman KR, Franco MA, Kuklin NA, Rott LS, Butcher EC, and Greenberg HB (2002). *J Immunol* 168, 2173–81.

Zabel BA, Agace WW, Campbell JJ, Heath HM, Parent D, Roberts AI, Ebert EC, Kassam N, Qin S, Zovko M, LaRosa GJ, Yang LL, Soler D, Butcher EC, Ponath PD, Parker CM, and Andrew DP (1999). *J Exp Med* 190, 1241–56.

IgA Adaptation to the Presence of Commensal Bacteria in the Intestine

A. J. Macpherson (✉)

Department of Medicine, McMaster University Medical Center, Room 3N51H, 1200 Main St. West, Hamilton Ontario, L8 N 3Z5, Canada
macpher@mcmaster.ca

1	**Introduction**	118
1.1	The Intestinal Bacterial Microflora—Complexity and Uncertainty	118
1.2	Tools to Investigate Mutualism Between Commensal Intestinal Bacteria and the Host Immune System	119
1.3	Mutual Adaptation of the Host and the Intestinal Bacterial Flora	120
2	**Immune Responses to Commensal Intestinal Bacteria**	121
2.1	Mucosal Immune Responses to Commensal Intestinal Microorganisms . .	121
2.2	Systemic Immune Ignorance of Commensal Intestinal Microorganisms . .	123
3	**Mechanisms of Mucosal IgA Induction to Commensal Intestinal Bacteria**	124
3.1	Regional Separation of Culturable Organisms After Challenge Doses of *Enterobacter cloacae*	124
3.2	Induction of IgA by Dendritic Cells Loaded with Live *Enterobacter cloacae*	126
3.3	Induction of IgA by Intestinal Conditioning of Mice In Vivo with Live *Enterobacter cloacae*	126
4	**Compartmentalisation of Mucosal Immune Responses to Commensal Bacteria**	128
4.1	Induction by Dendritic Cells Loaded with Commensal Bacteria Focuses the Process Within the Mucosal Immune System	128
4.2	Dendritic Cells Loaded with Commensal Bacteria Are Retained in the Mesenteric Lymph Nodes and Do Not Reach Systemic Secondary Lymphoid Structures	129
5	**Function of IgA in Mutual Adaptation to the Presence of Commensal Intestinal Bacteria**	130
References		131

Abstract The lower intestine of mammals is colonised by a dense flora composed mainly of non-pathogenic commensal bacteria. These intestinal bacteria have a wide-ranging impact on host immunity and physiology. One adaptation following intestinal colonisation is increased production and secretion of polyspecific intestinal IgA. In contrast to the strong mucosal immune response to bacterial colonisation, the systemic immune system remains ignorant of these organisms in pathogen-free mice. Small numbers of bacteria can penetrate the epithelial surface overlying Peyer's patches and survive in dendritic cells to induce IgA by T-dependent and T-independent mechanisms. These dendritic cells loaded with live commensal organisms can home to the mesenteric lymph nodes but do not reach systemic secondary lymphoid structures, so induction of mucosal responses is focused in mucosal lymphoid tissues. The secretion of antibodies across the intestinal epithelial surface in turn limits the penetration of commensal organisms, but this is one of many mechanisms which adapt the intestinal mucosa to co-existence with commensal bacteria.

1
Introduction

1.1
The Intestinal Bacterial Microflora—Complexity and Uncertainty

The lower intestine of mammals is a marvellous habitat for microorganisms. The temperature is a steady 34–40°C and there is a reliable supply of carbon sources, vitamins, minerals and water. It is therefore not surprising that immense numbers of bacteria inhabit the distal small intestine (ileum), the caecum, and the colon. Their densities range up to 10^{12} organisms/ml intestinal contents, so overall the bacteria that we carry outnumber our own cells, and within about 1,000 species present there are approximately 100 times as many genes as on our own chromosomes (Hooper et al. 2001). In normal circumstances, this habitat can never remain sterile for long, so we are colonised just after birth and carry these microbial passengers throughout life (Mackie et al. 1999).

This review summarises experiments carried out to examine the way in which the immune system has adapted to the presence of commensal intestinal bacteria for mutual co-existence, with an emphasis on the secretory IgA response.

The relationship with intestinal bacteria, and microbes that colonise other body surfaces, is usually mutually beneficial. In the intestine, bacteria salvage energy from carbon sources that cannot be digested by mammalian enzymes and supply the host with vitamin precursors. They also appear to compete effectively with pathogenic bacteria, leading to the use of commensal bacteria

(Tvede and Rask-Madsen 1989) or non-pathogenic *Saccharomyces* (McFarland et al. 1994) as therapeutic 'probiotics' to treat recurrent infections with toxigenic *Clostridium difficile* or some forms of relapsing inflammatory bowel disease (Cummings and Kong 2004). Although there is epidemiological evidence that these treatments work, the mechanisms are largely speculative because we understand so little about the complex consortia of bacteria that live in or adjacent to the mucus layer overlying the single-cell-thick sheet of epithelia cells. This has immense practical importance, because the bacteria that are seen by the immune system are probably mainly those intimately associated with the epithelium in biofilms. Conversely, we assume that mucosal immunity has an important effect on the composition and density of these biofilms, but there is very little information to show whether this is true in vivo. We still need much better information about the dynamics and plasticity of the commensal intestinal flora.

1.2
Tools to Investigate Mutualism Between Commensal Intestinal Bacteria and the Host Immune System

Three main different experimental setups have been used in our lab and others to study the bacterial-host interactions described in this article. First, we can take germ-free animals with no intestinal bacteria whatsoever and study the changes in the host mucosal and systemic immune systems as bacteria colonise the intestine: to recolonise germ-free animals it is only necessary to put a normal animal containing an intestinal flora in the same cage. Alternatively, animals may be selectively colonised by deliberate inoculation with one or more bacterial species. Second, we can deliberately challenge specific pathogen-free (SPF) animals with doses of live bacteria given into the stomach, or directly into the intestine. SPF animals have a simple flora of intestinal bacteria (Macpherson and Harris 2004), so challenging them with test doses of organisms increases the bacterial load (Macpherson and Uhr 2004). The test organism can, of course, be engineered to express a chimeric protein in order to measure specific immune responses (Macpherson et al. 2000). The third experimental setup is to compare the density and composition of the unmanipulated bacterial flora in animals with known genetic lesions with the flora in control animals (Fagarasan et al. 2002). These approaches are assumed to be giving complementary information, for example, that the changes occurring as an animal acquires a flora from the germ-free state are exaggerated when animals with an established flora are challenged with intestinal bacteria.

In general terms, it is necessary to do strictly in vivo studies, because we are investigating the interactions of at least two interacting complex supersystems:

host immunity and intestinal bacteria consortia. The availability of large numbers of mouse strains with distinct genetic lesions affecting immunity and the ability to manipulate their flora are key to the progress of this field, because mechanisms of immune adaptation to commensal intestinal bacteria can be dissected in vivo with experiments using different strain combinations.

1.3
Mutual Adaptation of the Host and the Intestinal Bacterial Flora

Interest in the relationships between animals and their intestinal bacteria has a long history (Cushing and Livingood 1900; Metchnikoff 1908). Classic observations established that nutrition has a profound influence on the composition of the intestinal flora [reviewed by Dubos and Schaedler (1960)], including the special medically important situation when formula feeding is substituted for breast feeding in human infants (Tissier 1905), causing the luminal content of lactobacilli to fall and gram-negative bacilli and clostridia to rise.

Pasteur considered that microbes would be essential to the viability of plants and animals (Pasteur 1885). It was nevertheless shown that life is possible without microbes by raising animals in an aseptic environment, initially for several weeks (Cohendy 1912, 1914) and later over a normal full life span. The programme to maintain a variety of laboratory rodents germ free long term started at Notre Dame University in 1928 (Reyniers 1959). Although germ-free animals are viable, the benefits of commensal bacteria to their host were shown by comparing animals kept in germ-free conditions with the same strain colonised with environmental bacteria. For example, animals kept in sterile conditions suffered nutritional (vitamin) deficiencies (Gustafsson 1959) and had immature lymphoid structures (Glimstedt 1936; Miyakawa 1959) and low levels of serum gamma globulins (Thorbecke 1959).

Subsequent investigations have shown that the germ-free animal has many other differences compared with the same strain colonised with bacteria. The germ-free mucosal immune system has only a sparse content of lamina propria IgA-secreting cells (Benveniste et al. 1971a, 1971b; Moreau et al. 1978), and the mucosal lymphoid structures—the Peyer's patches—are hypoplastic with few B cell follicles and germinal centres (Yamanaka et al. 2003). The content of some intestinal epithelial lymphocyte subsets, particularly those bearing the CD8αβ heterodimer and double-positive CD4+ CD8+ subsets, are also reduced (Guy-Grand et al. 1978; Helgeland et al. 1996, 1997; Takimoto et al. 1992; Umesaki et al. 1993). In the systemic immune system, isotype-switched immunoglobulins are generally at low levels, the secondary lymphoid structures are relatively poorly formed (Bauer et al. 1963; Manolios et al. 1988) and the high endothelial morphology is abnormal (Manolios et al. 1988). The immune response to immunisation appears to have a smaller non-specific (polyclonal) component (Bakker et al. 1995). The age-related diversification of the B cell repertoire also appears to be reduced (Williams et al. 2000). Where studied, these differences are shown to be reversed within weeks of introduction of a bacterial flora to a previously germ-free animal (Macpherson and Harris 2004; Shroff et al. 1995).

Adaptation to commensal intestinal bacteria is by no means restricted to the immune system. Elegant experiments on the gene expression profile of intestinal epithelial cells have shown that there is reprogramming in the presence of commensals (Hooper and Gordon 2001; Hooper et al. 2001, 2003). For example, there is upregulation of antimicrobial proteins including angiogenin 4 (Hooper et al. 2003), and signals that determine body metabolism are altered, such as the circulating lipoprotein lipase inhibitor Faif, which is suppressed by colonisation with intestinal bacteria (Backhed et al. 2004). Paradoxically, even the homeostasis of the epithelial cell barrier of the mucosa requires signalling from the intestinal bacterial molecule ligands for the Toll-like receptors, including TLR-2 and TLR-4 (Rakoff-Nahoum et al. 2004).

We can therefore conclude that many systems in the body are highly adapted to the presence of intestinal bacteria, although the functional consequences of most of these alterations are unclear.

2
Immune Responses to Commensal Intestinal Bacteria

2.1
Mucosal Immune Responses to Commensal Intestinal Microorganisms

As discussed in Sect. 1.3, it has long been clear that IgA is one of the most striking adaptations to the presence of intestinal bacteria (Benveniste et al. 1971a, 1971b). It is induced more than an order of magnitude 3–4 weeks after germ-free mice are recolonised (Shroff et al. 1995). This means that in colonised mammals IgA constitutes approximately 70% of all antibody production, and it is mostly secreted across mucous membranes. The requirements for class switch recombination to IgA have been studied in cell culture experiments and in a series of elegant in vivo studies using cholera toxin as a mucosal adjuvant [reviewed in Johansen and Brandtzaeg (2004)]. These (neutralising) exotoxin-induced IgA responses are highly T cell dependent (Gardby et al. 1998; Hörnquist et al. 1995; Lycke and Holmgren 1986; Vajdy et al. 1995).

Using Western blots of membrane protein preparations of *Enterobacter cloacae* (the principal aerobe in our colony of SPF mice in Zürich), we found that intestinal secretory IgA bound to many different bacterial proteins (Macpherson et al. 2000). Binding to other purified cell wall components was also seen in ELISA assays. Within this polyspecific IgA binding profile, no additional proteins were bound if the bacterial IgA preparations were isolated from wild-type animals containing T cells, rather than mice deficient in T cells as a result of targeted genetic lesions of both the β and δ T cell receptor chains (TCRβ$^{-/-}$δ$^{-/-}$; Macpherson et al. 2000). Moreover, although the total amount of IgA produced in TCRβ$^{-/-}$δ$^{-/-}$ mice was reduced to about a quarter of that in wild-type animals, there was still significant IgA production without T cell help (Macpherson et al. 2000).

We also studied strains deficient in lymphoid structure formation to examine the requirements for secondary lymphoid structures within the intestinal mucosa for IgA induction to take place. We found that IgA is normally produced in the p55 tumour necrosis factor receptor I-deficient strain, which lacks follicular dendritic cell (DC) networks and has few Peyer's patches that are highly disorganised structures with lymphocytes interspersed between epithelial cells (Pasparakis et al. 1997). In contrast, two strains of mice with generalised lymphoid structure deficiencies, including absent B cell structures in the intestine, lacked IgA. For example, the lymphotoxin α-deficient mouse (De Togni et al. 1994), which lacks most secondary lymphoid structures, including isolated lymphoid follicles and Peyer's patches, expresses no IgA. The other IgA-deficient strain studied was the alymphoblastic (aly/aly) mouse, which carries a spontaneous point mutation in an exon-intron splice site for NFκB-inducing kinase (Shinkura et al. 1999; Macpherson and Uhr 2003): this results in absent lymphoid structures (including Peyer's patches and isolated lymphoid follicles) apart from the spleen and thymus, which are disorganised (Hamada et al. 2002; Miyawaki et al. 1994). Even if the B cell defect in aly/aly mice (Karrer et al. 2000) is corrected by reconstitution with wild-type bone marrow, there is no reconstitution of intestinal IgA, although about half the serum IgA is recovered (Macpherson et al. 2001). Our interpretation of these results was that primitive disorganised lymphoid structures in the mucosa were sufficient for intestinal mucosal IgA induction to occur, whereas about half the serum IgA is independently expressed without intestinal induction. Fagarasan and her colleagues subsequently presented evidence for IgA switching outside the Peyer's patches within the lamina propria (Fagarasan et al. 2001), although these are very demanding experiments in which it is possible that there was a problem with contamination of the lamina propria leukocyte preparations with isolated lymphoid follicles (Shikina et al. 2004). Nonetheless, it is still unclear whether the vast majority of precursors for IgA-secreting intestinal plasma cells are IgA+ B cells induced in the Peyer's patches and recirculate through the mesenteric lymph and blood stream as described in classic experiments (Craig and Cebra 1971; Husband and Gowans 1978), or whether there are other pathways of in situ IgA switching or direct migration out of intestinal lymphoid structures without recirculation (Yamamoto et al. 2004).

By colonising SPF mice with recombinant bacteria-expressing novel chimeric proteins, it was possible to show that a proportion of the T-independent intestinal IgA response was antigen specific (Macpherson et al. 2000). As with most immune responses, this is certainly only a component of the total IgA response (Bos et al. 2001). It is probable that T cell-independent signalling for the IgA class switch reaction and response amplification also occurs independently of the B cell receptor (Casola et al. 2004), for example, by DC expression of the TNF family molecules BAFF and APRIL (Castigli et al. 2004, 2005; Litinskiy et al. 2002) or through TLR ligand stimulation.

The conclusion is that the secretory IgA immune response is a rather primitive system that is not dependent on cognate T cell help and probably does not require complex organisation of the secondary lymphoid structures containing B cells in the intestinal wall. This is supported by almost normal production of IgA in the MHC Class II-deficient mouse (Snider et al. 1999) and by the restricted diversity of $V_{H\alpha}$ sequences in both mouse (Stoel et al. 2005) and human (Holtmeier et al. 2000), without evidence for sequential accumulation of somatic mutations expected in a conventional germinal centre reaction to improve binding affinity. Within the complex secretory IgA repertoire we do not yet have good information about binding affinities, but we assume that the system is producing relatively low-affinity antibodies capable of binding a diverse range of redundant epitopes in the bacterial flora (Bouvet and Fischetti 1999; Macpherson et al. 2000).

2.2
Systemic Immune Ignorance of Commensal Intestinal Microorganisms

In contrast to the profound mucosal IgA responses that occur in unmanipulated mice, provided the animals are kept in pathogen-free (SPF) conditions the systemic immune system is ignorant of commensal organisms. This was shown by the lack of specific serum IgG binding in Western blot experiments with membrane proteins of the dominant aerobic commensal *E. cloacae* similar to those described in Sect. 2.1 for IgA. This was a true negative, because if the mice are deliberately infected intravenously (i.v.) with 10^4–10^6 c.f.u. *E. cloacae*, there is consistent induction of specific serum IgG 14 days later (Macpherson et al. 2000). Serum IgG responses are therefore a sensitive indicator of the penetration of commensal intestinal bacteria into systemic secondary lymphoid structures. Some spontaneous priming of anti-*E. cloacae*

IgG was seen in the aly/aly and IgA-deficient strains, suggesting that the secretion of antibodies at mucosal sites is required to protect against penetration of commensal organisms (Macpherson et al. 2000).

Healthy adult humans normally contain serum IgG antibodies against model commensal organisms, suggesting that they have responded to systemic penetration of commensal organisms to systemic lymphoid tissues at some point in the past (Macpherson et al. 1996). This is not surprising because of the many infections, drugs, foodstuffs and alcoholic drinks that have the potential to damage the intestinal permeability barrier (Bjarnason et al. 1995); however, this is still consistent with the observation in clean mice that powerful mucosal immune induction occurs in the face of systemic immune ignorance of commensal organisms. This geographical separation of the handling of commensal bacteria allows the systemic immune system only to respond as required, for example, when there is bacteriaemia or an infection from commensals, such as mastitis. In general, it is only necessary to induce systemic immune responses to commensals if they reach systemic secondary lymphoid structures in sufficient numbers, because innate mechanisms are normally sufficient to clear commensal bacteraemias (Shiloh et al. 1999).

3
Mechanisms of Mucosal IgA Induction to Commensal Intestinal Bacteria

3.1
Regional Separation of Culturable Organisms After Challenge Doses of *Enterobacter cloacae*

In an attempt to understand the way in which the mucosal immune system functionally protects the intestinal surface from the penetration of commensals, we challenged mice either by gavage (10^9 c.f.u.) or i.v. injection (10^7 c.f.u.) with *E. cloacae*. When the organism was administered i.v., not surprisingly, we found abundant culturable bacteria in splenocytes but very few in leukocytes from the mesenteric lymph nodes (MLN). Conversely, when the bacteria were given into the intestine, small numbers of culturable organisms were recovered from the MLN over approximately 60 h, whilst the spleen and other systemic secondary lymphoid structures remained sterile (Macpherson and Uhr 2004).

The reason for studying the MLN rather than mucosal tissues directly was that the latter were inevitably contaminated with culturable organisms from the intestinal lumen when tissues were disrupted in leukocyte extraction protocols. This can be experimentally overcome by incubating tissue fragments in antibiotics before disruption to kill extracellular but not intracellular bacteria. With this method (with MLN fragments treated similarly) the uptake of live bacteria was shown to start in the Peyer's patches 5–9 h after the intestinal dose, after which lower numbers of organisms were detected in the mesenteric leukocytes after 12 h (Macpherson and Uhr 2004).

To determine which cell type contained the bacteria we carried out sorting experiments with magnetic beads or flow cytometry 18 h after administering the bacteria (Macpherson and Uhr 2004). The results were essentially identical, but the flow cytometry data have been described because the purities were always far better (>98%). Our intention had been to measure the live bacterial load in CD11b$^+$ CD11c$^-$ macrophages according to whether or not mice secreted intestinal antibodies, but it was the CD11b$^+$ CD11c$^+$ DC compartment that contained the live bacteria. Using ex vivo assays of macrophage killing of bacteria, we found that this could be explained by the fact that killing was almost complete within the 4–6 h that it took us to isolate the leukocytes, run the cell sort and plate out the cell fractions for bacterial culture. In contrast, DC have relatively poor microbiocidal mechanisms (Delamarre et al. 2005). Different subsets of DC have been described in the Peyer's patches (Kelsall and Strober 1996) and the intestinal lamina propria (Becker et al. 2003; Huang et al. 2000; Niess et al. 2005), but we found similar recoveries of live bacteria from CD11c+ mesenteric leukocytes in both the CD8$^+$ and the CD8$^-$ fractions.

The data showing sampling of luminal bacterial material by DC could be reproduced in standard flow cytometry, by transforming *E. cloacae* to express green fluorescent protein (GFP) under the control of the constitutive rpsM (ribosomal protein) promoter (Macpherson and Uhr 2004). In this case we were not dependent on live culture as a readout, and green fluorescence could also be seen in the macrophage fractions. GFP could also be seen directly within Peyer's patch CD11c+ DC with immunofluorescence. We did not see significant numbers of organisms either by live culture or by FACS in lamina propria DC, although evidence has been presented by two other groups (Becker et al. 2003; Niess et al. 2005) of sampling of luminal commensal bacteria by subepithelial DC in the ileum (distal part of the small intestine). The tissue in most of our experiments was usually taken over the entire length of the small intestine, diluting the signal on a regional effect, and our technique of pulsing the intestine with bacteria may have allowed easier access to DC in the Peyer's patches because the mucus covering and surface glycocalyx are thinner. Despite these caveats, our data suggest that the Peyer's patches and isolated lymphoid follicles are probably the predominant site for sampling luminal intestinal bacteria, whereas small numbers of bacteria that reside beneath the mucus close to the surface epithelial cells can be sampled by subepithelial DC subsets of the lamina propria (Becker et al. 2003; Niess et al. 2005).

3.2
Induction of IgA by Dendritic Cells Loaded with Live *Enterobacter cloacae*

To examine the function of DC loaded with commensal bacteria, we set up cultures of B220+ B cells and CD4+ T cells purified from mesenteric leukocytes of SPF C57BL/6 mice that had not been challenged with *E. cloacae* with CD11c+ cells purified from the Peyer's patches of C57BL/6 mice gavaged with live *E. cloacae*. Similar B and T cell cultures from unchallenged C57BL/6 mice were set up with CD11c+ cells purified from Peyer's patches of mice challenged with heat-killed *E. cloacae* (Macpherson and Uhr 2004). The results were that the addition of DC from mice gavaged with live *E. cloacae* caused a population of IgA$^+$ B cells (1.9±0.6%) and the production of supernatant IgA (950±90 ng/ml) absent from cultures incubated with DC from the Peyer's patches of mice treated in vivo with heat-killed *E. cloacae* (0.09±0.04%; <50 ng/ml).

We also found that the addition of purified CD11c+ cells from the Peyer's patches of animals that had been treated with live *E. cloacae* also induced IgA$^+$ B cells (1.2±0.3%; 610±65 ng/ml) and production of supernatant IgA when T cells were omitted from the cultures. This was shown not to be due to low level contamination with T cells, because the IgA induction with DC loaded with live bacteria also worked when B cells were purified from animals deficient in T cells as a result of targeted genetic lesions of the β and δ T cell receptor chains (TCRβ$^{-/-}$δ$^{-/--}$).

DC have previously been shown in spontaneous ex vivo culture experiments to be a key cell type required for the class switch recombination reaction to express IgA (Fayette et al. 1997; Schrader and Cebra 1993). In our experiments the translocation of live commensal bacteria, and their uptake by DC, has been shown to promote this effect, but we do not know whether the mechanism is a consequence of signalling from bacterial surface molecular patterns through Toll-like receptors on DC or by direct stimulation of B cells (for example, after regurgitation of whole bacteria by the DC) to provide bacterial surface molecular arrays which would potentially be able to bind even low-affinity Ig binding sites. We also do not yet know whether heat-killed *E. cloacae* are not effectively taken up by intestinal DC, or whether live bacteria are required at a cellular level for the response.

3.3
Induction of IgA by Intestinal Conditioning of Mice In Vivo with Live *Enterobacter cloacae*

To determine whether the induction of IgA by the protocol of loading live commensal bacteria worked in vivo we repeatedly challenged wild-type SPF C57BL/6 mice with *E. cloacae* in the intestine by giving gavage doses of

10^7 organisms every third day for a month (Macpherson and Uhr 2004). These SPF mice already contained a simple flora of intestinal bacteria, and the protocol was designed and shown to increase intestinal bacterial density. Seven days after the last dose we found that there was a four- to fivefold increased number of IgA-producing cells in the intestinal lamina propria over sham-treated animals both by ELISPOT analysis and by immunohistochemistry. The serum IgA level was also increased five- to tenfold. Induction of IgA through this mechanism was not T cell dependent because it worked (at lower levels) in T cell-deficient (TCR$\beta^{-/-}\delta^{-/-}$) animals, but it did require gavaging with live bacteria, because the response was absent in groups in mice treated with the same preparation of *E. cloacae* that had been split and heat-treated before administration.

The in vivo IgA induction protocol with live commensal bacteria also worked when *Enterobacter faecalis*, *Bacillus puminatus* and *Staphylococcus saprophyticus* (Macpherson and Uhr 2004) were used in place of *E. cloacae*. It is also important to note that intestinal bacterial conditioning is very effective at inducing total intestinal and serum IgA, yet the response is isotype specific— unlike induction of IgA with intestinal administration of cholera toxin (Elson and Ealding 1984a, b; Snider et al. 1994), there is no increase in serum IgM, IgG or IgE. In addition to the substantial increase in total IgA, use of recombinant bacteria expressing a specific chimeric protein at a high level indicates that a proportion of this IgA response is bacterial antigen specific (Macpherson et al. 2000).

Just as the colonisation of germ-free mice leads to substantial induction of IgA during adaptation to the presence of intestinal bacteria, so repeated challenge of SPF mice already containing a commensal flora with experimental doses of live bacteria given into the intestine leads to selective IgA induction. In the latter case, the mechanism can be shown to be dependent on the uptake of live commensal bacteria which have penetrated the epithelial layer by DC and subsequent stimulation of B (and probably T) cell responses. However, it is still an assumption that the in vivo repeated challenge protocol accurately models the spontaneous induction from the germ-free to the colonised state, because measurement of the low levels of spontaneous penetration of commensal bacteria is at the limit of current detection methods.

4 Compartmentalisation of Mucosal Immune Responses to Commensal Bacteria

4.1 Induction by Dendritic Cells Loaded with Commensal Bacteria Focuses the Process Within the Mucosal Immune System

As described in Sect. 2.1, the systemic immune system of SPF mice remains ignorant of their commensal intestinal flora, but specific serum IgG responses can easily be induced by administration of 10^4–10^6 live organisms into the tail vein. On one hand, it makes good sense that the systemic immune system is not repeatedly primed to commensal organisms, because the diverse responses (which would be largely superfluous since innate mechanisms are very effective at killing these bacteria) could potentially trigger allergy or autoimmunity. On the other, it is important not to be generally tolerant of commensal bacteria, as this may lead to an inability to mount neutralising responses against pathogenic bacterial epitopes. The question is, how can a powerful mucosal immune response be achieved while maintaining systemic ignorance of commensals?

It was striking that administration of challenge doses of *E. cloacae* or other intestinal bacteria led to penetration of a small proportion ($\approx$0.001%) of the live bacteria as far as the MLN, but not to the spleen or other systemic secondary lymphoid structures. To show that this penetration was within migrating DC rather than as free bacteria we carried out experiments in which two segments of small intestine were disconnected from the main intestinal stream and each was separately attached with a stoma to the skin surface so bacteria could be injected into the loop. The vascular and lymphatic supplies to these segments of intestine were not disturbed, and the remaining ends of the small intestine (from which the loops had been removed) were anastomosed with microsurgical techniques to restore intestinal continuity and allow the animal to feed normally. Once the animal had recovered from surgery, we challenged one loop with *E. cloacae* which had been made stably naladixic acid resistant as a bacterial chromosomal mutation and the other loop with *E. cloacae* that had been made rifampicin resistant. After 18 h we isolated mesenteric leukocytes and plated them on bacterial growth medium. If we lysed the mesenteric leukocytes before plating we found that there was a 20±7% increase in the number of bacterial colonies, indicating that a proportion of the leukocytes (shown by the flow cytometric sorting experiments described earlier to be DC) contained more than one bacterium. The question now was whether those DC containing multiple bacteria always had organisms of a single antibiotic resistance (in which case the DC would have picked up the bacteria and carried them to the MLN) or whether both antibiotic resistances were present (when free bacteria would have penetrated and been taken up by DC in the MLN). After plating out the mesenteric leukocytes on unselective nutrient bacterial agar and then using this as a master plate for replica plating on antibiotic-containing selective growth medium, we showed that only a single antibiotic resistance was ever present in colonies arising from the leukocytes. If both Nal^R *E. cloacae* and Rif^R *E. cloacae* were both injected into a single loop, the replica plating experiment showed that approximately 12% of colonies on the master plate had both antibiotic resistances.

Because the *E. cloacae* surface was identical whether it carried the Nal^R or Rif^R marker, the only way to keep the different antibiotic resistances separated within different cells would be if the bacteria had been taken up by the DC in the intestinal loops (where each isolated intestinal segment was injected with *E. cloacae* carrying only one distinct antibiotic resistance) and carried from there within the DC to the MLN. Additional evidence for carriage within DC was that virtually no bacteria were recovered from the MLN of CCR 7-deficient mice (Forster et al. 1999), in which lymph node homing signals are disrupted by a targetted genetic deficiency. The bacteria that do reach the MLN within DC in wild-type animals do not penetrate further to reach the spleen or other systemic secondary lymphoid structures (Macpherson and Harris 2004). This is probably because DC are relatively short-lived, and once they die, local macrophages take up and kill any residual bacteria.

4.2
Dendritic Cells Loaded with Commensal Bacteria Are Retained in the Mesenteric Lymph Nodes and Do Not Reach Systemic Secondary Lymphoid Structures

The concept that the MLN are an important barrier for translocated bacteria within DC was addressed experimentally by examining the results of intestinal bacterial challenge and serial intestinal bacterial conditioning in C57BL/6 mice without MLN (Macpherson and Uhr 2004). If MLN were surgically removed by dissecting along the superior mesenteric artery, it could be shown that the lymphatics had reanastomosed after a month during healing by gavaging a mouse with olive oil and seeing the resultant brilliant white lymphatic vessels containing chylomicrons, but without MLN present. After such mesenteric adenectomy the conditioning protocol was carried out as described in Sect. 3.3: Giving SPF C57BL/6 mice gavage doses of 10^7 *E. cloacae* organisms every third day for a month induced IgA normally, but at the end of the experiment there was massive splenomegaly in the MLN^- animals with priming of specific systemic IgG responses. A single challenge dose of *E. cloacae* also resulted in culturable organisms in the spleen of MLN^- animals.

The conclusion from these experiments is that small numbers of live commensal bacteria can penetrate the surface epithelium, especially the M cells overlying Peyer's patches and isolated lymphoid follicles. These live bacteria are confined to the mucosal immune system because they are rapidly killed if taken up by macrophages and can only survive in low numbers within intestinal DC, which do not penetrate further into the body than the MLN.

5
Function of IgA in Mutual Adaptation to the Presence of Commensal Intestinal Bacteria

Although secretory IgA constitutes the bulk of our bodily antibody output, we have only limited information about its function. Selective IgA deficiency in either mouse or human has a relatively benign phenotype, but this is probably because IgM can substitute for IgA in both species. For either IgA or IgM to be transported through the surface epithelial cells into the intestinal lumen, they must be in polymeric form, containing J chain, and undergo transcytosis bound to the polymeric immunoglobulin receptor (Brandtzaeg 1973, 1974). Mice deficient for this pIgR show a protein losing enteropathy, indicative of low-grade intestinal inflammation (Johansen et al. 1999).

To address the function of secretory immunoglobulin in protecting the mucosa against commensal bacteria we performed two different sorts of experiments (Macpherson and Uhr 2004). The first was to follow recolonisation of germ-free C57BL/6 (wild type) and $J_H^{-/-}$ (antibody deficient) animals in parallel as they acquired an SPF flora from a sentinel animal. In the first 48 h of the experiment there was overgrowth of both aerobic and anaerobic organisms, which then settled to steady-state levels with no significant differences between the strains. However, the penetration of culturable aerobes from the lumen to the MLN was greater in the $J_H^{-/-}$ strain and persisted longer (from *day 5* until *day 42*). Because the MLN do become sterile after a delay in the $J_H^{-/-}$ strain, secreted antibodies are only part of the adaptation mechanism to commensal bacteria; they are not essential. In a different experimental setup we challenged SPF C57BL/6 wild-type mice and SPF $J_H^{-/-}$ antibody-deficient animals (already containing an SPF flora) with graded doses of *E. cloacae* and compared the levels of live bacterial penetration to the MLN 18 h later. This experiment also showed that the antibody-deficient strain had slightly higher levels of penetration at each dose compared with the wild-type control. In contrast, wild-type animals that had been conditioned with *E. cloacae* for a month and then rested for 7 days before challenge (resulting in a substantial increase in IgA levels as described in Sect. 3.3) had lower levels at every challenge dose compared with wild-type controls that had not been conditioned. Therefore, secreted antibodies appear to protect the mucosa overall from bacterial penetration beneath the epithelial surface.

Other experiments show that the function of IgA is probably not just immune exclusion. Studies of the activation-induced cytidine deaminase (AID) knockout strain, which is deficient in both isotype class switch recombination and affinity maturation, have shown that there is overgrowth of anaerobes and lymphonodular hyperplasia in the ileum (Fagarasan et al. 2002; Suzuki et al. 2004). This can be corrected by reconstituting IgA expression (Suzuki et al. 2004). A third possible functional consequence of IgA coating of intestinal bacteria may even be to increase the uptake via specialised IgA receptors on epithelial M cells overlying the Peyer's patches (Mantis et al. 2002; Roy and Varvayanis 1987; Weltzin et al. 1989), facilitating sampling of luminal bacteria.

The overall functional consequence of IgA expression is to limit penetration of bacteria beneath the intestinal epithelial surface. The IgA system therefore can work by negative feedback, whereby increased penetration of commensals into DC leads to IgA induction, which in turn limits bacterial translocation through the mucosa. Although secretory IgA is a protective mechanism against commensal bacteria, it is not essential—evolution has ensured that there are a number of protective responses against damage by the immunostimulatory molecules in the luxuriant intestinal commensal bacterial flora (Sansonetti 2004).

References

Backhed F, Ding H, Wang T, Hooper LV, Koh GY, Nagy A, Semenkovich CF, Gordon JI (2004) The gut microbiota as an environmental factor that regulates fat storage. Proc Natl Acad Sci USA 101:15718–15723.

Bakker R, Lasonder E, Bos NA (1995) Measurement of affinity in serum samples of antigen-free, germ-free and conventional mice after hyperimmunization with 2,4-dinitrophenyl keyhole limpet hemocyanin, using surface plasmon resonance. Eur J Immunol 25:1680–1686.

Bauer H, Horowitz RE, Levenson SM, Popper H (1963) The response of lymphatic tissue to the microbial flora. Studies on germfree mice. Am J Pathol 42:471–479.

Becker C, Wirtz S, Blessing M, Pirhonen J, Strand D, Bechthold O, Frick J, Galle PR, Autenrieth I, Neurath MF (2003) Constitutive p40 promoter activation and IL-23 production in the terminal ileum mediated by dendritic cells. J Clin Invest 112:693–706.

Benveniste J, Lespinats G, Adam C, Salomon, J. C. 1971a. Immunoglobulins in intact, immunized, and contaminated axenic mice: study of serum IgA. J Immunol 107:1647–1655.

Benveniste J, Lespinats G, Salomon, J. 1971b. Serum and secretory IgA in axenic and holoxenic mice. J Immunol 107:1656–1662.

Bjarnason I, Macpherson AJ, Hollander D (1995) Intestinal permeability: an overview. Gastroenterology 108:1566–1581.

Bos NA, Jiang HQ, Cebra JJ (2001) T cell control of the gut IgA response against commensal bacteria. Gut 48:762–764.

Bouvet JP, Fischetti VA (1999) Diversity of antibody-mediated immunity at the mucosal barrier. Infect Immun 67:2687–2691.

Brandtzaeg P (1973) Two types of IgA immunocytes in man. Nat New Biol 243:142–143.

Brandtzaeg P (1974) Presence of J chain in human immunocytes containing various immunoglobulin classes. Nature 252:418–420.

Casola S, Otipoby KL, Alimzhanov M, Humme S, Uyttersprot N, Kutok JL, Carroll MC, Rajewsky K (2004) B cell receptor signal strength determines B cell fate. Nat Immunol 5:317–327.

Castigli E, Scott S, Dedeoglu F, Bryce P, Jabara H, Bhan AK, Mizoguchi E, Geha RS (2004) Impaired IgA class switching in APRIL-deficient mice. Proc Natl Acad Sci USA 101:3903–3908.

Castigli E, Wilson SA, Scott S, Dedeoglu F, Xu S, Lam KP, Bram RJ, Jabara H, Geha RS (2005) TACI and BAFF-R mediate isotype switching in B cells. J Exp Med 201:35–39.

Cohendy M (1912) Experiencecs sur la vie sans microbes. Compt rend 154:533–536.

Cohendy M (1914) Experiences sur la vie sans microbes, élevage aseptique de cobages. Compt rend 158:1283–1284.

Craig SW, Cebra JJ (1971) Peyer's patches: an enriched source of precursors for IgA-producing immunocytes in the rabbit. J Exp Med 134:188–200.

Cummings JH, Kong SC (2004) Probiotics, prebiotics and antibiotics in inflammatory bowel disease. Novartis Found Symp 263:99–111; discussion 111–114, 211–118.

Cushing H, Livingood LE (1900) Johns Hopkins Hospital Reports 9:543–549.

De Togni P, Goellner J, Ruddle NH, Streeter PR, Fick A, Mariathasan S, Smith SC, Carlson R, Shornick LP, Strauss-Schoenberger J, et al. 1994. Abnormal development of peripheral lymphoid organs in mice deficient in lymphotoxin. Science 264:703–707.

Delamarre L, Pack M, Chang H, Mellman I, Trombetta ES (2005) Differential lysosomal proteolysis in antigen-presenting cells determines antigen fate. Science 307:1630–1634.

Dubos R, Schaedler RW (1960) The effect of the intestinal flora on the growth rate of mice, and on their susceptibility to experimental infections. J Exp Med 111:407–411.

Elson CO, Ealding, W. 1984a. Cholera toxin feeding did not induce oral tolerance in mice and abrogated oral tolerance to an unrelated protein antigen. J Immunol 133:2892–2897.

Elson CO, Ealding, W. 1984b. Generalized systemic and mucosal immunity in mice after mucosal stimulation with cholera toxin. J Immunol 132:2736–2741.

Fagarasan S, Kinoshita K, Muramatsu M, Ikuta K, Honjo T (2001) In situ class switching and differentiation to IgA-producing cells in the gut lamina propria. Nature 413:639–643.

Fagarasan S, Muramatsu M, Suzuki K, Nagaoka H, Hiai H, Honjo T (2002) Critical roles of activation-induced cytidine deaminase in the homeostasis of gut flora. Science 298:1424–1427.

Fayette J, Dubois B, Vandenabeele S, Bridon JM, Vanbervliet B, Durand I, Banchereau J, Caux C, Briere F (1997) Human dendritic cells skew isotype switching of CD40-activated naive B cells towards IgA1 and IgA2. J Exp Med 185:1909–1918.

Forster R, Schubel A, Breitfeld D, Kremmer E, Renner-Muller I, Wolf E, Lipp M (1999) CCR7 coordinates the primary immune response by establishing functional microenvironments in secondary lymphoid organs. Cell 99:23–33.

Gardby E, Lane P, Lycke NY (1998) Requirements for B7-CD28 costimulation in mucosal IgA responses: paradoxes observed in CTLA4-Hγ1 transgenic mice. J Immunol 161:49–59.

Glimstedt G (1936) Bakterienfrei Meerschweinchen. Aufzucht, Lebensfähigkeit und Wachstum, nebst Untersuchung über das lymphatische Gewebe. Acta Pathol Microbiol Scand Suppl 30:1–295.

Gustafsson BE (1959) Vitamin K deficiency in germfree rats. Ann NY Acad Sci 78:166–174.

Guy-Grand D, Griscelli C, Vassalli P (1978) The mouse gut T lymphocyte, a novel type of T cell. Nature, origin, and traffic in mice in normal and graft-versus-host conditions. J Exp Med 148:1661–1677.

Hamada H, Hiroi T, Nishiyama Y, Takahashi H, Masunaga Y, Hachimura S, Kaminogawa S, Takahashi-Iwanaga H, Iwanaga T, Kiyono H, Yamamoto H, Ishikawa H (2002) Identification of multiple isolated lymphoid follicles on the antimesenteric wall of the mouse small intestine. J Immunol 168:57–64.

Helgeland L, Vaage JT, Rolstad B, Halstensen TS, Midtvedt T, Brandtzaeg P (1997) Regional phenotypic specialization of intraepithelial lymphocytes in the rat intestine does not depend on microbial colonization. Scand J Immunol 46:349–357.

Helgeland L, Vaage JT, Rolstad B, Midtvedt T, Brandtzaeg P (1996) Microbial colonization influences composition and T-cell receptor Vβrepertoire of intraepithelial lymphocytes in rat intestine. Immunology 89:494–501.

Holtmeier W, Hennemann A, Caspary WF (2000) IgA and IgM V_H repertoires in human colon: evidence for clonally expanded B cells that are widely disseminated. Gastroenterology 119:1253–1266.

Hooper LV, Gordon JI (2001) Commensal host-bacterial relationships in the gut. Science 292:1115–1118.

Hooper LV, Stappenbeck TS, Hong CV, Gordon JI (2003) Angiogenins: a new class of microbicidal proteins involved in innate immunity. Nat Immunol 4:269–273.

Hooper LV, Wong MH, Thelin A, Hansson L, Falk PG, Gordon JI (2001) Molecular analysis of commensal host-microbial relationships in the intestine (cites personal communication from Joshua Lederberg). Science 291:881–884.

Hörnquist CE, Ekman L, Grdic KD, Schön K, Lycke NY (1995) Paradoxical IgA immunity in CD4-deficient mice. J Immunol 155:2877–2887.

Huang, F.-P., Platt N, Wykes M, Major JR, Powell TJ, Jenkins CD, MacPherson GG (2000) A discrete subpopulation of dendritic cells transports apoptotic intestinal epithelial cells to T cell areas of mesenteric lymph nodes. J Exp Med 191:435–444.

Husband AJ, Gowans JL (1978) The origin and antigen-dependent distribution of IgA-containing cells in the intestine. J Exp Med 148:1146–1160.

Johansen FE, Brandtzaeg P (2004) Transcriptional regulation of the mucosal IgA system. Trends Immunol 25:150–157.

Johansen FE, Pekna M, Norderhaug IN, Haneberg B, Hietala MA, Krajci P, Betsholtz C, Brandtzaeg P (1999) Absence of epithelial immunoglobulin A transport, with increased mucosal leakiness, in polymeric immunoglobulin Receptor/Secretory component-deficient mice. J Exp Med 190:915–922.

Karrer U, Althage A, Odermatt B, Hengartner H, Zinkernagel RM (2000) Immunodeficiency of alymphoplasia mice (aly/aly) in vivo: structural defect of secondary lymphoid organs and functional B cell defect. Eur J Immunol 30:2799–2807.

Kelsall B, Strober W (1996) Distinct populations of dendritic cells are present in the subepithelial dome and T cell regions of the murine Peyer's patch. J Exp Med 183:237–247.

Litinskiy MB, Nardelli B, Hilbert DM, Schaffer A, Casali P, Cerutti A (2002) Antigen presenting cells induce CD40-independent immunoglobulin class switching through BLyS and APRIL. Nat Immunol 3:822–829.

Lycke N, Holmgren J (1986) Intestinal mucosal memory and presence of memory cells in lamina propria and Peyer's patches in mice 2 years after oral immunization with cholera toxin. Scand J Immunol 23:611–616.

Mackie R, Sghir A, Gaskins HR (1999) Developmental microbial ecology of the neonatal gastrointestinal tract. Am J Clin Nutr 69:1035S-1045S.

Macpherson A, Khoo UY, Forgacs I, Philpott-Howard J, Bjarnason I (1996) Mucosal antibodies in inflammatory bowel disease are directed against intestinal bacteria. Gut 38:365–375.

Macpherson AJ, Gatto D, Sainsbury E, Harriman GR, Hengartner H, Zinkernagel RM (2000) A primitive T cell-independent mechanism of intestinal mucosal IgA responses to commensal bacteria. Science 288:2222–2226.

Macpherson AJ, Harris N (2004) Interactions between commensal intestinal bacteria and the immune system. Nat Rev Immunol 4:478–485.

Macpherson AJ, Lamarre A, McCoy K, Dougan G, Harriman G, Hengartner H, Zinkernagel R (2001) IgA B cell and IgA antibody production in the absence of μ and δ heavy chain expression early in B cell ontogeny. Nat Immunol 2:625–631.

Macpherson AJ, Uhr T (2003) The genomic sequence of the murine alymphoplasia (aly/aly) shows a donor splice site mutation in NFκB-inducing kinase. Immunogenetics 54:693–698.

Macpherson AJ, Uhr T (2004) Induction of protective IgA by intestinal dendritic cells carrying commensal bacteria. Science 303:1662–1665.

Manolios N, Geczy CL, Schrieber L (1988) High endothelial venule morphology and function are inducible in germ-free mice: a possible role for interferon-γ. Cell Immunol 117:136–151.

Mantis NJ, Cheung MC, Chintalacharuvu KR, Rey J, Corthesy B, Neutra MR (2002) Selective adherence of IgA to murine Peyer's patch M cells: evidence for a novel IgA receptor. J Immunol 169:1844–1851.

McFarland LV, Surawicz CM, Greenberg RN, Fekety R, Elmer GW, Moyer KA, Melcher SA, Bowen KE, Cox JL, Noorani Z, et al. 1994. A randomized placebo-controlled trial of *Saccharomyces boulardii* in combination with standard antibiotics for *Clostridium difficile* disease. JAMA 271:1913–1918.

Metchnikoff E (1908) The prolongation of life. Putman & Sons (reprinted 2003, Springer Publishing Company).

2. IgA$^+$ B cell development is dependent on antigenic stimulation and T cell help, which induces germinal center (GC) formation.
3. PP GC are intrinsically different to other GC, owing to the presence of special T cells (CD4$^+$) and dendritic cells (DC) that promote class-switching specifically to IgA.
4. There is a preferential homing of IgA$^+$ B cells but not IgM$^+$ or IgG$^+$ B cells to the mucosal tissues, because of special adhesion molecules as well as factors derived from local environments that selectively attract the circulating precursors of mucosal IgA plasma cells.
5. IgA provides protection against bacterial, parasitic, and viral mucosal pathogens.

These conclusions represent a solid foundation that allowed further scientific quests into the complexity, diversity, and dynamism of the immune responses and reciprocal relationships between bacteria and the immune system.

In this chapter we attempt to combine the classic view of the mucosal immune system with recent developments that have revealed new layers of complexity relating to the sites, mechanisms, and function of gut IgA. We discuss the contribution of intestinal bacteria to development of the gut immune system and emphasize the key role of IgA in shaping the gut microbiota and, as such, in regulation of local and systemic immune responses.

2
Generation of Mucosal IgA in Organized Follicular Structures

The GALT, which is the main site for generation of mucosal immune responses, is generally divided into two compartments: inductive sites, represented by organized follicular structures, and effector sites, represented by diffuse tissue of the intestinal LP (Brandtzaeg et al. 1999; Fagarasan and Honjo 2003). The major inductive sites in the small intestine are PP and solitary follicles that are scattered throughout the intestine, called isolated lymphoid follicles (ILF) (Hamada et al. 2002), which develop before and after birth, respectively. Their organization requires multiple interactions between inducer cells of hematopoietic origin and organizer mesenchymal cells (Nishikawa et al. 2003). Among the key events absolutely necessary for PP and ILF formation is the expression of LTα1β2 on CD3$^-$CD4$^+$IL-7R$^+$ inducer cells on stimulation through IL-7R and its interaction with LTβR$^+$ organizer cells (Honda et al. 2001; Lorenz et al. 2003; McDonald et al. 2005; Yoshida et al. 2002). Several feedback loops necessary for PP and ILF formation involve chemokines and adhesion molecules such as CXCR5-CXCL13 and CXCR5-induced α4β1-VCAM-1 interactions (Finke et al. 2002).

Cellular studies suggested that bone marrow-derived precursors for IgA$^+$ plasma cells are mainly generated in the PP (Cebra and Shroff 1994; Tseng 1981, 1984), and a clonal relationship between IgA$^+$ B cells in the PP and IgA plasma cells in the (LP has been demonstrated (Dunn-Walters et al., 1997; Stoel et al., 2005).

It is generally accepted that IgA B cell development depends on the antigenic stimulation and induction of GC, a microenvironment that allows strong interactions between B cells, antigens trapped on follicular dendritic cells (FDC) and local CD4 T cells, that facilitate B cell proliferation, class switch recombination (CSR) and somatic hypermutation (SHM) and affinity maturation which are necessary for efficient humoral responses (Butcher et al. 1982; Strobel et al. 2005; Weinstein and Cebra 1991).

Indeed, neonatal mice or germ-free mice are almost completely devoid of IgA$^+$ B cells in gut. However, gut IgA$^+$ B cells are detected after bacterial colonization, around the peak of the GC reaction in PP, and these IgAs commonly have specificities against molecules such as phosphocholine, β2-1 fructosyl and β galactosyl groups associated with bacteria present in the intestine (Cebra 1999).

In conventionally reared mice, PP as well as ILF, which are induced to develop by bacterial stimulation (see later discussion), continuously exhibit GC and contain the highest proportion of actively dividing IgA$^+$ B cells as compared with GC from spleen or peripheral lymph nodes, in which the predominant switched isotype is IgG (Cebra 1999).

The IgA$^+$ B cells in PP or ILF are generated by in situ switching of IgM$^+$ B cells after antigenic stimulation. This is demonstrated by the presence of large amounts of AID, the master molecule for CSR and SHM (Muramatsu et al. 2000), in IgM$^+$ B cells from PP (Fagarasan et al., 2001). Furthermore, footprints for recent switching can be detected in PP IgA$^+$ B cells. These are short-lived transcripts, known as α circle-transcripts (αCT), which are initiated from the Iα promoter located in the circular DNA that is looped out during IgA switching (Fagarasan et al. 2001; Kinoshita et al. 2001). This preferential switching to IgA in PP led to the proposal that PP GC are intrinsically different from other GC, most likely because of the constant antigenic stimulation, the presence of special regulatory T cells and dendritic cells (DC) that through costimulatory molecules (CD40-CD40L, CD80/CD86-CD28) and Th2 cytokines would promote efficient switching to IgA (Cebra and Shroff 1994; Lycke 1998).

3
Generation of Mucosal IgA Outside Organized Follicular Structures

Multiple studies in genetically manipulated mice, however, revealed a poor correlation between the presence of GC, organized follicular structures such as PP and IgA plasma cells in the LP, implying the existence of multiple, intricate pathways for IgA B cell development in gut. For example, fully functional, somatically mutated gut IgA against T-dependent antigens does not necessarily require the presence of GC. $CD28^{-/-}$ mice that lack GC and have an impaired systemic response show normal mucosal IgA responses to a T-dependent antigen (Gardby et al. 2003). This would imply that T cell activation by the B7-CD28 signaling pathway that is essential for serum IgA (and IgG) responses can be complemented by an alternative, mucosa-specific, and GC-independent mechanism.

Peritoneal B1 cells, which are known to be unable to migrate to GC in PP, generate large amounts of gut IgA, at least in mice (Fagarasan and Honjo 2000; Fagarasan et al. 2000; Kroese et al. 1989). Unlike the IgA generated in the PP, IgA production by B1 cells appears to be independent of T cell help, and functionally the B1-derived IgAs appear to be fully capable of preventing systemic invasion of intestinal bacteria (Fagarasan and Honjo 2000; Macpherson et al. 2000).

Furthermore, mice deficient for inhibitor of bHLH transcription factor (Id2), retinoic acid-related orphan receptor (ROR) $\gamma t^{-/-}$ mice, or bone marrow (BM)-reconstituted $LT\alpha^{-/-}$ or $TNF-LT\alpha^{-/-}$ mice, which lack PP, mesenteric lymph nodes (MLN), or any other gut follicular structures including ILF, do have IgA plasma cells in the intestine, although their number varies depending on the mouse background and rearing conditions. These observations clearly indicate that gut IgAs can be also generated outside GC or gut organized follicular structures (Eberl and Littman 2004; Kang et al. 2002; Ryffel et al. 1998).

4
Homing of IgA$^+$ B Cells from the Inductive to the Effector Sites

It is still generally accepted that from PP IgA$^+$ B cells migrate to the draining MLN, where they further proliferate and differentiate into plasmablasts, which, via the thoracic duct and blood, home preferentially to the gut LP (Guy-Grand et al. 1974; McWilliams et al. 1977). The tissue specificity of IgA$^+$ B cell homing is the result of complex interactions between receptors present on the lymphocytes and their ligands expressed on the vascular endothelium of the target tissues (Youngman et al. 2005). The selective migration to gut

LP is principally achieved through downregulation of L-selectin and strong induction of integrin $\alpha 4\beta 7$, which allows a preferential interaction of intestinal lymphocytes with vascular addressin molecule MadCAM-1, abundantly expressed by postcapillary venules in the gut LP (Berlin et al. 1993). The preferential homing of IgA^+ but not IgM^+ or IgG^+ B cells to the gut LP in normal mice is explained by the selective response of the former to TECK/CCL25, a chemokine expressed within the small intestine, especially in the epithelial crypts (Bowman et al. 2002; Kunkel et al. 2000). Further migration into the LP of the villi is proposed to depend on CXCL12, as IgA^+ B cells (as well as IgM^+ and IgG^+ cells) respond to CXCL12, and this chemokine is also expressed in the gut (Cyster 2003).

5
Recruitment of IgM$^+$ B Cells to the Gut LP

Generation of IgA plasma cells independent of GALT and the presence of IgM^+ B cells in the LP suggest that some IgM^+ B cells are able to directly migrate to the LP. Recent studies revealed that functional LTβR signaling on LP stromal cells is crucial for the presence of IgM^+ B cells and IgA plasma cells in the gut LP.

Indeed, LT$\beta R^{-/-}$ mice and *aly/aly* mice, which have impaired signaling through LTβR because of a point mutation in the downstream signaling molecule nuclear factor-κB-inducing kinase (NIK) (Shinkura et al. 1999), are completely devoid of IgM^+ B cells and IgA plasma cells in the gut LP (Fagarasan et al. 2000; Kang et al. 2002). Reconstitution of *aly/aly* or LT$\beta R^{-/-}$ with BM cells fails to restore the number of B cells and IgA plasma cells in the gut, unless coinjected with NIK-sufficient gut stromal cells or transplanted with a segment of normal small intestine (Kang et al. 2002; Suzuki et al. 2005). These facts, together with the observation that administration of LTβR antagonists after birth causes a marked decrease in the number of LP B cells and plasma cells (Newberry et al. 2002), demonstrate the essential role of permanent signaling through LTβR/NIK on gut stromal cells for the B cell recruitment to gut. Although the impaired LTα-LTβR interaction is suggested to affect the local concentration of adhesion molecules such as MadCAM-1 and homeostatic chemokines (Fagarasan et al. 2000; Kang et al. 2002), the cellular and molecular mechanisms by which defects in LTβR and/or NIK signaling in gut stromal cells selectively affect B cell recruitment still remain to be elucidated.

However, unlike naive BM B cells, migration of gut-activated B cells appears to be independent of gut stromal cells with a functional NIK. This is supported by the observation that IgM^+ B cells from PP or naive BM B cells that had been allowed to experience a normal gut environment (after short-term parabiosis of BM reconstituted *aly* with RAG-2$^{-/-}$ mice) can migrate to LP of *aly/aly* mice (Suzuki et al. 2005).

Together these observations imply that naive and gut-activated B cells have different requirements for migration to the gut and strongly suggest that normal gut environment imprints not only T cells but also B cells with gut-seeking properties (Iwata et al. 2004; Johansson-Lindbom et al. 2003; Krivacic and Levine 2003; Mora et al. 2003; Suzuki et al. 2005).

6
IgA Switching and Generation of IgA Plasma Cells in the Gut LP

Thus IgM$^+$ B cells present in the LP can be either gut-experienced cells emigrating from the PP and ILF or naive B cells recruited from the blood by LTβR/ NIK-sufficient gut stromal cells. Although is it extremely difficult to estimate the extent to which these two pathways participate in recruitment of IgM$^+$ B cells to LP in a normal gut, it is likely that IgA generated in GALT-deficient mice must be derived from the IgM$^+$ B cells that were recruited in a NIK-dependent manner, switched in situ to IgA$^+$ B cells, and further differentiated to IgA plasma cells in the LP. Indeed, activated IgM$^+$ B cells expressing large amounts of AID and α-germline transcripts, as well as IgA$^+$ cells, can be detected in LP preparations of GALT-deficient mice, namely, in LP of *aly/aly* after double reconstitution with BM and NIK-sufficient gut stromal cells (Suzuki et al. 2005). Furthermore, stromal cells isolated from the gut LP appear to support preferential switching to IgA$^+$ B cells and differentiation to IgA plasma cells of activated IgM$^+$ B cells regardless of their provenience (PP, MLN, or spleen), even in the absence of T cells (Fagarasan et al. 2001). IgA switch-inducing activity of LP stromal cells is due to their capacity to produce and secrete large amounts of active TGF-β, because anti-TGF-β antibodies drastically decrease the efficiency of switching to IgA. Further differentiation of IgA$^+$ B cells to plasma cells is supported by IL-6, IL-10, and probably other cytokines or chemokines produced by LP stromal cells (Fagarasan et al. 2001). Thus gut stromal cells are capable not only of supporting recruitment of IgM$^+$ B cells but also of facilitating their local differentiation to IgA plasma cells.

7
Biological Relevance of Gut IgA for Immune Homeostasis

The almost exclusive predominance of IgA in the gut as well as the existence of multiple pathways for its generation, independent of T cell help or follicular organization, makes pertinent the proposal that IgA is a constitutive Ig isotype in the gut that represents an evolutionarily primitive form of the adaptive immunity. Then what has led to the evolution of such a system that generates almost under any conditions large amounts of IgA in the intestine? In other words, what is the physiological importance of IgA secretion in the gut?

Numerous studies in animal models and in humans have provided evidence that oral immunization confers protection against various mucosal pathogens (Russell and Kilian 2005). However, mice unable to produce IgA (because of deletion of the Cα gene) or unable to assemble and transport polymeric Ig (because of the J chain gene deletion) have yielded conflicting results with regards to susceptibility to mucosal pathogens (Harriman et al. 1999; Lycke et al. 1999).

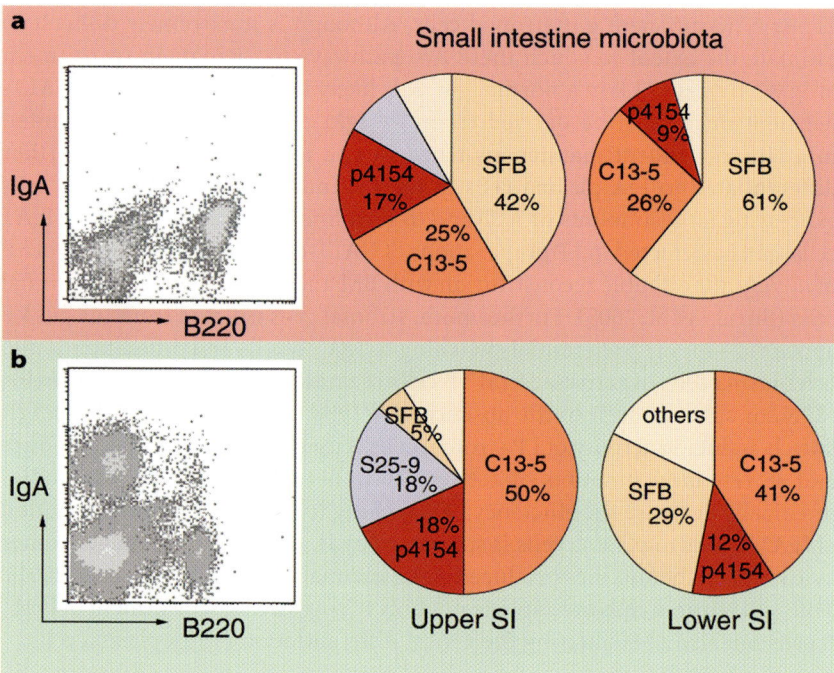

Fig. 1a, b Regulation of gut bacterial communities by IgA. FACS profiles of lamina propria cells, and composition of small intestine microbiota from AID$^{-/-}$ mice (**a**) without and (**b**) with B220$^-$IgA$^+$ plasma cells, reconstituted after parabiosis with normal mice. Intestinal flora in the biopsies from upper and lower segments of the small intestine of aged matched AID$^{-/-}$ mice was analyzed based on culture-independent 16S rRNA sequence analyses

Our own studies on mice deficient for AID, which have a complete block of CSR and SHM and thus are able to produce and secrete only nonmutated IgM in gut, clearly indicate that hypermutated mucosal IgAs are critical for regulation of bacterial composition in gut. The absence of IgA leads to an abnormal expansion of anaerobic bacteria in all segments of the small intestine. Among the bacteria expanded, uncultured anaerobes originally designated as segmented filamentous bacteria (SFB), strongly adherent to the epithelium of the small intestine, are the dominant population (Fig. 1). Significantly, reconstitution of AID$^{-/-}$ mice with normal IgA (by long-term parabiosis with normal animals) leads to a retreat of SFB to the large intestine and a complete normalization of composition of microbiota in the small intestine (Suzuki et al. 2004) (Fig. 1). A similar anaerobic expansion is observed in immunodeficient mice, such as RAG-2$^{-/-}$ mice, raised under specific pathogen-free conditions. This anaerobic shift in RAG-2$^{-/-}$ small intestine persists after their reconstitution with BM from AID$^{-/-}$ mice but is abolished by transfer of BM from normal mice, in concomitance with normalization of IgA levels in intestinal secretions (Suzuki et al. 2004). A delay in colonization of the

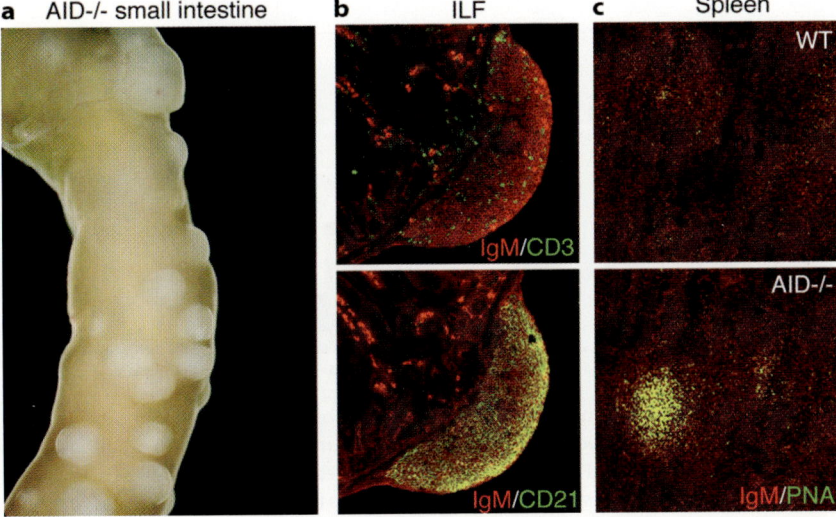

Fig. 2a–c IgA deficiency leads to mucosal and systemic B cell hyperplasia. **a** Duodenal segment of the small intestine of AID$^{-/-}$ mouse, showing hypertrophy of Peyer's patch and isolated lymphoid follicles (*ILF*). **b** ILF consist of IgM$^+$ B cells, and a few scattered CD3$^+$ T cells, assembling on a CD21$^+$ follicular dendritic cell (*FDC*) network. Note the presence of many IgM$^+$ plasma cells in the lamina propria of AID$^{-/-}$ mice. **c** Germinal center in spleens of nonimmunized wild-type and AID$^{-/-}$ mice

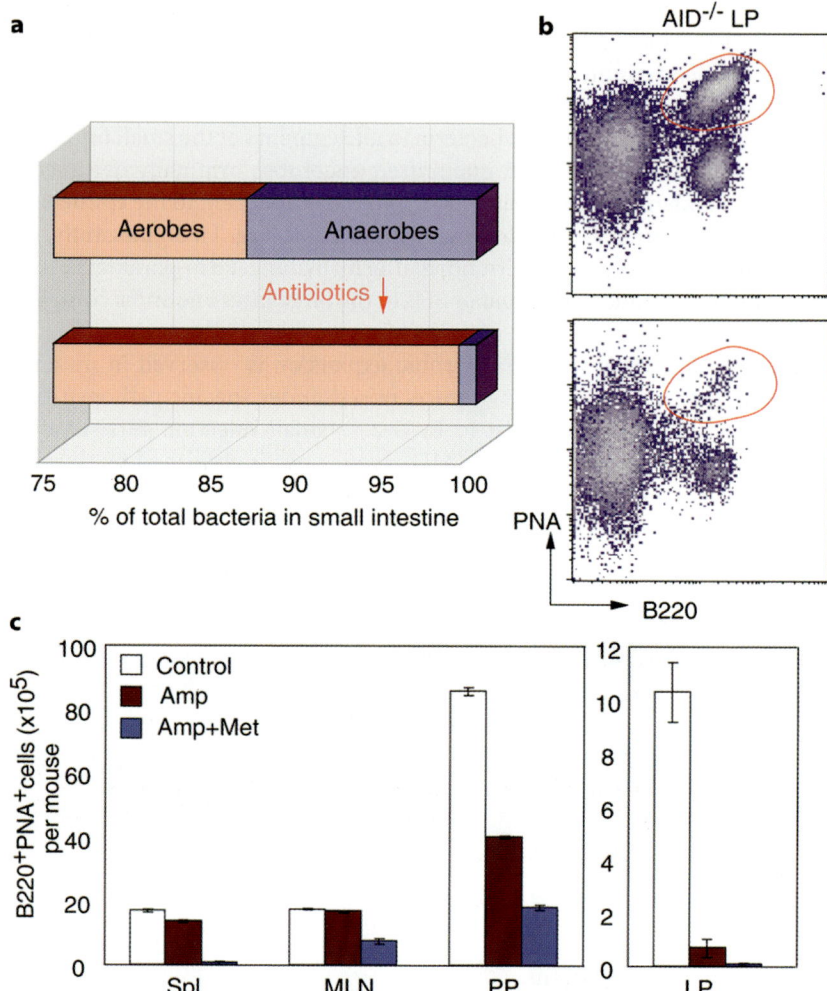

Fig. 3a–c Antibiotic treatment decreases the anaerobic expansion and abolishes B cell hyperplasia in AID$^{-/-}$ mice. **a** Composition of cultured microbiota in small intestine of AID$^{-/-}$ mice before and 2 weeks after antibiotic treatment. **b** The change in bacterial composition after administration of antibiotics leads to a drastic reduction of germinal center B cells (B220$^+$PNA$^+$ cells) in the lamina propria of treated mice. **c** Total number of B220$^+$PNA$^+$ cells in control and antibiotic-treated AID$^{-/-}$ mice. One set of mice received a mixture containing ampicillin, imipenem, and neomycin for 2 weeks (*brown bars*). Another set of mice received the same mixture for 1 week, followed by 1 week of metronidazole (*blue bars*). Although both treatments decreased the numbers of GC B cells in gut, only the anaerobic-specific treatment abolished systemic activation

small intestine with SFB and the retreat of SFB to the large intestine were also reported in mice neonates in relation with the presence of IgA, acquired by passive transfer or later generated by IgA plasma cells in the LP (Jiang et al. 2001).

The anaerobic shift of the gut microbiota has a profound effect on the immune system. Persistent activation by strongly adherent anaerobic bacteria causes an enhanced recruitment of IgM$^+$ B cells in the small intestine, as demonstrated in AID$^{-/-}$ mice, in which LP IgM$^+$ B cell number is increased by a factor of 10 compared with wild-type littermates. IgM$^+$ B cells accumulated in ILF anlagen, leading to organization and ultimately to hypertrophy of ILF as well as induction and accumulation of GC B cells (Fig. 2a, b). The IgM B cell hyperplasia is, however, not restricted to the gut LP, as accumulation of IgM$^+$B cells with a GC phenotype can be seen essentially in all lymphoid tissues (Fagarasan et al. 2002) (Fig. 2c). This hyperactivated phenotype is also observed in patients with AID deficiency or those with common variable immunodeficiency syndrome (CVID), which have enlarged GC in lymph nodes and develop nodular lymphoid hyperplasia of the small intestine (Bastlein et al. 1988; Burt and Jacoby 1999). In both mice and humans, an antibiotic treatment that decreases the gut bacterial load, particularly anaerobes, results in loss of intestinal hyperplasia and a drastic reduction of mucosal and systemic GC B cells (Fig. 3). The same results are obtained after reconstitution of normal IgA levels in the intestine, which leads to normalization of gut microbiota, followed by disappearance of lymphoid hyperplasia (Suzuki et al. 2004). These observations established the relevance of IgA present in the gut, which are clearly important for regulation of the intestinal bacterial community, and maintenance of an appropriate "geographical" distribution of bacteria in intestinal segments.

8
Conclusions and Perspectives

Taken together, the new advances in the mucosal immunity field, briefly presented in this chapter and summarized in Fig. 4, would imply the following amendments to the classic concepts for mucosal IgA synthesis:

1. Intestinal IgA plasma cells are generated by multiple, intricate pathways in both organized (PP, ILF, MLN) as well as nonorganized (LP) gut structures.

2. IgA represent a constitutive Ig isotype in gut, and IgA B cell development is dependent on microbial colonization but does not necessarily require T cell help and GC formation.

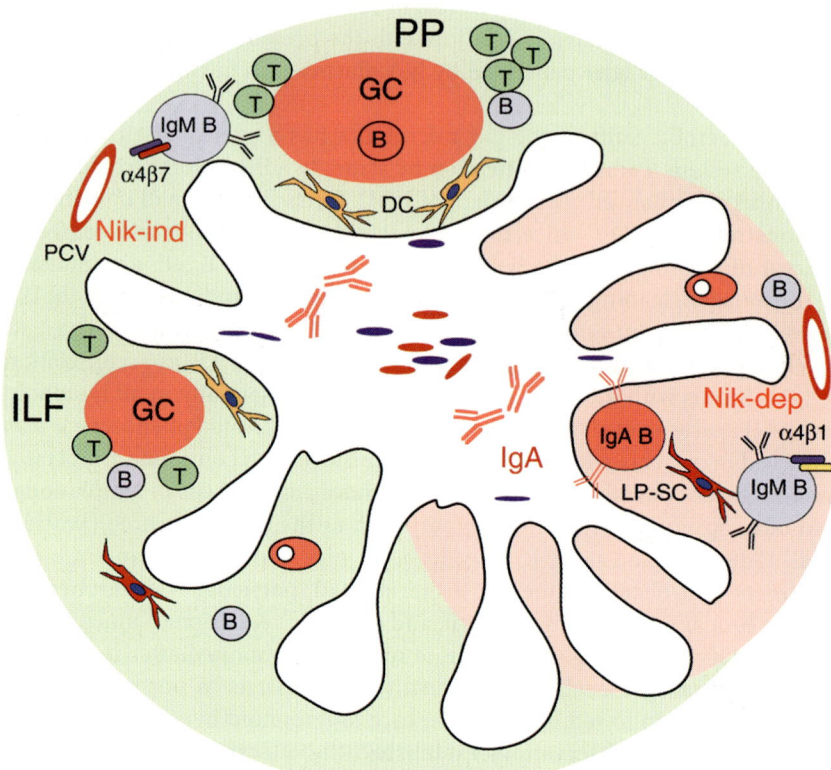

Fig. 4 Multiple pathways for generation of IgA in gut. Schematic representation of gut, with organized lymphoid structures, Peyer's patches (*PP*) and isolated lymphoid follicles (*ILF*), and diffuse tissues of lamina propria (*LP*). PP and ILF are composed of a subepithelial dome rich in dendritic cells (*DCs*), T cells, and B-cell follicle(s) that contain germinal centers (*GCs*). In these organized follicular structures B cells undergo efficient class switch recombination to IgA and somatic hypermutation and acquire gut-seeking properties through activation of integrin α4β7. Migration of both IgM$^+$ and IgA$^+$ B cells into the intestinal villi takes place through MadCAM-1$^+$ postcapillary venules (*PCV*) and does not require NIK-dependent activation of NF-κB in LP stromal cells (*LP-SC*). In the absence of PP or ILF, IgA plasma cells are generated by an alternative pathway and require NIK-dependent activation of LP-SC. NIK-signaling in LP-SC is necessary for recruitment of naive α4β1$^+$ IgM$^+$ B cells into the gut, which will switch and differentiate to IgA plasma cells in situ in the LP. IgA secreted into the intestinal lumen regulates both composition and appropriate segmental distribution of gut microbiota. T cell- and follicular-dependent pathway for IgA generation is shown in *green*. The alternative, T cell and/or follicular-independent pathway, is depicted in *pink*

3. There is a preferential homing of not only IgA$^+$ but also IgM$^+$ gut-activated B cells to the LP. The gut-seeking properties of IgM$^+$ B cells are most likely acquired in organized follicular structures of the gut. By contrast, naive IgM$^+$ B cell migration to LP and generation of IgA plasma cells require a LTβR/NIK-sufficient gut stromal compartment.

4. Intestinal IgA, besides providing protection against mucosal pathogens, plays a key role in selection and maintenance of a spatially diversified gut bacterial community.

There is now strong evidence that regulation of microbial composition through IgA in gut is required for initiation and maintenance of the fitness of our immune system. The absence of IgA homeostatic control results in a disregulation of gut microbiota, which in turn causes hyperactivation of the whole immune system.

The challenges for understanding molecular foundations for immune fitness, with multiple feedback and feed-forward controls involving both bacteria and immune cells, are great. The rewards for tackling such a complex issue certainly should include new insights into genetic strategies that our immune system has adopted over the last 250 million years of evolution, understanding of commensal tolerance, and new approaches for the prevention and therapy of mucosal disorders involving the immune system.

References

Backhed F, Ley RE, Sonnenburg JL, Peterson DA, Gordon JI (2005). Host-bacterial mutualism in the human intestine. Science 307:1915–1920

Bastlein C, Burlefinger R, Holzberg E, Voeth C, Garbrecht M, Ottenjann R (1988). Common variable immunodeficiency syndrome and nodular lymphoid hyperplasia in the small intestine. Endoscopy 20:272–275

Berlin C, Berg EL, Briskin MJ, Andrew DP, Kilshaw PJ, Holzmann B, Weissman IL, Hamann A, Butcher EC (1993). α4β7 Integrin mediates lymphocyte binding to the mucosal vascular addressin MAdCAM-1. Cell 74:185–185

Bowman EP, Kuklin NA, Youngman KR, Lazarus NH, Kunkel EJ, Pan J, Greenberg HB, Butcher EC (2002). The intestinal chemokine thymus-expressed chemokine (CCL25) attracts IgA antibody-secreting cells. J Exp Med 195:269–275

Brandtzaeg P, Baekkevold ES, Farstad IN, Jahnsen FL, Johansen FE, Nilsen EM, Yamanaka T (1999). Regional specialization in the mucosal immune system: what happens in the microcompartments? Immunol Today 20:141–151

Burt RW, Jacoby RF (1999). Polyposis Syndromes. In Textbook of Gastroenterology, Yamada T, Alpers D, Laine L, Owyang C, and Powell D, eds. (Philadelphia, Lippincott Williams & Wilkins), pp. 1995–2022

Butcher EC, Rouse RV, Coffman RL, Nottenburg CN, Hardy RR, Weissman IL (1982). Surface phenotype of Peyer's patch germinal center cells: implications for the role of germinal centers in B cell differentiation. J Immunol 129:2698–2707

Cebra JJ (1999). Influences of microbiota on intestinal immune system development. Am J Clin Nutr 69:1046S-1051S

Cebra JJ, Shroff KE (1994). Peyer's patches as inductive sites for IgA commitment. In Handbook of Mucosal Immunology, Ogra P, Mestecky J, Lamm M, Strobel W, McGhee J, and Bienenstock J, eds. (San Diego, Academic Press), pp. 151–157

Craig SW, Cebra JJ (1971). Peyer's patches: an enriched source of precursors for IgA-producing immunocytes in the rabbit. J Exp Med 134:188–200

Cyster JG (2003). Homing of antibody secreting cells. Immunol Rev 194:48–60

Dunn-Walters DK, Isaacson PG, Spencer J (1997). Sequence analysis of human IgVH genes indicates that ileal lamina propria plasma cells are derived from Peyer's patches. Eur J Immunol 27:463–467

Eberl G, Littman DR (2004). Thymic origin of intestinal $\alpha\beta$ T cells revealed by fate mapping of RORγt+ Cells. Science 305:248–251

Fagarasan S, Honjo T (2000). T-Independent immune response: new aspects of B cell biology. Science 290:89–92

Fagarasan S, Honjo T (2003). Intestinal IgA synthesis: regulation of front-line body defences. Nat Rev Immunol 3:63–72

Fagarasan S, Kinoshita K, Muramatsu M, Ikuta K, Honjo T (2001). In situ class switching and differentiation to IgA-producing cells in the gut lamina propria. Nature 413:639–643

Fagarasan S, Shinkura R, Kamata T, Nogaki F, Ikuta K, Tashiro K, Honjo T (2000). Alymphoplasia (aly)-type nuclear factor κB-inducing kinase (NIK) causes defects in secondary lymphoid tissue chemokine receptor signaling and homing of peritoneal cells to the gut-associated lymphatic tissue system. J Exp Med 191:1477–1486

Finke D, Acha-Orbea H, Mattis A, Lipp M, Kraehenbuhl J (2002). CD4+CD3− cells induce Peyer's patch development: role of $\alpha 4\beta 1$ integrin activation by CXCR5. Immunity 17:363–373

Gardby E, Wrammert J, Schon K, Ekman L, Leanderson T, Lycke N (2003). Strong differential regulation of serum and mucosal IgA responses as revealed in CD28-deficient mice using cholera toxin adjuvant. J Immunol 170:55–63

Guy-Grand D, Griscelli C, Vassalli P (1974). The gut-associated lymphoid system: nature and properties of the large dividing cells. Eur J Immunol 4:435–443

Hamada H, Hiroi T, Nishiyama Y, Takahashi H, Masunaga Y, Hachimura S, Kaminogawa S, Takahashi-Iwanaga H, Iwanaga T, Kiyono, H., *et al.* (2002). Identification of multiple isolated lymphoid follicles on the antimesenteric wall of the mouse small intestine. J Immunol 168:57–64

Harriman GR, Bogue M, Rogers P, Finegold M, Pacheco S, Bradley A, Zhang Y, Mbawuike IN (1999). Targeted deletion of the IgA constant region in mice leads to IgA deficiency with alterations in expression of other Ig isotypes. J Immunol 162:2521–2529

Honda K, Nakano H, Yoshida H, Nishikawa S, Rennert P, Ikuta K, Tamechika M, Yamaguchi K, Fukumoto T, Chiba T, Nishikawa SI (2001). Molecular basis for hematopoietic/mesenchymal interaction during initiation of Peyer's patch organogenesis. J Exp Med 193:621–630

Hooper LV, Gordon JI (2001). Commensal host-bacterial relationships in the gut. Science 292:1115–1118

Iwata M, Hirakiyama A, Eshima Y, Kagechika H, Kato C, Song SY (2004). Retinoic acid imprints gut-homing specificity on T cells. Immunity 21:527–538

Jiang HQ, Bos NA, Cebra JJ (2001). Timing, localization, and persistence of colonization by segmented filamentous bacteria in the neonatal mouse gut depend on immune status of mothers and pups. Infect Immun 69:3611–3617

Johansson-Lindbom B, Svensson M, Wurbel MA, Malissen B, Marquez G, Agace W (2003). Selective generation of gut tropic T cells in gut-associated lymphoid tissue (GALT): requirement for GALT dendritic cells and adjuvant. J Exp Med 198:963–969

Kang HS, Chin RK, Wang Y, Yu P, Wang J, Newell KA, Fu YX (2002). Signaling via LTβR on the lamina propria stromal cells of the gut is required for IgA production. Nat Immunol 3:576–582

Kinoshita K, Harigai M, Fagarasan S, Muramatsu M, Honjo T (2001). A hallmark of active class switch recombination: transcripts directed by I promoters on looped-out circular DNAs. Proc Natl Acad Sci USA 98:12620–12623

Krivacic KA, Levine AD (2003). Extracellular matrix conditions T cells for adhesion to tissue interstitium. J Immunol 170:5034–5044

Kroese FG, Butcher EC, Stall AM, Lalor PA, Adams S, Herzenberg LA (1989). Many of the IgA producing plasma cells in murine gut are derived from self-replenishing precursors in the peritoneal cavity. Int Immunol 1:75–84

Kunkel EJ, Campbell JJ, Haraldsen G, Pan J, Boisvert J, Roberts AI, Ebert EC, Vierra MA, Goodman SB, Genovese, M. C., et al. (2000). Lymphocyte CC chemokine receptor 9 and epithelial thymus-expressed chemokine (TECK) expression distinguish the small intestinal immune compartment: epithelial expression of tissue-specific chemokines as an organizing principle in regional immunity. J Exp Med 192:761–768

Lorenz RG, Chaplin DD, McDonald KG, McDonough JS, Newberry RD (2003). Isolated lymphoid follicle formation is inducible and dependent upon lymphotoxin-sufficient B lymphocytes, lymphotoxin β receptor, and TNF receptor I function. J Immunol 170:5475–5482

Lycke N (1998). T cell and cytokine regulation of the IgA response. In Mucosal T cells, MacDonald T, ed. (Basel, Karger), pp. 209–234

Lycke N, Erlandsson L, Ekman L, Schon K, Leanderson T (1999). Lack of J chain inhibits the transport of gut IgA and abrogates the development of intestinal antitoxic protection. J Immunol 163:913–919

Macpherson AJ, Gatto D, Sainsbury E, Harriman GR, Hengartner H, Zinkernagel RM (2000). A primitive T cell-independent mechanism of intestinal mucosal IgA responses to commensal bacteria. Science 288:2222–2226

McDonald KG, McDonough JS, Newberry RD (2005). Adaptive immune responses are dispensable for isolated lymphoid follicle formation: antigen-naive, lymphotoxin-sufficient B lymphocytes drive the formation of mature isolated lymphoid follicles. J Immunol 174:5720–5728

McWilliams M, Phillips-Quagliata JM, Lamm ME (1977). Mesenteric lymph node B lymphoblasts which home to the small intestine are precommitted to IgA synthesis. J Exp Med 145:866–875

Mora JR, Bono MR, Manjunath N, Weninger W, Cavanagh LL, Rosemblatt M, Von Andrian UH (2003). Selective imprinting of gut-homing T cells by Peyer's patch dendritic cells. Nature 424:88–93

Mostov KE (1994). Transepithelial transport of immunoglobulins. Annu Rev Immunol 12:63–84

Muramatsu M, Kinoshita K, Fagarasan S, Yamada S, Shinkai Y, Honjo T (2000). Class switch recombination and hypermutation require activation-induced cytidine deaminase (AID), a potential RNA editing enzyme. Cell 102:553–563

Newberry RD, McDonough JS, McDonald KG, Lorenz RG (2002). Postgestational lymphotoxin/lymphotoxin β receptor interactions are essential for the presence of intestinal B lymphocytes. J Immunol 168:4988–4997

Nishikawa S, Honda K, Vieira P, Yoshida H (2003). Organogenesis of peripheral lymphoid organs. Immunol Rev 195:72–80

Russell M, Kilian M (2005). Biological activities of IgA. In Mucosal immunology, Mestecky J, Lamm M, McGhee J, Bienenstock J, Mayer L, and Strobel W, eds. (San Diego, Academic Press), pp. 267–289

Ryffel B, Le Hir M, Muller M, Eugster HP (1998). Correction of the TNF-LTα-deficient phenotype by bone marrow transplantation. Dev Immunol 6:253–260

Shinkura R, Kitada K, Matsuda F, Tashiro K, Ikuta K, Suzuki M, Kogishi K, Serikawa T, Honjo T (1999). Alymphoplasia is caused by a point mutation in the mouse gene encoding NF-κb-inducing kinase. Nat Genet 22:74–77

Sonnenburg JL, Angenent LT, Gordon JI (2004). Getting a grip on things: how do communities of bacterial symbionts become established in our intestine? Nat Immunol 5:569–573

Stoel M, Jiang HQ, van Diemen CC, Bun JC, Dammers PM, Thurnheer MC, Kroese FG, Cebra JJ, Bos NA (2005). Restricted IgA repertoire in both B-1 and B-2 cell-derived gut plasmablasts. J Immunol 174:1046–1054

Strobel W, Fagarasan S, Lycke N (2005). IgA B cell development. In Mucosal immunology, Mestecky J, Lamm M, McGhee J, Bienenstock J, Mayer L, and Strobel W, eds. (San Diego, Academic Press), pp. 583–616

Suzuki K, Meek B, Doi Y, Honjo T, Fagarasan S (2005). Two distinctive pathways for recruitment of naive and primed IgM+ B cells to the gut lamina propria. Proc Natl Acad Sci USA 102:2482–2486

Suzuki K, Meek B, Doi Y, Muramatsu M, Chiba T, Honjo T, Fagarasan S (2004). Aberrant expansion of segmented filamentous bacteria in IgA-deficient gut. Proc Natl Acad Sci USA 101:1981–1986

Tseng J (1981). Transfer of lymphocytes of Peyer's patches between immunoglobulin allotype congenic mice: repopulation of the IgA plasma cells in the gut lamina propria. J Immunol 127:2039–2043

Tseng J (1984). A population of resting IgM-IgD double-bearing lymphocytes in Peyer's patches: the major precursor cells for IgA plasma cells in the gut lamina propria. J Immunol 132:2730–2735

van der Heijden PJ, Stok W, Bianchi AT (1987). Contribution of immunoglobulin-secreting cells in the murine small intestine to the total 'background' immunoglobulin production. Immunology 62:551-555

van Egmond M, Damen CA, van Spriel AB, Vidarsson G, van Garderen E, and van de Winkel JG (2001). IgA and the IgA Fc receptor. Trends Immunol 22:205–211

Weinstein PD, Cebra JJ (1991). The preference for switching to IgA expression by Peyer's patch germinal center B cells is likely due to the intrinsic influence of their microenvironment. J Immunol 147:4126–4135

Yoshida H, Naito A, Inoue J, Satoh M, Santee-Cooper SM, Ware CF, Togawa A, Nishikawa S (2002). Different cytokines induce surface lymphotoxin-$\alpha\beta$ on IL-7 receptor-α cells that differentially engender lymph nodes and Peyer's patches. Immunity 17:823–833

Youngman K, Lazarus N, Butcher E (2005). Lymphocyte homing: chemokines and adhesion molecules in T cell and IgA plasma cell localization in the mucosal immune system. In Mucosal immunology, Mestecky J, Lamm M, McGhee J, Bienenstock J, Mayer L, and Strobel W, eds. (San Diego, Academic Press), pp. 667–680

B Cell Recruitment and Selection in Mouse GALT Germinal Centers

S. Casola (✉) · K. Rajewsky

The CBR Institute for Biomedical Research, Harvard Medical School,
Boston, MA 02115, USA
stefan.casola@ifom-ieo-campus.it

1	Introduction 156
2	LMP2A Knock-in Mice: A Tool to Study the Role of BCR-Mediated Antigen Recognition in GALT GC Responses 158
2.1	LMP2A Drives B Cell Differentiation in the Absence of BCR Expression . . 158
2.2	Spontaneous GALT GC in BCR-Deficient LMP2A Mice 160
3	Spontaneous GC Responses in GALT of Mice with a Limited Repertoire of Antibody Specificities 161
4	Role of the Intestinal Microflora in GALT GC Responses 162
5	Involvement of Complement Activation and Toll-Like Receptor Signaling in GALT GC Responses 163
6	T Cell Control of GALT GC Responses 164
7	Principles of B Cell Selection in GALT GC 167
References	168

Abstract In conventionally reared mice germinal centers (GCs) are chronically induced in Peyer's patches (PP), mesenteric lymph node (MLN), and isolated lymphoid follicles (ILF) of gut-associated lymphoid tissues (GALT), as a result of continuous B cell stimulation by commensal bacteria. It is generally thought that BCR-mediated antigen recognition controls the recruitment and thus selection of B cells within GALT GCs. However, recent results challenge this view and suggest that engagement of innate immune receptors by microbial antigens promotes B cell recruitment to, and maintenance within, the GC, irrespective of BCR specificity. We propose a scenario in which microbial determinants presented by follicular dendritic cells (FDCs) to innate receptors on B cells within the GC support the survival and concomitant expansion of somatically mutated, IgA-class-switched B cell clones expressing a variety of BCR specificities. From this pool, B cell mutants recognizing gut-derived antigens through their BCR are either, in GCs, drawn into the process of affinity maturation, or, in the lamina propria (LP) of the gut, locally selected to differentiate into plasmablasts, thus contributing to the continuous production of IgA antibodies required for an efficient protection against commensal and pathogenic microorganisms.

1
Introduction

A functional antibody system depends on the presence of a pool of B lymphocytes expressing a diversified repertoire of immunoglobulin (Ig) receptors. In humans and mice, diversification of the primary antibody repertoire is generated through the rearrangement of multiple V, D, and J segments occurring in the bone marrow as a life-long process (Rajewsky 1996). In other species including rabbit, sheep, and chicken (also called 'GALT species'), combinatorial diversity is limited and the preimmune antibody repertoire is largely determined by postrearrangement processes including gene conversion (chicken and rabbit; Becker and Knight 1990; Reynaud et al. 1987; Thompson and Neiman 1987) and somatic hypermutation (sheep and rabbit; Reynaud et al. 1991; Weinstein et al. 1994) that occur in GALT (Reynaud and Weill 1996). Diversification of the antibody repertoire in the GALT is accompanied by intense B cell proliferation in primary B cell follicles or germinal centers (GCs) (Pospisil and Mage 1998), is triggered by recognition of self- or foreign antigens, and occurs in specific anatomical sites during a restricted time window of pre- and/or postnatal life (Pospisil and Mage 1998; Reynaud et al. 1991, 1994).

In mice, the GALT represent sites of intense B cell activation, proliferation, and terminal differentiation in response to foreign antigens, in particular of bacterial origin. The major function of the GALT is to protect the organism from the attack of microorganisms present in the gut lumen. This is mainly achieved through the production of large amounts of secretory IgA (sIgA) by plasma cells residing in the LP of the intestine. sIgA is actively transported to the gut lumen in a dimeric or polymeric form (Kraehenbuhl and Neutra 1992). Although its precise role in the gut lumen is still unknown, it is thought that, by coating commensal and pathogenic bacteria, sIgA prevents their adhesion to the intestinal epithelia and hence penetration of luminal microorganisms through the intestinal wall. Luminal sIgA bound to opsonized bacteria may also be transported back to the subepithelial region of Peyer's patches (PP) through specialized epithelial microfold (M) cells, thereby facilitating the induction of local humoral response against specific microorganisms (Weltzin et al. 1989).

Production of sIgA is dependent on the presence of the commensal flora (Shroff et al. 1995) and, to a large extent, on the induction of GC responses in PP, ILF (Shikina et al. 2004) and mesenteric lymph nodes (MLN) (Cebra 1999; Talham et al. 1999). Here, chronic GC responses are triggered as a result of the continuous stimulation of B cells with antigens derived from a spectrum of commensal bacteria transported through the epithelia by M cells and delivered to the subepithelial region of PP and ILF, rich in B cells, T cells, and dendritic cells (DCs). Sampling of bacterial antigens from the gut lumen may also take place through specialized LP DCs extending dendrites between the epithelial cells of the small intestine (Rescigno et al., 2001). Recent work has shown that LP DCs can also engulf and transport live commensal bacteria, delivered to them by M cells, to the draining MLN where bacterial antigens are processed and presented to T cells (Macpherson and Uhr 2004). Somatically mutated, surface IgA$^+$ B cells, generated in GALT GCs, migrate to the draining MLN and, via the thoracic duct lymph and the blood, reach the intestinal LP, where they undergo terminal differentiation into plasmablasts on antigen re-encounter (Craig and Cebra 1971; Husband and Gowans 1978). Direct IgA isotype switching in LP by IgM$^+$ B cells followed by terminal differentiation in response to stimulation by microbial antigens in the presence of a specific cytokine milieu produced by DCs and stromal cells has been also proposed (Fagarasan et al. 2001).

Two major subsets of mature B cells contribute to the generation of IgA-secreting plasma cells in mouse GALT. Conventional B cells (also called B-2 cells) are predominantly recruited into GALT GCs, where they undergo Ig somatic mutation and class switch recombination to become IgA$^+$ B cells. Another subset of B cells that can give rise in mice to IgA-secreting plasma cells consists of B-1 cells (Kroese et al. 1989). Located in the peritoneal and pleural cavities, these cells can migrate to GALT to undergo terminal differentiation upon encounter with microbial antigens, presumably in a T cell-independent manner (Fagarasan et al. 2000; Macpherson et al. 2000). In general, B-1 cells do not participate in GALT GC responses. However, IgA$^+$ gut plasmablasts derived from these cells carry frequently somatically mutated Ig genes (Bos et al. 1996; Stoel et al. 2005). The contribution of B-1 cells to the generation of "natural" and antigen-specific mucosal IgA responses in immunoproficient mice has recently been questioned (Thurnheer et al. 2003).

It is generally assumed that specific antigen recognition through the B cell antigen receptor (BCR) is an essential condition for the recruitment and subsequent selection of GC B cells (MacLennan 1994). However, studies performed in the rabbit have suggested that GALT GC represent sites for antigenindependent diversification of the preimmune antibody repertoire (Lanning et al. 2000).

What is the contribution of antigen in mouse GALT GC responses? On which basis are B cells recruited and selected in mouse GALT GCs? What are the contributions of the commensal flora and of innate immune receptors to these responses? Which T cell subset supports B cells in GC responses, and by which mechanism is T cell help delivered?

In the remaining part of this review we discuss a series of recent findings that address these long-standing questions, with special emphasis on the role of BCR-mediated antigen recognition in the recruitment and selection of GC B cells.

2
LMP2A Knock-in Mice: A Tool to Study the Role of BCR-Mediated Antigen Recognition in GALT GC Responses

2.1
LMP2A Drives B Cell Differentiation in the Absence of BCR Expression

The Epstein-Barr virus (EBV)-encoded latent membrane protein (LMP) 2A is a multispanning transmembrane protein expressed in latently infected human B lymphocytes and in tumor cells of several malignancies including Hodgkin disease and nasopharyngeal carcinoma (Thorley-Lawson 2001). With Igα and Igβ, the signaling subunits of the BCR complex, LMP2A shares in its cytoplasmic domain the immunoreceptor tyrosine activation motif (ITAM) that is constitutively phosphorylated in EBV-infected B cells (Fruehling and Longnecker 1997). Through the phosphorylated ITAMs, LMP2A recruits non-receptor tyrosine kinases and adaptor proteins, many of which are also critical for BCR signaling (Miller et al. 1995). Thus it was suggested that LMP2A acts as a BCR surrogate. Studies in vivo with LMP2A transgenic mice have confirmed this hypothesis, showing that LMP2A can support survival of B cells lacking BCR expression (Caldwell et al. 1998).

In an effort to develop a mouse model of Hodgkin lymphoma to study the contribution of LMP2A to the transformation process, we generated knock-in animals in which expression of the viral protein is induced in a cell-type and stage-specific manner by the Cre/loxP recombination system (Casola et al. 2004). The conditional LMP2A allele was inserted into the IgH genomic locus, replacing the J_H segments (Fig. 1). As a result, homozygous LMP2A mice are unable to rearrange the IgH chain variable region genes and are thus BCR deficient. Two independent lines of IgH knock-in mice expressing different levels of LMP2A, as a result of different promoter usage, were generated (Fig. 1). In homozygous mutant mice of both these lines, Cre-dependent expression of the viral protein starting from the early B cell precursors led

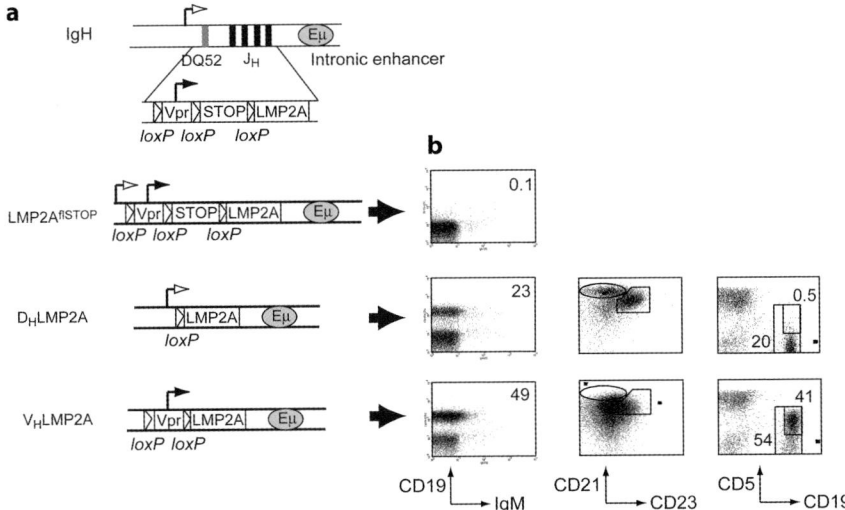

Fig. 1a, b **a** A conditional LMP2A transgene (LMP2A^{flSTOP}) was inserted into the IgH locus replacing the J$_H$ segments. On Cre-mediated deletion of a loxP-flanked transcription and translation STOP cassette, expression of LMP2A is driven from two alternative promoters. In D$_H$LMP2A mice, LMP2A expression is under the control of the weak promoter of the DQ52 gene segment. In V$_H$LMP2A mice, expression of the transgene is under the control of a stronger promoter isolated from the V$_H$186.2 variable region gene. **b** Flow cytometric analyses of splenocytes isolated from mice homozygous for the different LMP2A alleles. Staining of CD19$^+$ gated B cells for CD21 and CD23 reveals the follicular B (CD21$^+$CD23$^+$) and marginal zone B (CD21^{hi}CD23^{lo}) cell subsets. Coexpression of CD19 and CD5 on splenic B cells identifies B-1a B cells. *Numbers* indicate percentages of B cells and/or B cell subsets falling within the lymphocyte gate

to a significant accumulation of BCR-less B cells in peripheral lymphoid organs. A phenotypic analysis of these cells indicated similarities with those belonging to the major subsets of mature B cells of wild-type mice. Specifically, D$_H$LMP2A knock-in mice expressing low levels of LMP2A developed B-2 and marginal zone (MZ) B cells and lacked peritoneal B-1 cells. In contrast, mice with high expression levels of LMP2A (V$_H$LMP2A) limited B cell development exclusively to the B-1 subset (Fig. 1). These studies suggested that LMP2A promotes differentiation as well as survival of BCR-deficient B cells and, most importantly, that expression levels and thus signal strength through the viral BCR surrogate determines the fate of the developing B cells (Casola et al. 2004).

2.2
Spontaneous GALT GC in BCR-Deficient LMP2A Mice

The availability of LMP2A knock-in mice gave us the unique chance to study the contribution of BCR-mediated antigen recognition to the induction of GC responses. Intraperitoneal immunization of LMP2A mice with T cell-dependent (TD) antigens revealed a lack of GCs in the spleen of these mice (Casola et al. 2004). The same result was obtained regardless of whether the B-2 and MZ or the B-1 B cell subsets constituted the majority of B cells present in the different LMP2A strains. This indicated that GC responses induced during conventional TD immune responses are strictly dependent on specific antigen recognition through the BCR.

Surprisingly, when LMP2A mice were analyzed for the occurrence of spontaneous GCs in PP and MLN, a normal fraction of GC B cells showing the typical increased surface expression of the death receptor Fas and of the receptor for peanut agglutinin (PNA) was identified by flow cytometric analysis. The GC identity was confirmed by histological analysis demonstrating areas of intense staining for the GC B cell-specific marker BCL-6 within PP and MLN (Fig. 2). Functionally, GALT GC B cells in LMP2A mice resembled those of wild-type animals in that they underwent somatic hypermutation of rearranged IgL chain variable region genes and Ig class switch recombination as a result of induction of expression of activation-induced cytidine deaminase (AID), which is required for both processes (Casola et al. 2004, Muramatsu et al. 2000).

B-2 cells represent the major subset of B cells recruited into GCs of the GALT in mice and humans. In accordance with this notion, normal numbers of GC, of normal size, were observed in PP and MLN of the LMP2A strain that developed B-2 and MZ B cells. In contrast, LMP2A mice whose B cells were predominantly of the B-1 phenotype lacked spontaneous GCs in MLN and only occasionally had some in PP. Thus, when B-2 cells are missing, B-1 cells can occasionally participate to GCs reactions in PP (Fig. 2).

Together, these results indicated that the special microenvironment of the GALT supports the induction of GC responses in the absence of specific antigen recognition through the BCR and thus BCR-mediated antigen presentation. This predicts the existence in B cells of an alternative (non-specific) mechanism of antigen internalization that would allow its subsequent processing and presentation via major histocompatibility complex (MHC)-class II molecules to antigen-specific T cells to obtain the required costimulation for the induction of a GC response (see Sect. 6). Alternatively, T cell-help could derive from bystander T cells that become activated in response to gut-derived antigens presented to them by LP/PP DC (see Sect. 6).

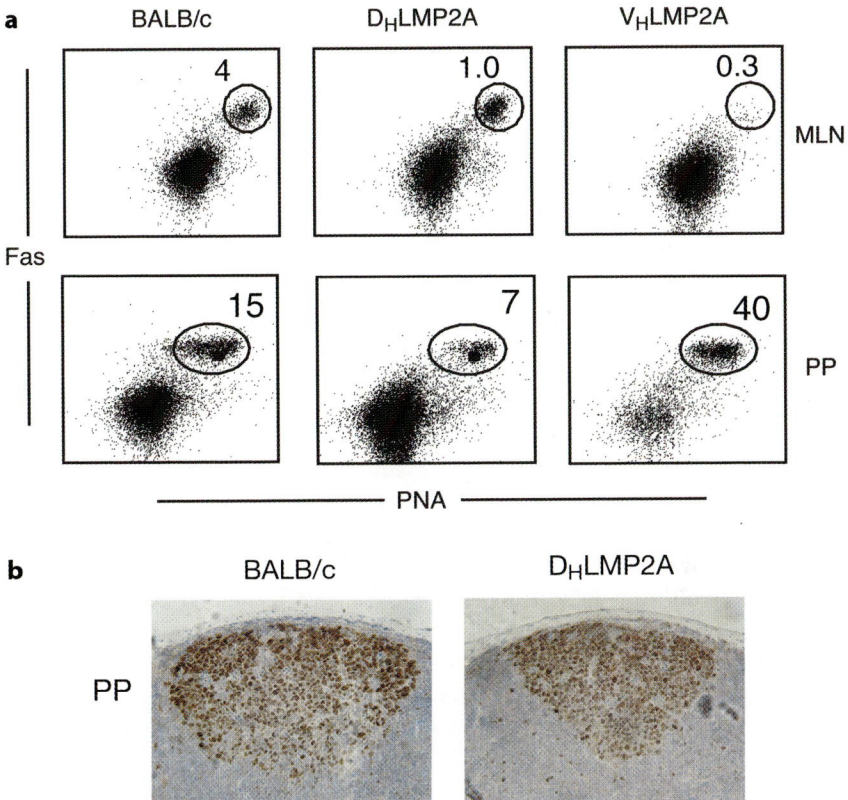

Fig. 2a, b Spontaneous GC formation in GALT of V_H and D_HLMP2A homozygous knock-in mice (both on a BALB/c genetic background) as revealed by flow cytometric analyses (**a**) and histology (**b**). GC B cells are defined as CD19$^+$ gated B cells that express high levels of Fas and the peanut agglutinin (*PNA*) receptor. For V_HLMP2A mice, a case is displayed in which a high percentage of GC B cells was observed in PP. GC B cells in PP of D_HLMP2A mice resemble those found in wild-type BALB/c mice as they express high levels of the GC-B cell-specific marker BCL-6 (stained in *brown*) (**b**). Numbers indicate percentages of B cells falling within the GC B cell boxed gate

3
Spontaneous GC Responses in GALT of Mice with a Limited Repertoire of Antibody Specificities

The spontaneous recruitment of B cells into GCs of the GALT in LMP2A mice predicts that B cells can be driven into these structures in the absence of specific antigen recognition. To test this hypothesis, we analyzed three inde-

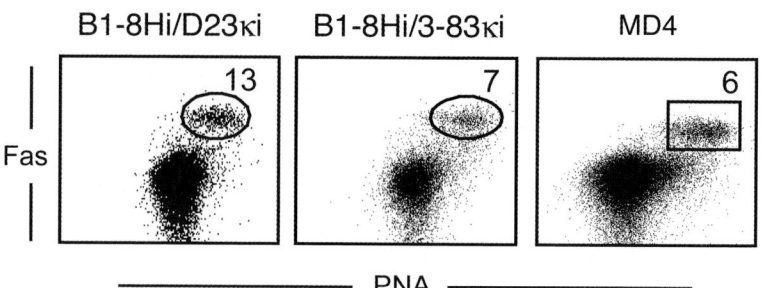

Fig. 3 Spontaneous GCs in PP of three independent BCR transgenic mice as revealed by flow cytometric analyses. Shown are CD19⁺ gated B cells. Percentages of boxed GC B cells within the CD19⁺ B cell gate are indicated

pendent transgenic mouse strains expressing non-autoreactive prerearranged IgH + IgL chain genes (Casola et al. 2004). In one strain of mice (MD4) the specificity of the BCR receptor is known (hen egg lysozyme), in the other two (B1-8Hi;3-83κi, and B1-8Hi;D23κi) no specific antigen has been so far identified. In all three BCR transgenic mouse strains the vast majority of the peripheral B cells expressed the original BCR specificity. Spontaneous GCs were observed in PP and MLN of all three transgenic strains (Fig. 3). The fraction of GC B cells was comparable to that of wild-type mice. Importantly, molecular analysis of sorted GC and non-GC B cells of PP of the three transgenic strains excluded the possibility that B cells in the GALT GCs of these animals were selected on the basis of the expression of a second BCR generated through secondary IgL chain rearrangements (Casola et al. 2004). These results support the concept that efficient recruitment of B cells into GALT GCs can occur in the absence of antigen recognition through the BCR.

4
Role of the Intestinal Microflora in GALT GC Responses

Commensal bacteria are essential to induce GALT GC responses and to promote both antigen-specific and natural IgA antibody titers. Germ-free animals lack spontaneous GCs in PP and in other GALT sites, and IgA antibody titers are strongly diminished in these mice (Shroff and Cebra 1995). Colonization of the gut of germ-free mice with a single commensal strain leads to a rapid induction of GALT GC responses resulting in a vigorous IgA antibody response (Talham et al. 1999). The molecular mechanisms responsible for the induction of GALT GCs by the intestinal microflora are still largely unknown, although BCR-mediated antigen recognition of bacterial antigens has been suggested.

To test the latter hypothesis, we studied the contribution of commensal bacteria to GALT GC responses of BCR-deficient LMP2A mice. Specifically, 3-week old LMP2A mice received for 2 weeks in the drinking water a cocktail of antibiotics against a spectrum of both aerobic and anaerobic Gr^+ and Gr^- bacteria. Flow cytometric analysis of single-cell suspensions from PP and MLN of LMP2A mice revealed a significant and selective reduction in the fraction of GC B cells in treated animals, compared with their littermate controls kept on antibiotic-free water (Casola et al. 2004). These results suggest that GCs in GALT of LMP2A mice are, as in wild-type animals, dependent on the presence of the intestinal microflora. Thus we conclude that bacterial stimulation can recruit B cells into GALT GCs irrespective of their BCR specificity, possibly through the engagement of innate immune receptors. A similar mechanism may also account for the induction of GC responses in the rabbit appendix undergoing primary diversification of the antibody repertoire as a result of postnatal encounter with commensal bacteria of the intestinal flora (Rhee et al. 2004).

5
Involvement of Complement Activation and Toll-Like Receptor Signaling in GALT GC Responses

Transport across the epithelial barrier operated by M cells provides the underlying B cell follicles of PP and ILF with a rich source of microorganisms. We hypothesized that direct activation of the complement cascade on the surface of the bacteria in these sites may lead to their presentation to B cells by FDC that express high levels of the complement receptors Cr1/Cr2. Indeed, we could show deposition of active complement fragments on the FDC network present within GCs in PP of wild-type and LMP2A mice. In addition, as the latter animals lack any form of immunoglobulin, activation of complement in these sites is likely to have occurred on the surface of the microorganisms through the alternative or mannose lectin-binding pathway (Walport 2001).

In search for the mechanisms responsible for BCR-independent recruitment of B cells into GALT GCs, we postulated that engagement of Toll-like receptors (TLR) on B cells by microbial ligands, potent activators of B cell proliferation and terminal differentiation (Kearney and Lawton 1975; Krieg et al. 1995), could play an important role in this context. For this purpose we recently analyzed GALT GC responses in LMP2A mice lacking the adaptor protein MyD88, which is essential for signaling through most TLR (Akira and Takeda, 2004). Preliminary experiments revealed a strong reduction of spontaneous GC in PP of the compound mouse mutant strains (S. Casola and K. Rajewsky, unpublished results). The contribution of TLR signaling to GALT GC responses may extend beyond a direct effect on B cells. DC play a major role in the homeostasis of the GALT. By sorting, processing, and thus presenting microbial antigens to different T cell subsets, LP/PP DCs are essential for a rapid and efficient induction of a local immune response against commensal bacteria, thereby limiting their ability to disseminate systemically (Macpherson and Uhr, 2004). As TLR greatly enhance the antigen presentation properties of DCs and their ability to secrete cytokines, they may facilitate DC-dependent activation of T cells, which are essential to provide help to B cells in the GC response through cell-to-cell interactions and/or production of specific cytokines (see below).

6
T Cell Control of GALT GC Responses

Previous reports have indicated that spontaneous GCs in mouse GALT are strictly dependent on T cell help provided by $\alpha\beta$ and/or $\gamma\delta$ T cells (Koni and Flavell 1999; Macpherson et al. 2000). An absolute requirement for T cells was also observed for the induction of spontaneous GALT GC responses in the BCR transgenics and LMP2A knock-in animals that we have tested (Fig. 4 and Casola et al. 2004). The latter result suggests that the cross talk between B and T cells required to induce and sustain GC responses in PP and MLN can occur in the absence of BCR-dependent antigen presentation. This result led us to investigate whether MHC-II-restricted antigen presentation was essential for triggering GALT GC responses in mice. To our surprise, 30% of MHC-II deficient animals (Madsen et al. 1999) had a normal representation of GC B cells within the pool of B cells in PP and MLN (Fig. 5 and S. Casola and K. Rajewsky, unpublished results). In support of this observation, a recent report showed that on intranasal infection of mice with Influenza virus, normal antigen-specific mucosal IgA titers were produced in the absence of direct interactions between antigen-specific B cells and CD4$^+$ T cells through the MHC class II-TCR complex (Sangster et al. 2003).These results suggest that T cells other than conventional CD4$^+$ T-helper cells can support GC responses in the GALT. A possible candidate is represented by natural killer-T (NK-T) cells, which play a critical role in the regulation of both adaptive and innate immune responses in mice and humans (Kronenberg 2004). They represent a subset of thymus-derived, double-negative or CD4$^+$, T cells expressing a semi-invariant TCR repertoire selected by self-antigens (Zhou

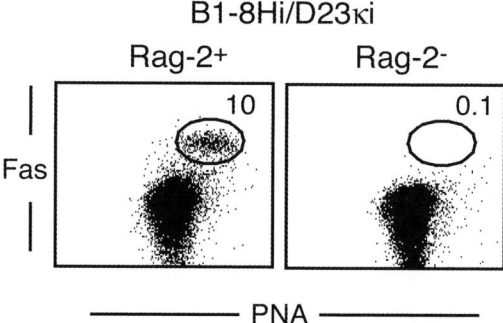

Fig. 4 Flow cytometric analysis of spontaneous GC responses in PP of B1-8Hi/3-83Ki BCR transgenic mice on either a Rag-2 proficient (rag-2$^+$) or deficient (rag-2$^-$) genetic background. Percentages of boxed GC B cells falling within the CD19$^+$ B cell gate are indicated

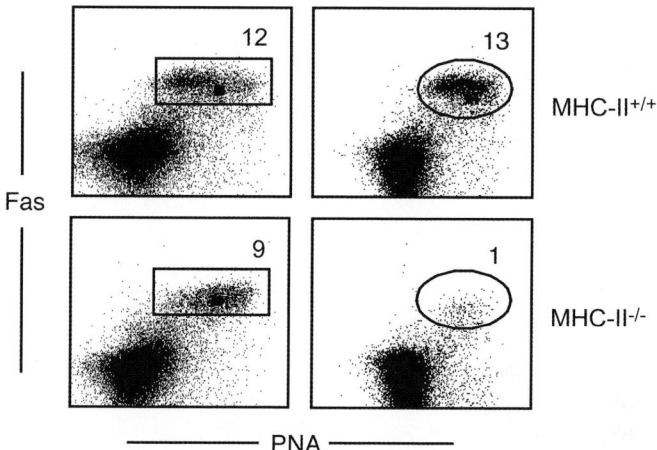

Fig. 5 Flow cytometric analysis of spontaneous GCs in GALT of MHC-class II deficient mice. Shown are PP CD19$^+$ gated B cells from representative cases of MHC class II mutant animals (on a C57BL/6 genetic background), either lacking or retaining a significant fraction of boxed GC B cells. Wild-type C57BL/6 mice obtained from the same animal husbandry were used as controls. *Numbers* indicate percentages of GC B cells falling within the CD19$^+$ B cell gate

et al. 2004) presented on the invariant MHC-class Ib molecule, CD1 (Brigl and Brenner 2004). A large fraction of NK-T cells is consistently found within the mucosal sites of the intestine (Kaser et al. 2004). Here, NK-T cells may become activated on recognition of self-ligands and/or microbial antigens presented by several CD1d-expressing cell types including DC, B cells, and enterocytes (Brigl et al. 2003; Kaser et al. 2004; Mattner et al. 2005). Experiments to analyze the contribution of NK-T cells in GALT GC responses are in progress.

The so-called mucosa-associated invariant T (MAIT) cells represent another subset of invariant T cells found in mucosal sites of the intestine (Treiner et al. 2005). MAIT cells originate in the thymus and are selected on the MHC-class I-like molecule MR1. Interestingly, the development of MAIT cells is strictly dependent on the commensal flora and on MR1-mediated antigen presentation by B cells (Treiner et al. 2005). So far no MR1-restricted self-ligand(s) has been identified. Future studies on MR1-deficient mice will determine whether MAIT cells contribute to GALT GC responses.

Thus, extrapolating from our own work and that of others, B cells in the GALT may receive T cell help through distinct, non-mutually exclusive mechanisms. GCs may be initiated upon conventional T-B cell interactions after BCR-mediated recognition, internalization, processing, and presentation of antigen to antigen-specific T cells by MHC class II molecules. This interaction likely involves conventional CD4$^+$ T helper cells. Alternatively, B cells may receive help from bystander T cells (CD4$^+$ T helper and/or NK-T, MAIT cells) activated in MLN and PP upon recognition of microbial antigens and/or self ligands presented to them by DC via MHC class II and/or MHC class I-like (CD1d, MR1) molecules. Activated T cells in GALT may trigger B cell re-

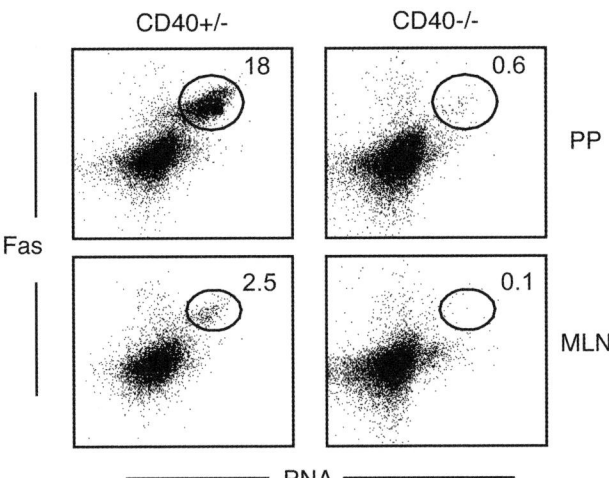

Fig. 6 CD40 deficiency leads to impairment of GALT GC responses. *Numbers* indicate percentages of GC B cells falling within the CD19$^+$ B cell gate as determined by flow cytometric analyses

cruitment into GCs by releasing Th$_2$-type cytokines such as IL-4, essential for GALT GC responses (Vajdy et al. 1995) and/ or by interacting with B cells through several costimulatory receptors including CD40L. A critical role for the CD40-CD40L interaction in the induction of GALT GCs is supported by the significant impairment in GALT GC responses observed in CD40-deficient mice (Fig. 6).

7
Principles of B Cell Selection in GALT GC

Within GCs, B cells undergo an initial stage of intense proliferation that is associated with the onset of somatic hypermutation (SHM) of IgH and IgL chain variable region genes. In response to cytokines produced by different cell types including T cells and DCs, a large fraction of GC B cells also activate germline transcription of IgH constant region genes downstream of Cμ and Cδ. In GALT, local production of TGF-β by T cells and other cell types drives GC B cells to transcribe preferentially the Cα locus, thus leading to IgA isotype switching (Cazac and Roes 2000; Weinstein et al. 1991).

What is the fate of the of B cells generated in the GC that express mutated BCRs?

In conventional T cell-dependent immune responses, a stringent selection process involving interactions with FDCs and T cells favors the survival of a limited set of mutated B cells, expressing antigen-specific, high-affinity BCRs. The remaining GC B cells that either lack a functional BCR or whose BCR has lost antigen specificity because of SHM die by apoptosis (MacLennan 1994).

In GALT GCs, the nature and extent of microbial stimulation, together with the particular cytokine milieu produced by activated B, T, DCs, and epithelial cells, may significantly interfere with clonal selection of high-affinity mutants. Rather, the continuous availability of non-limiting amounts of gut-derived microbial determinants, exposed on the surface of FDC, may support the survival and expansion of B cells within GCs in the absence of antigen-driven affinity maturation, through interactions with innate immune receptors. In this context, a "tonic" BCR signal is likely still essential for the survival of the cells (Kraus et al. 2004), such that only BCR-positive, potentially functional cells persist. Alternatively, poly/oligoclonal expansion of somatically mutated B cells in GALT GCs may result from signals originating from BCR interactions with bacterial or self-encoded superantigens through V$_H$ framework regions, as recently suggested (Rhee et al. 2005). The existence of a putative superantigen of self or bacterial origin in mouse GALT GCs remains to be demonstrated. This general scenario predicts that B cells leaving GCs in the GALT express a broad repertoire of somatically mutated BCRs, whose specificities would only partly be generated through classic affinity maturation, although it is still possible that antigen recognition through the BCR is required for the cells to transit into a post-GC compartment. A further step of selection of the cells on the basis of antigen recognition could be their "trapping" in the LP of the gut, where plasmablasts expressing somatically mutated IgA antibodies of a restricted repertoire are indeed found (Stoel et al. 2005). Thus the LP, in addition to the GC light zone, may serve as a site of B cell positive selection, where GALT GC emigrants [which specifically migrate into this location (Craig and Cebra 1971)] are selected by an ever-changing antigenic environment that originates from the gut flora, and where cells expressing "useless" BCRs are eliminated (Husband and Gowans 1978), like T cells lacking specificity for self in the thymus. Overall, an efficient system of antibody-based defense against gut-borne infections would result, in which invading pathogens would encounter both a polyclonal population of B cells expanding in GC and ready to undergo rapid affinity maturation in response to the infection and, potentially, post-GC IgA$^+$ B cells in the LP selected on the basis of a previous encounter of the same or a cross-reacting pathogen. This system would also be able to contain the commensal flora in the gut such that it peacefully coexists with the host. Indeed, antibodies against commensal bacteria of the gut are present in the "natural" sIgA produced by B cells in the GALT (Macpherson et al. 2000).

Acknowledgements This work was supported by the National Institutes of Health (RO1-CA 098285001A1 and RO1-A1054636-01). S. Casola was supported in part by the Human Frontier Science Program and the Cancer Research Institute.

References

Akira S, Takeda K (2004). Toll-like receptor signalling. Nat Rev Immunol 4, 499–511.

Becker RS, Knight KL (1990). Somatic diversification of immunoglobulin heavy chain VDJ genes: evidence for somatic gene conversion in rabbits. Cell 63, 987–997.

Bos NA, Bun JC, Popma SH, Cebra ER, Deenen GJ, van der Cammen MJ, Kroese FG, Cebra JJ (1996). Monoclonal immunoglobulin A derived from peritoneal B cells is encoded by both germ line and somatically mutated VH genes and is reactive with commensal bacteria. Infect Immun 64, 616–623.

Brigl M, Brenner MB (2004). CD1: antigen presentation and T cell function. Annu Rev Immunol 22, 817–890.

Brigl M, Bry L, Kent SC, Gumperz JE, Brenner MB (2003). Mechanism of CD1d-restricted natural killer T cell activation during microbial infection. Nat Immunol 4, 1230–1237.

Caldwell RG, Wilson JB, Anderson SJ, Longnecker R (1998). Epstein-Barr virus LMP2A drives B cell development and survival in the absence of normal B cell receptor signals. Immunity 9, 405–411.
Casola S, Otipoby KL, Alimzhanov M, Humme S, Uyttersprot N, Kutok JL, Carroll MC, Rajewsky K (2004). B cell receptor signal strength determines B cell fate. Nat Immunol 5, 317–327.
Cazac BB, Roes J (2000). TGF-β receptor controls B cell responsiveness and induction of IgA in vivo. Immunity 13, 443–451.
Cebra JJ (1999). Influences of microbiota on intestinal immune system development. Am J Clin Nutr 69, 1046S-1051S.
Craig SW, Cebra JJ (1971). Peyer's patches: an enriched source of precursors for IgA-producing immunocytes in the rabbit. J Exp Med 134, 188–200.
Fagarasan S, Kinoshita K, Muramatsu M, Ikuta K, Honjo T (2001). In situ class switching and differentiation to IgA-producing cells in the gut lamina propria. Nature 413, 639–643.
Fagarasan S, Shinkura R, Kamata T, Nogaki F, Ikuta K, Honjo T (2000). Mechanism of B1 cell differentiation and migration in GALT. Curr Top Microbiol Immunol 252, 221–229.
Fruehling S, Longnecker R (1997). The immunoreceptor tyrosine-based activation motif of Epstein-Barr virus LMP2A is essential for blocking BCR-mediated signal transduction. Virology 235, 241–251.
Husband AJ, Gowans JL (1978). The origin and antigen-dependent distribution of IgA-containing cells in the intestine. J Exp Med 148, 1146–1160.
Kaser A, Nieuwenhuis EE, Strober W, Mayer L, Fuss I, Colgan S, Blumberg RS (2004). Natural killer T cells in mucosal homeostasis. Ann N Y Acad Sci 1029, 154–168.
Kearney JF, Lawton AR (1975). B lymphocyte differentiation induced by lipopolysaccharide. I. Generation of cells synthesizing four major immunoglobulin classes. J Immunol 115, 671–676.
Koni PA, Flavell RA (1999). Lymph node germinal centers form in the absence of follicular dendritic cell networks. J Exp Med 189, 855–864.
Kraehenbuhl JP, Neutra MR (1992). Transepithelial transport and mucosal defence II: secretion of IgA. Trends Cell Biol 2, 170–174.
Kraus M, Alimzhanov MB, Rajewsky N, Rajewsky K (2004). Survival of resting mature B lymphocytes depends on BCR signaling via the Igα/β heterodimer. Cell 117, 787–800.
Krieg AM, Yi AK, Matson S, Waldschmidt TJ, Bishop GA, Teasdale R, Koretzky GA, Klinman DM (1995). CpG motifs in bacterial DNA trigger direct B-cell activation. Nature 374, 546–549.
Kroese FG, Butcher EC, Stall AM, Lalor PA, Adams S, Herzenberg LA (1989). Many of the IgA producing plasma cells in murine gut are derived from self-replenishing precursors in the peritoneal cavity. Int Immunol 1, 75–84.
Kronenberg M (2004). Toward an understanding of NKT cell biology: progress and paradoxes. Annu Rev Immunol.
Lanning D, Zhu X, Zhai SK, Knight KL (2000). Development of the antibody repertoire in rabbit: gut-associated lymphoid tissue, microbes, and selection. Immunol Rev 175, 214–228.
MacLennan IC (1994). Germinal centers. Annu Rev Immunol 12, 117–139.

Macpherson AJ, Gatto D, Sainsbury E, Harriman GR, Hengartner H, Zinkernagel RM (2000). A primitive T cell-independent mechanism of intestinal mucosal IgA responses to commensal bacteria. Science 288, 2222–2226.

Macpherson AJ, Uhr T (2004). Induction of protective IgA by intestinal dendritic cells carrying commensal bacteria. Science 303, 1662–1665.

Madsen L, Labrecque N, Engberg J, Dierich A, Svejgaard A, Benoist C, Mathis D, Fugger L (1999). Mice lacking all conventional MHC class II genes. Proc Natl Acad Sci USA 96, 10338–10343.

Mattner J, Debord KL, Ismail N, Goff RD, Cantu C, 3rd, Zhou D, Saint-Mezard P, Wang V, Gao Y, Yin, N., et al. (2005). Exogenous and endogenous glycolipid antigens activate NKT cells during microbial infections. Nature 434, 525–529.

Miller CL, Burkhardt AL, Lee JH, Stealey B, Longnecker R, Bolen JB, Kieff E (1995). Integral membrane protein 2 of Epstein-Barr virus regulates reactivation from latency through dominant negative effects on protein-tyrosine kinases. Immunity 2, 155–166.

Muramatsu M, Kinoshita K, Fagarasan S, Yamada S, Shinkai Y, Honjo T (2000). Class switch recombination and hypermutation require activation-induced cytidine deaminase (AID), a potential RNA editing enzyme. Cell 102, 553–563.

Pospisil R, Mage RG (1998). Rabbit appendix: a site of development and selection of the B cell repertoire. Curr Top Microbiol Immunol 229, 59–70.

Rajewsky K (1996). Clonal selection and learning in the antibody system. Nature 381, 751–758.

Rescigno M, Urbano M, Valzasina B, Francolini M, Rotta G, Bonasio R, Granucci F, Kraehenbuhl JP, Ricciardi-Castagnoli P (2001). Dendritic cells express tight junction proteins and penetrate gut epithelial monolayers to sample bacteria. Nat Immunol 2, 361–367.

Reynaud CA, Anquez V, Grimal H, Weill JC (1987). A hyperconversion mechanism generates the chicken light chain preimmune repertoire. Cell 48, 379–388.

Reynaud CA, Bertocci B, Dahan A, Weill JC (1994). Formation of the chicken B-cell repertoire: ontogenesis, regulation of Ig gene rearrangement, and diversification by gene conversion. Adv Immunol 57, 353–378.

Reynaud CA, Mackay CR, Muller RG, Weill JC (1991). Somatic generation of diversity in a mammalian primary lymphoid organ: the sheep ileal Peyer's patches. Cell 64, 995–1005.

Reynaud CA, Weill JC (1996). Postrearrangement diversification processes in gut-associated lymphoid tissues. Curr Top Microbiol Immunol 212, 7–15.

Rhee KJ, Jasper PJ, Sethupathi P, Shanmugam M, Lanning D, Knight KL (2005). Positive selection of the peripheral B cell repertoire in gut-associated lymphoid tissues. J Exp Med 201, 55–62.

Rhee KJ, Sethupathi P, Driks A, Lanning DK, Knight KL (2004). Role of commensal bacteria in development of gut-associated lymphoid tissues and preimmune antibody repertoire. J Immunol 172, 1118–1124.

Sangster MY, Riberdy JM, Gonzalez M, Topham DJ, Baumgarth N, Doherty PC (2003). An early CD4+ T cell-dependent immunoglobulin A response to influenza infection in the absence of key cognate T-B interactions. J Exp Med 198, 1011–1021.

Shikina T, Hiroi T, Iwatani K, Jang MH, Fukuyama S, Tamura M, Kubo T, Ishikawa H, Kiyono H (2004). IgA class switch occurs in the organized nasopharynx- and gut-associated lymphoid tissue, but not in the diffuse lamina propria of airways and gut. J Immunol *172*, 6259–6264.

Shroff KE, Cebra JJ (1995). Development of mucosal humoral immune responses in germ-free (GF) mice. Adv Exp Med Biol *371A*, 441–446.

Shroff KE, Meslin K, Cebra JJ (1995). Commensal enteric bacteria engender a self-limiting humoral mucosal immune response while permanently colonizing the gut. Infect Immun *63*, 3904–3913.

Stoel M, Jiang HQ, van Diemen CC, Bun JC, Dammers PM, Thurnheer MC, Kroese FG, Cebra JJ, Bos NA (2005). Restricted IgA repertoire in both B-1 and B-2 cell-derived gut plasmablasts. J Immunol *174*, 1046–1054.

Talham GL, Jiang HQ, Bos NA, Cebra JJ (1999). Segmented filamentous bacteria are potent stimuli of a physiologically normal state of the murine gut mucosal immune system. Infect Immun *67*, 1992–2000.

Thompson CB, Neiman PE (1987). Somatic diversification of the chicken immunoglobulin light chain gene is limited to the rearranged variable gene segment. Cell *48*, 369–378.

Thorley-Lawson DA (2001). Epstein-Barr virus: exploiting the immune system. Nat Rev Immunol *1*, 75–82.

Thurnheer MC, Zuercher AW, Cebra JJ, Bos NA (2003). B1 cells contribute to serum IgM, but not to intestinal IgA, production in gnotobiotic Ig allotype chimeric mice. J Immunol *170*, 4564–4571.

Treiner E, Duban L, Moura IC, Hansen T, Gilfillan S, Lantz O (2005). Mucosal-associated invariant T (MAIT) cells: an evolutionarily conserved T cell subset. Microbes Infect, in press.

Vajdy M, Kosco-Vilbois MH, Kopf M, Kohler G, Lycke N (1995). Impaired mucosal immune responses in interleukin 4-targeted mice. J Exp Med *181*, 41–53.

Walport MJ (2001). Complement. First of two parts. N Engl J Med *344*, 1058–1066.

Weinstein PD, Anderson AO, Mage RG (1994). Rabbit IgH sequences in appendix germinal centers: VH diversification by gene conversion-like and hypermutation mechanisms. Immunity *1*, 647–659.

Weinstein PD, Schweitzer PA, Cebra-Thomas JA, Cebra JJ (1991). Molecular genetic features reflecting the preference for isotype switching to IgA expression by Peyer's patch germinal center B cells. Int Immunol *3*, 1253–1263.

Weltzin R, Lucia-Jandris P, Michetti P, Fields BN, Kraehenbuhl JP, Neutra MR (1989). Binding and transepithelial transport of immunoglobulins by intestinal M cells: demonstration using monoclonal IgA antibodies against enteric viral proteins. J Cell Biol *108*, 1673–1685.

Zhou D, Mattner J, Cantu C, 3rd, Schrantz N, Yin N, Gao Y, Sagiv Y, Hudspeth K, Wu YP, Yamashita T, et al. (2004). Lysosomal glycosphingolipid recognition by NKT cells. Science *306*, 1786–1789.

Structural Insights into Antibody-Mediated Mucosal Immunity

A. E. Hamburger[1] · P. J. Bjorkman[1,2] · A. B. Herr[3] (✉)

[1]Division of Biology, California Institute of Technology, 114-96, Pasadena, CA 91125, USA

[2]Howard Hughes Medical Institute, California Institute of Technology, Pasadena, CA 91125, USA

[3]Department of Molecular Genetics, Biochemistry and Microbiology, University of Cincinnati College of Medicine, 231 Albert Sabin Way, Cincinnati, OH 45267-0524, USA
Andrew.Herr@UC.edu

1	Introduction	174
2	**Antibody Structure and Function**	176
2.1	Antibody Structures	176
2.2	Antibodies of the Mucosae	177
2.3	IgA Structure	179
2.4	Polymeric IgA and IgM	183
2.5	Joining (J) Chain	186
3	**Fc Receptors Implicated in Mucosal Immunity**	187
3.1	pIgR Function	187
3.2	pIgR D1 Structure	189
3.3	IgA–Receptor Interactions: Implications for Signaling	191
4	**Pathogen Evasion of Host Mucosal Immunity**	192
4.1	IgA1 Proteases	192
4.2	IgA-Binding Proteins	193
4.3	pIgR-Binding Proteins	194
5	**Future Directions**	195
References		195

Abstract The mucosal regions of the body are responsible for defense against environmental pathogens. Particularly in the lumen of the gut, antibody-mediated immune responses are critical for preventing invasion by pathogens. In this chapter, we review structural studies that have illuminated various aspects of mucosal immunity. Crystal structures of IgA1-Fc and IgA-binding fragments of the polymeric immunoglobulin receptor and FcαRI, combined with models of intact IgA and IgM from solution scattering studies, reveal potential mechanisms for immune exclusion and induction of inflammatory responses. Other recent structures yield insights into bacterial mechanisms for evasion of the host immune response.

Abbreviations

SIgA	Secretory IgA
SIgM	Secretory IgM
Ig	Immunoglobulin
pIgR	Polymeric Ig receptor
SC	Secretory component
Fab	Antigen-binding fragment
Fc	Crystallizable fragment
Fcγ	Fc fragment of IgG
Fcε	Fc fragment of IgE
pIgA	Polymeric IgA
J chain	Joining chain
ADCC	Antibody-dependent cell-mediated cytotoxicity
FcR	Fc receptor
ITAM	Immunoreceptor tyrosine activation motif
Fcα	Fc fragment of IgA
pIg	Polymeric Ig
dIgA	Dimeric IgA
Fcμ	Fc fragment of IgM
MDCK	Madin-Darby canine kidney
CD	Circular dichroism
cDNA	Complementary DNA
D1	Domain 1
CDR	Complementarity-determining region
KIR	Killer cell Ig-like receptor
LIR	Leukocyte Ig-like receptor
FcRn	Neonatal Fc receptor
SSL7	Staphylococcal superantigen-like protein 7
OB	Oligonucleotide/oligosaccharide-binding
CbpA	Choline-binding protein A
EBV	Epstein-Barr virus
NMR	Nuclear magnetic resonance

1
Introduction

In humans, the mucosal regions of the body represent the first line of defense against many pathogens, including those that are ingested or inhaled. The mucosae form an intermediate zone in the body that separates the external environment from the internal systems of the body. The unique requirements of this boundary zone dictate certain characteristics of the mucosal immune response. Rather than mounting a robust inflammatory response, the primary goal in the mucosae is preventing pathogens from adhering to and invading the thin mucosal epithelial layer that protects the interior region of the body. This distinction is particularly critical in the gut, which contains a high bacterial load, encompassing pathogens as well as benign commensal bacteria. A chronic inflammatory response to commensal bacteria would itself compromise the integrity of the mucosal epithelial barrier. The mucosal immune response is therefore a specialized subset of the immune system capable of meeting these varied requirements. Mucosal immunity, particularly in the lumen of the gut, is primarily mediated by humoral rather than cellular responses, and important roles are played by secretory IgA (SIgA) and IgM (SIgM) antibodies.

SIgA and SIgM are produced via specific transcytosis of polymeric forms of IgA and IgM across the mucosal epithelium by the polymeric Ig receptor (pIgR) (Mostov 1994). Once transcytosed, the pIgR ectodomain (called secretory component, SC) is cleaved, releasing the SC-bound antibody, known as secretory Ig, into mucosal secretions (Norderhaug et al. 1999). In addition to its role in transcytosis of pIgs, SC protects secretory antibodies from proteolytic cleavage in the harsh environment of the mucosae (Crottet and Corthesy 1998) and anchors SIgA within the mucus layer overlaying epithelial cells, which facilitates immune exclusion of bacterial pathogens (Fernandez et al. 2003). SIgA and, to some extent, SIgM function as the immune system's first line of defense in mucosal secretions by binding to pathogens and sterically blocking their adherence to, and invasion of, mucosal epithelial cells, a process known as immune exclusion (Brandtzaeg et al. 1999; Monteiro and van de Winkel 2003). SIgA also plays an important role in antigen sampling in the gut by delivering intestinal antigens to submucosal gut-associated lymphoid tissue via an IgA2-specific M cell receptor in Peyer's patches (Mantis et al. 2002). Despite steric hindrance resulting from binding SIgA, pathogens do occasionally breach the mucosal epithelium; in these cases, serum IgA, as well as other antibody isotypes, can recognize the pathogen and trigger a robust inflammatory response. Pathogen-bound serum IgA antibodies, which lack SC, can activate potent inflammatory responses via the IgA-specific receptor FcαRI (Monteiro et al. 1990; van Egmond et al. 2000). In contrast, SIgA antibodies do not trigger FcαRI except in the presence of an integrin coreceptor, consistent with the primarily passive role SIgA plays in immune exclusion (van Egmond et al. 2000; van Spriel et al. 2001; Vidarsson et al. 2001). Bacteria have evolved several mechanisms to evade IgA-mediated immune responses, both in the gut and in the serum. These include the secretion of IgA1-specific proteases by several bacterial genera (Plaut et al. 1975), release of IgA-binding proteins that mask the FcαRI-binding site by *Streptococcus* and *Staphylococcus* species (Pleass et al. 2001; Langley et al. 2005), and expression of a choline-binding protein by *Streptococcus pneumoniae* that binds to the pIgR ectodomain and allows *S. pneumoniae* to hijack its way into the mucosal epithelium (Zhang et al. 2000).

High-resolution structures of IgG, IgE, IgA, and IgM antibody fragments and even intact IgG antibodies have been known for several years. Until recently, however, there was a paucity of information on structural aspects of mucosal immunity. In the last few years, there have been several advances in the structural biology of IgA, Fc receptors, and bacterial proteins involved in evasion of the IgA-mediated immune response. This review focuses on these recent structural studies that have illuminated important aspects of antibody-mediated mucosal immune responses and bacterial evasion of host mucosal immunity.

2
Antibody Structure and Function

2.1
Antibody Structures

All antibodies exhibit a similar basic architecture, with two light chains and two heavy chains. Each light chain contains an N-terminal variable and a C-terminal constant region, whereas the heavy chain contains one N-terminal variable and three or four C-terminal regions. In simple terms, the conformation of most antibodies can be thought of as a capital letter Y, in which each of the two arms of the Y corresponds to an antigen-binding fragment (Fab) and the base of the Y corresponds to the Fc region (called the crystallizable fragment, based on the propensity of IgG-Fc to form crystals). Each Fab is composed of a light chain and the two N-terminal Ig domains of a heavy chain and is connected by a hinge region to the Fc, which is a dimer of the two C-terminal domains of each heavy chain. Regions of highly variable sequence within the light and heavy chains in each Fab combine to form a specific antigen-binding site, whereas the Fc region is comprised of constant regions of the heavy chains and interacts with isotype-specific Fc receptors. Fc receptors are responsible for a number of important biological processes including activation of immune effector functions, transport of antibodies to specific cellular locations, and protection of secretory antibodies from proteolytic degradation. The five human classes of antibody (IgG, IgE, IgD, IgM, and IgA) are defined by the features of their heavy chains, which differ in their sequences, the number and position of their disulfide bonds, the number and type of carbohydrates attached, the length of their hinge regions, and the number of C-terminal domains (Janeway et al. 1999). High-resolution structures of intact IgG (Harris et al. 1992, 1998) and fragments of IgG (Huber et al. 1976; Matsushima et al. 1978), IgA (Satow et al. 1986; Suh et al. 1986; Herr et al. 2003), IgM (Corper et al. 1997), and IgE (Wurzburg et al. 2000; Wan et al. 2002) have been solved by X-ray crystallography, as well as low-resolution structures of intact IgA1 (Boehm et al. 1999), IgA2 (Furtado et al. 2004), and IgM (Perkins et al. 1991) by small-angle X-ray and neutron scattering.

IgG, the most abundant serum Ig, was the first antibody isotype for which high-resolution structural information became available. Crystal structures of IgG Fab fragments and Fab-antigen complexes revealed a four-domain β-barrel arrangement and showed that, in some cases, the antibody combining site is a concave pocket into which the antigen binds. In other cases, portions of the antibody protrude into the antigen (reviewed in Wilson et al. 1991). IgG-Fc fragments (called Fcγ) also have four β-barrel Ig domains with extensive contact surface between the Cγ3 domains and no protein-protein contacts between the Cγ2 domains (Huber et al. 1976). An N-linked carbohydrate attached to the inner surface of the Cγ2 domain interacts with the domain through both polar and hydrophobic residues (Deisenhofer 1981). The N-glycans attached to each heavy chain occupy the space between the Cγ2 domains and mediate the proper domain orientation required for binding to Fcγ receptors (Fig. 2a). Intact IgG structures have provided several snapshots of these flexible molecules with an overall Y or T shape but each with an asymmetric arrangement of the Fab and Fc fragments, consistent with the flexible nature of antibodies (Harris et al. 199, 1998). Another antibody isotype, IgE, is present at low concentrations in serum and primarily targets parasites. The interaction of IgE with its receptor is responsible for inflammation and allergic reactions. The crystal structure of IgE-Fc (Fcε) revealed that the overall structure is very similar to Fcγ, including the position of the N-linked carbohydrate between the Cε3 domains, which is an analogous location to the carbohydrate on Cγ2 in IgG (Garman et al. 2000; Wurzburg et al. 2000). However, IgE (and IgM) contain an Ig domain in place of the flexible hinge region, and the crystal structure of Fcε containing this hingelike Ig domain revealed that it is folded back onto the surface of the Fc region, presumably introducing a pronounced bend in the intact IgE structure (Wan et al. 2002).

2.2
Antibodies of the Mucosae

IgA is found in both serum and mucosal secretions and is the most abundant human Ig isotype overall, as well as the principal mucosal antibody (Kerr 1990). Indeed, more IgA is produced in adult humans per day than all other antibody isotypes combined (Monteiro and van de Winkel 2003). IgA in mucosal secretions has been described as the "first line of defense" of the immune system against pathogens, and serum IgA forms a "second line of defense" against those pathogens that have penetrated the epithelial barrier (van Egmond et al. 2000). Serum IgA is predominantly found in the so-called monomeric form (actually a heterotetramer of two heavy and two light chains), although approximately five to ten percent of serum IgA is polymeric. Polymeric IgA (pIgA) is composed of two or more IgA monomers linked by disulfide bonds between a small protein called J ("joining") chain and C-terminal extensions called the tailpieces on each IgA monomer. Polymeric IgA is delivered to mucosal secretions by pIgR, a receptor that actively transcytoses J chain-containing pIgs from the basolateral side to the apical surface of epithelial cells (Mostov 1994). Once in secretions, SIgA binds pathogens and their toxins and prevents their attachment to, and invasion of, the host. SIgA can neutralize pathogens by directly blocking interactions between bacterial adhesins and their cellular receptors or by inhibiting the movement of the bacteria by cross-linking them or interacting with their flagella (reviewed in Lamm 1997). Binding can occur specifically to defined antigens by the IgA antigen-binding site (Outlaw and Dimmock 1990; Armstrong and Dimmock 1992; Lamm 1997) or nonspecifically to bacterial lectins by carbohydrate moieties in the hinge region of IgA1 or on pIgR (Wold et al. 1990). In addition to its barrier function in mucosal secretions, SIgA is also a major component in human breast milk and provides passive immunization to newborns (reviewed in Brandtzaeg 2003; van de Perre 2003; Cleary 2004).

IgA has long been considered noninflammatory because it does not bind and activate complement by the classic pathway (Russell et al. 1989; Kaetzel et al. 1991). However, many studies have now shown that aggregated serum IgA triggers cellular functions similar to IgG such as phagocytosis, antibody-dependent cell-mediated cytotoxicity (ADCC), degranulation, and respiratory burst after binding to its receptor, FcαRI (reviewed in Monteiro and van de Winkel 2003). Intracellular signaling by IgA, IgG, and IgE receptors is transduced via the same coreceptor, the FcR γ chain, which contains a cytoplasmic immunoreceptor tyrosine activation motif (ITAM) that recruits SH2-containing signaling molecules (Monteiro and van de Winkel 2003). Monomeric and dimeric forms of IgA, but not SIgA, can elicit strong inflammatory responses via FcαRI; however, SIgA is unable to trigger FcαRI except in the presence of an integrin coreceptor (van Egmond et al. 2000; van Spriel et al. 2001; Vidarsson et al. 2001). As described above, the main function of SIgA is immune exclusion at mucosal surfaces, where the body is in constant contact with antigens from pathogens but also commensal bacteria and ingested food. Therefore, it would actually be disadvantageous for SIgA to elicit inflammatory signals to foreign substances because the body would be in a constant state of mucosal inflammation, which would eventually damage the protective barrier of the epithelial lining. However, the ability of serum IgA to trigger these cellular functions when pathogens have breached the epithelium provides additional protection in the serum. Recent work has indicated that FcαRI itself is able to mediate both inflammatory and noninflammatory responses, depending on the extent of receptor clustering. Transient crosslinking of FcαRI leads to recruitment of the tyrosine phosphatase SHP-1 and inhibition of FcγR and FcεRI signaling, whereas prolonged FcαRI clustering due to multivalent interactions with antigen-bound IgA recruits the Syk kinase, displacing SHP-1 and triggering downstream inflammatory responses (Pasquier et al. 2005). The structural basis for the ability of monomeric and dimeric IgA but not SIgA to initiate phagocytosis is described below.

IgM, the first antibody produced in the humoral response to infection, is present in both serum and mucosal secretions (Janeway et al. 1999). Although SIgA is the primary Ig in secretions, SIgM is also present at lower concentrations and clears pathogens via similar mechanisms (Norderhaug et al. 1999). Serum IgM is able to activate the classic complement pathway very effectively, whereas SIgM in mucosal secretions does not (Davis et al. 1988; Randall et al. 1990; Wiersma et al. 1998). In patients with IgA deficiency, IgM is thought to substitute for the function of IgA (Brandtzaeg et al. 1987). A small percentage of plasma cells in the lamina propria secrete IgG. Although there is no known active transport of IgG to mucosal secretions in humans, damage to the epithelial layer can result in passively transferred IgG molecules, particularly at mucosal surfaces with low proteolytic activity such as the respiratory and reproductive tracts. Therefore, IgG provides some, albeit minimal, protection at mucosal surfaces (Lamm 1997; Norderhaug et al. 1999).

2.3
IgA Structure

IgA has two subclasses, IgA1 and IgA2, that differ from each other in the number of N-linked oligosaccharide attachment sites and in the length of the hinge region. IgA1 contains a heavily O-glycosylated 23-residue hinge region and two N-linked glycosylation sites, whereas IgA2 has a 13-residue deletion, including the five O-linked glycosylation sites, in the hinge region compared to IgA1 and contains additional N-linked oligosaccharide attachment sites. Serum IgA is predominantly monomeric IgA1, whereas mucosal IgA is mainly dimeric with a relative increase in IgA2 (Kett et al. 1986; Mestecky and McGhee 1987; Kerr 1990). Early electron microscopic studies of IgA revealed a domain arrangement of Fab and Fc fragments similar to that of IgG (Svehag and Bloth

1970). More recently, structural models derived from small-angle X-ray and neutron solution scattering experiments have provided more detailed information about the orientation of the Fab and Fc domains in both IgA1 (Boehm et al. 1999) and IgA2 (Furtado et al. 2004). Interestingly, the best-fit model of IgA1 has a significantly extended conformation for the hinge region (Boehm et al. 1999) (Fig. 1a). As described below, the hinge region of IgA1 is a target of a number of bacterial IgA1-specific proteases. Consistent with the 13-residue deletion in the IgA2 hinge region, the solution structure of IgA2 reveals a more compact structure than seen for IgA1 (Furtado et al. 2004) (Fig. 1b). The difference in hinge regions between IgA1 and IgA2 results in significantly different spacing and orientation of the two Fab regions of the two antibody subtypes (Fig. 1c). This may allow IgA1 and IgA2 to recognize a wider range of antigens on the surface of different pathogens, such as viruses and bacteria (Furtado et al. 2004). The solution scattering studies also indicated that the best fit to the data was obtained when the C-terminal 18-residue extension (the tailpiece) in both IgA1 and IgA2 is folded up against the Cα3 domain rather than extended from the base of the Fc region (Boehm et al. 1999; Furtado et al. 2004).

Although a high-resolution crystal structure of intact IgA is not presently available, crystal structures of Fab and Fc fragments from IgA have been solved. Murine Fab fragment crystal structures confirmed the β-sandwich conformation expected, similar to a number of IgG Fab structures (Satow et al. 1986; Suh et al. 1986). A recent crystal structure of IgA1-Fc (Fcα), however, has revealed notable differences between Fcα and previously determined structures of Fcγ and Fcε (Fig. 2a,b) (Herr et al. 2003). It should be noted that the structure of free Fcα has not yet been reported; the Fcα structure described here was extracted from the cocrystal structure of Fcα in complex with the FcαRI receptor (Herr et al. 2003). The overall architectures of Fcα, Fcγ, and Fcε are very similar: like Fcγ and Fcε, the Fcα region is formed by two heavy chains comprised of Ig domains, called Cα2 and Cα3. As with all known Fc structures, the Cα3 domains at the base of the Fc region form an extensive noncovalent dimer interface, which buries over 2,000 Å^2 of accessible surface area. However, the location of N-linked glycans in Fcα is significantly different from that observed in Fcγ and Fcε. Both Fcγ and Fcε have a conserved N-linked glycosylation site on each heavy chain (at Asn297 on the Cγ2 domain of Fcγ or the analogous residue Asn394 on the Cε3 domain of Fcε). The N-glycans from each heavy chain are located in the interior cavity between the Cγ2 (or Cε3) domains, preventing these domains from coming into direct contact (Fig. 2a). Indeed, the separation of these domains mediated by the N-glycans is necessary for binding of Fcγ or Fcε to their cognate Fc receptors, as seen in the crystal structures of Fcγ bound to FcγRIII (Sondermann et al. 2000) and Fcε bound to FcεRI (Garman et al. 2000). In contrast, the N-linked glycosylation

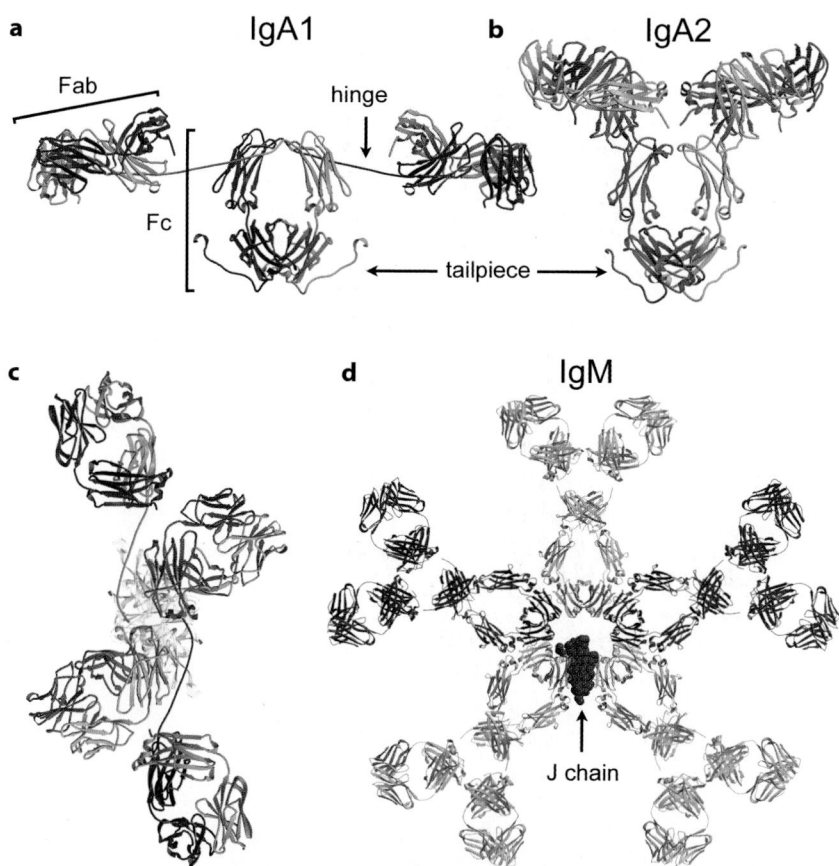

Fig. 1a–d Solution structures of intact IgA and IgM. **a** Structure of IgA1 determined by solution scattering (Boehm et al. 1999). Note the extended hinge region and the wide separation of Fab regions. **b** Structure of IgA2 determined by solution scattering (Furtado et al. 2004). **c** Top view of IgA1 (*blue/magenta*) and IgA2 (*tan/green*) after superposition of their Fc regions. Note the distinct Fab positions in the two IgA isotypes. **d** Solution structure of pentameric IgM with J chain (Perkins et al. 1991). Alternating IgM monomers are colored *blue* and *green*, and the J chain model is shown as *red spheres*

site on Fcα is at Asn263, which is located on the exterior surface of the Cα2 domain (Fig. 2b). The N-glycan extends downward from the Cα2 domain and contacts the Cα3 domain as well, unlike the glycans of Fcγ and Fcε. Because of their unusual location, the N-glycans of IgA are solvent accessible and would easily be able to interact with other macromolecules. This is consistent with reports that IgA can activate the lectin complement pathway (Roos et al. 2001)

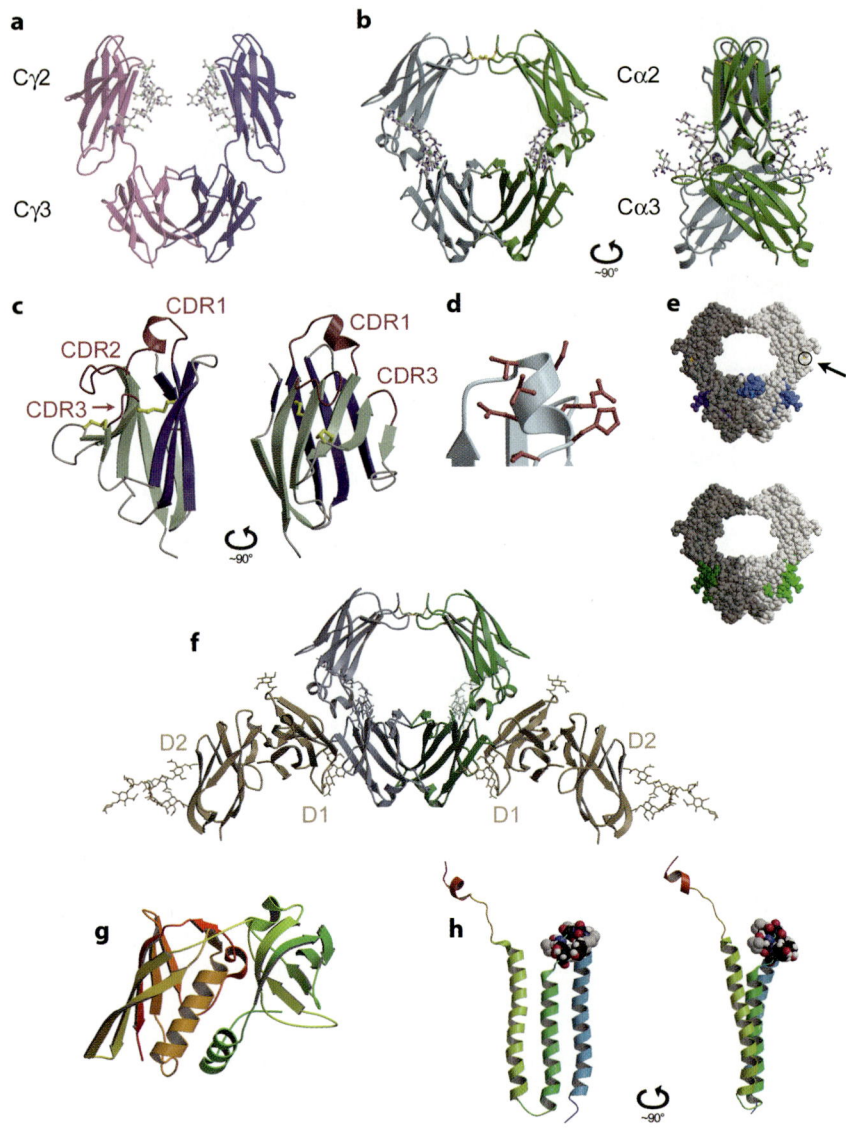

Fig. 2a–h Crystal structures of proteins involved in mucosal immunity. **a** Crystal structure of Fcγ (DeLano et al. 2000). Note the position of N-linked glycans between the Cγ2 domains. **b** Crystal structure of Fcα taken from the FcαRI-Fcα complex (Herr et al. 2003), shown in front and side views. Note the external location of the N-linked glycans and the disulfide bonds tethering the Cα2 domains. **c** Crystal structure of pIgR D1, with the CDR loops shown in *red* (Hamburger et al. 2004). **d** CDR1 residues of pIgR D1 implicated in binding to dIgA. **e** Binding sites for pIgR (*blue*) and FcαRI (*green*) mapped onto the surface of Fcα (*gray*). Note that the two binding sites overlap, specifically in the FG loop region. The *arrow* indicates the location of Cys311, which forms a disulfide bond with D5 of SC in SIgA. **f** Crystal structure of the FcαRI-Fcα complex (Herr et al. 2003). Two FcαRI molecules bind the Fcα dimer, one at each Cα2-Cα3 interface. **g** Crystal structure of SSL7, a staphylococcal IgA-binding protein (Al-Shangiti et al. 2004). The N-terminal OB domain is shown in *green*, and the C-terminal β-grasp domain is shown in red/orange. The putative IgA- or C5-binding site is found on the external surface of the OB domain (Langley et al. 2005). **h** NMR solution structure of the R2 repeat of *S. pneumoniae* CbpA, which binds pIgR and mediates invasion by reverse transcytosis (Luo et al. 2004). Residues in the hexapeptide motif that contribute to formation of the hydrophobic cluster implicated in pIgR binding are shown as *spheres*

and that N-glycans are important for IgA1 binding to the transferrin receptor (Moura et al. 2004). Residue 299 of Fcα, which is analogous to Asn297 of Fcγ (to which the N-glycans attach), is instead a cysteine. Cys299 of each IgA heavy chain forms an interdomain disulfide bond with Cys242 of the opposite heavy chain, resulting in two interchain disulfide bonds that tether the Cα2 domains together to form a small Cα2-Cα2 interface (275 Å^2 total buried surface area). The tethered orientation of the two Cα2 domains is in contrast to the separation of the Cγ2 and the counterpart Cε3 domains required for binding to the FcγRIII and FcεRI receptors; it is perhaps no surprise then that the primary IgA-specific inflammatory Fc receptor, FcαRI, uses a different binding mode for IgA recognition (Herr et al. 2003), as described below. Although there are additional differences between IgA and IgG or IgE in the hinge and tailpiece regions, the Fcα construct crystallized did not include either the tailpiece or the hinge, so detailed information on the conformation of these regions awaits further structural developments.

2.4
Polymeric IgA and IgM

IgA and IgM, unlike IgG, IgD and IgE, are unique in that they can form higher-order oligomers. Serum IgA is predominantly monomeric along with a small percentage of J chain-linked polymeric species (Monteiro and van de Winkel

2003). In contrast, mucosal IgA is predominantly dimeric, and higher-ordered trimers and tetramers have also been isolated (Vaerman et al. 1995). Serum IgM is primarily composed of J chain-containing pentamers with low levels of a J chain-free hexameric form, whereas mucosal IgM is pentameric (Davis et al. 1988; Niles et al. 1995). Because they are multivalent, pIgs can effectively cross-link several pathogens at once to limit their mobility and facilitate their clearance (Lamm 1997). The Fabs of polymeric Igs (pIgs), especially IgM, bind their antigens with relatively low affinities, an effect that is compensated for by the high avidity resulting from the presence of four identical binding sites in the case of dIgA and ten recognition sites in pIgM. Polymerization of IgA and pentameric IgM is dependent on covalent interactions between the tailpieces on the antibody heavy chains and the J chain. The tailpiece sequences in human IgA and IgM differ at seven amino acid positions (Yoo et al. 1999), but both contain a penultimate cysteine residue that is essential for efficient polymerization as well as a highly conserved N-linked glycosylation site that is required for efficient polymer assembly (Atkin et al. 1996; Wiersma et al. 1997). Besides the tailpiece, additional structural elements within the Cα3, and to a lesser extent Cα2, domains of IgA and the analogous Cμ4 and Cμ3 domains of IgM are required for J chain incorporation and polymer formation (Yoo et al. 1999).

Based on mutagenesis experiments and electron microscopy, a model for dIgA structure has been proposed (Feinstein et al. 1971; Garcia-Pardo et al. 1981; Bastian et al. 1995; Krugmann et al. 1997). One J chain molecule covalently bridges two IgA molecules arranged in an end-to end configuration (Garcia-Pardo et al. 1981). J chain Cys15 forms a disulfide bond with tailpiece Cys471 in the first Fcα homodimer, and J chain Cys69 forms a second disulfide bond with Cys471 in the tailpiece from the second Fcα homodimer. The two remaining tailpieces, one from each homodimer, are linked directly to each other by a disulfide bond between their penultimate cysteine residues (Bastian et al. 1995; Krugmann et al. 1997) (Fig. 3a). Pentameric IgM contains J chain (Fig. 3b) and, like pIgA, is actively transported to mucosal secretions by pIgR, but hexameric IgM lacks J chain and therefore does not bind to or get secreted by pIgR (Randall et al. 1990). The polymerization state of IgM depends on the amount of J chain, as IgM is secreted as hexamers in the absence of J chain and increased J chain production favors secretion of pentameric IgM (Niles et al. 1995). J chain is not found in small IgM assembly intermediates, suggesting that it does not get incorporated until late in the assembly (Randall et al. 1990; Brewer and Corley 1997). Pentameric IgM appears to be the substrate for J chain incorporation. A model proposes that five IgM molecules are joined by J chain, excluding a sixth IgM molecule that would normally be added to form hexameric IgM in the absence of J chain (Brewer and Corley 1997).

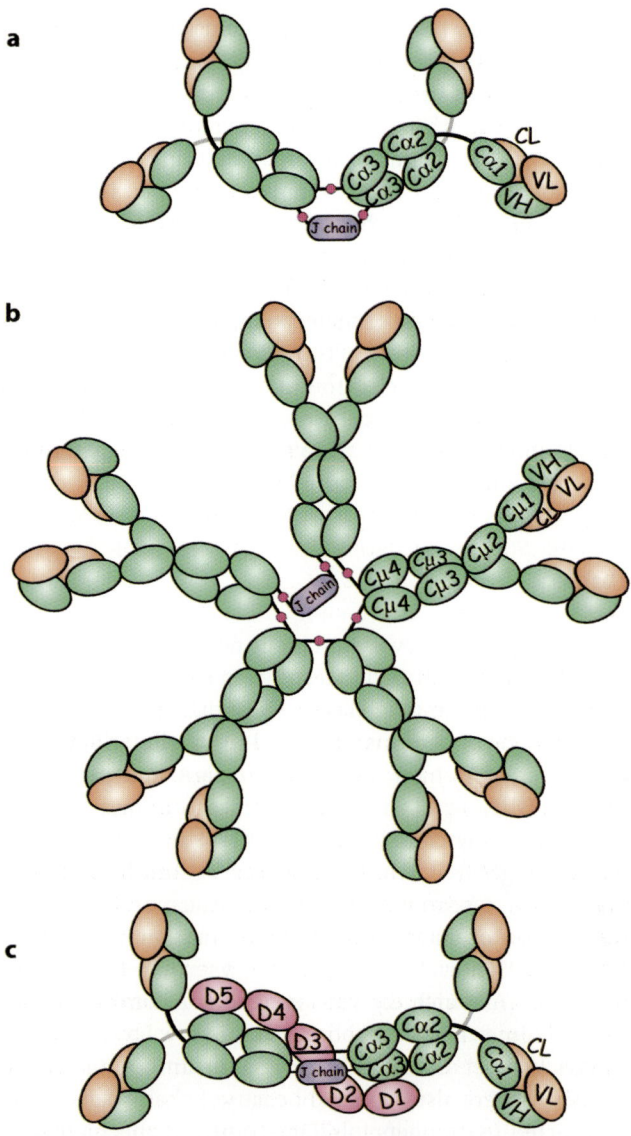

Fig. 3a–c Cartoon diagrams of polymeric IgA and IgM, and secretory IgA. **a** Diagram of dimeric IgA, illustrating the disulfide bonds (*magenta spheres*) between IgA monomers and J chain. **b** Diagram of polymeric IgM with J chain. Compare this figure with the solution structure of IgM in Fig. 1d. **c** Diagram of SIgA, showing a dimeric IgA complexed with pIgR D1-D5 (secretory component, SC). This model shows one possibility for the orientation of SC in SIgA, with D1 bound to the Cα3 domain of one IgA molecule and D5 forming a disulfide bond with the Cα2 domain of the other IgA molecule

Perkins and colleagues have reported the solution structure of intact pentameric IgM by X-ray and neutron scattering (Perkins et al. 1991). As with the solution structures of IgA1 and IgA2 (Boehm et al. 1999; Furtado et al. 2004), this approach allows accurate placement of individual domains but not detail at the level of side chains or atomic positions. The structure of IgM forms approximately a flat pseudo-pentameric star (Fig. 1d) in which the Fcμ regions form an inner ring with the insertion of a single J chain between two Fcμ regions. The authors tested a number of different orientations of the Fab regions and found that moderate (up to 45°) rotations of the Fab regions either side-to-side or out of the plane of the Fcμ ring were consistent with the data but more pronounced (90°) tilting of the Fab regions out of the plane was not. These data are consistent with electron microscopy results showing a planar form of free IgM, which is distinct from the antigen-bound "staple" conformation of IgM (Feinstein and Munn 1969) that is capable of C1q binding and complement activation (Janeway et al. 1999).

2.5
Joining (J) Chain

J chain, a 15-kDa polypeptide, was first identified as a component of SIgA and SIgM (Halpern and Koshland 1970; Mestecky et al. 1971). J chain is expressed by B cells that secrete various Ig classes (Brandtzaeg 1974); however, in the absence of IgA or IgM, J chain is degraded intracellularly (Mosmann et al. 1978). The number of J chain molecules in dIgA and pIgM is commonly accepted to be one (Zikan et al. 1986); however, early immunochemical studies suggested that dIgA may contain two and pIgM may contain three to four J chains (Brandtzaeg 1975). Although the exact function of J chain is not clear, it appears to be essential for the specific transport of pIgs by pIgR, and although it facilitates or stabilizes polymer formation, it is not essential for Ig polymerization (Hendrickson et al. 1995; Vaerman et al. 1998; Johansen et al. 2001). In mice in which the J chain gene was disrupted, a higher ratio of monomeric to dimeric IgA was observed, but low levels of dIgA were still present (Hendrickson et al. 1995). Increased serum IgA and reduced biliary and fecal IgA levels were also reported because J chain-deficient IgA are not actively transported by the hepatobiliary transport mechanism in rodents, and the lack of transfer of IgA from J chain-null mice was confirmed in vitro in Madin-Darby canine kidney (MDCK) cells (Hendrickson et al. 1995). Further analyses of these mice showed that SC was not associated with IgA and although IgA levels were decreased in bile and feces, they were unaffected in mucosal and glandular secretions, suggesting the possibility of an alternative mechanism for the transport of J chain-deficient IgA from wild-type IgA

(Hendrickson et al. 1996). J chain-null mice showed no change in serum IgM levels in one study (Hendrickson et al. 1995), but a reduction in serum IgM with impaired ability to activate complement was observed in another study (Erlandsson et al. 1998).

Mature human J chain contains 137 amino acids including eight cysteine residues (Max and Korsmeyer 1985), of which six are involved in intramolecular disulfide bonds and two form disulfide bonds to the tailpiece penultimate cysteine in pIgs (Bastian et al. 1992; Frutiger et al. 1992; Bastian et al. 1995). J chain also has an N-linked oligosaccharide attachment site, which appears to be important for the efficient assembly of dIgA (Krugmann et al. 1997). The three-dimensional structure of J chain remains elusive. Although the sequence of J chain does not resemble any known protein, several models have been proposed for its secondary structure. In the first model, a two-domain structure was proposed in which the N-terminal domain was predicted to contain a β-sheet followed by a mixture of α-helical, β-sheet, and random coil structures in the C-terminal domain (Cann et al. 1982). In the second model, J chain was suggested to form an eight-stranded β-sandwich based on its circular dichroism (CD) spectra and amino acid profiles for β-sheet propensity and hydrophobicity (Zikan et al. 1985), despite having only a low degree of sequence identity with other Ig domains. However, the proposed intramolecular disulfide bonds in this model were later shown to be incorrect (Frutiger et al. 1992). A third model based on conserved sequence features and the inter- and intramolecular disulfide bond pattern of J chain was also proposed (Frutiger et al. 1992). In this model, J chain contains two antiparallel β-sheets held together by two disulfide bonds, which is associated with a hairpin-like region composed of an α-helix and two β-strands (Frutiger et al. 1992). A similar two-domain model has recently been proposed, predominantly containing β-strands along with extended coils and two short α-helices (Johansen et al. 2001).

3
Fc Receptors Implicated in Mucosal Immunity

3.1
pIgR Function

The most extensively studied IgA and IgM receptor is pIgR, which was identified almost 40 years ago as a component of pIgA isolated from mucosal secretions. This glycoprotein expressed by secretory epithelial cells was shown to occur in both a transmembrane and a secreted free form (Tomasi et al.

1965; Brandtzaeg 1974). Since that time, pIgR transport of J chain-containing pIgs has been demonstrated both in vivo and in vitro. Expression of either rabbit or human pIgR cDNA in polarized MDCK cells, which normally do not express pIgR, results in the basolateral localization of pIgR and transport of the receptor to the apical surface in a ligand-independent manner (Mostov and Deitcher 1986; Tamer et al. 1995). Although pIgR transcytosis is constitutive, binding by dIgA stimulates increased transcytosis (Song et al. 1994). Disrupting the mouse pIgR gene results in a drastic increase of serum IgA, a slight increase in serum IgG and IgE, but unchanged IgM levels (Shimada et al. 1999). Additionally, IgA levels were reduced but not negligible in bile, feces, and intestinal secretions, further suggesting that dIgA is mainly transported by pIgR although a small amount may be secreted via an alternative pathway (Shimada et al. 1999).

pIgR is a type I transmembrane glycoprotein consisting of a 620-residue extracellular region arranged as five tandem Ig-like domains, a 23-residue transmembrane anchor, and a 103-residue cytoplasmic region. Human pIgA and pIgM bind to the extracellular region of pIgR (SC) with an affinity of approximately 10 nM (Natvig et al. 1997; Roe et al. 1999). Binding of human pIgR to dIgA takes place in two steps. In the first step, the pIgR N-terminal domain (D1), which contains loops analogous to the three antigen-binding complementarity determining regions (CDRs) Ig variable domains, binds the Cα3, and possibly Cα2, domains of dIgA (Frutiger et al. 1986; Geneste et al. 1986). In the second step, Cys467 of the human pIgR domain 5 (D5) forms a disulfide bridge with Cys311 in the Cα2 domain of the second IgA molecule in dIgA (Fallgreen-Gebauer et al. 1993) in a late transcytotic compartment (Chintalacharuvu et al. 1994). Unlike dIgA, pIgM does not become covalently bound to human pIgR (Brandtzaeg 1975). Mutagenesis and peptide binding experiments have been used to localize the pIgR D1 regions responsible for binding pIgA and pIgM. For pIgA binding, all three pIgR D1 CDR loops were shown to be essential, as was the EF loop, which is located on the opposite side of the domain from the CDRs (Coyne et al. 1994) (Fig. 2c). In binding of pIgR to pIgM, pIgR D1 CDR2 appears most critical for the interaction, although the CDR1 and CDR3 loops are also required for maximal affinity (Roe et al. 1999). Peptide binding studies have identified residues in pIgA that participate in binding to pIgR. The potential binding sites are in the Cα3 domain of pIgA and involve residues 402–410 in the DE loop and residues 430–443 in the FG loop (Hexham et al. 1999; White and Capra 2002) (Fig. 2e). Because J chain-containing pIgs are preferentially bound and transcytosed by pIgR (Vaerman et al. 1998), J chain may also contact pIgR directly.

The intracellular trafficking of pIgR and SIgA has been studied extensively (Rojas and Apodaca 2002). The 103-residue cytoplasmic tail of pIgR contains a number of cellular sorting signals. Deletion of the cytoplasmic tail results in a truncated pIgR that is able to bind ligand but is transported from the Golgi apparatus directly to the apical surface where it can be cleaved to SC (Mostov et al. 1986). Newly synthesized wild-type protein is targeted from the *trans*-Golgi network to the basolateral surface of epithelial cells via a 17-residue signal immediately C-terminal to the transmembrane region (Casanova et al. 1991). pIgR-pIg complexes are initially internalized by clathrin-coated pits and delivered to basolateral early endosomes (Mostov 1994). After sorting in this compartment, the pIgR-pIg complexes are targeted to common recycling endosomes. The complexes are then delivered to the apical surface, either directly from the common recycling endosome or via apical recycling (Mostov 1994), where pIgR is cleaved from the cell by an unidentified protease, releasing free SC or SIg. Multiple C-terminal truncations of released pIgR have been identified, indicating that multiple cleavage sites exist (Eiffert et al. 1984; Asano et al. 2004). Some pIgR escapes cleavage, however, and is internalized and delivered to apical early endosomes and recycled to either the apical surface or the basolateral surface by reverse transcytosis (Rojas and Apodaca 2002).

Protection from pathogens has been proposed to occur at several different stages during pIgR-mediated transport of dIgA (Monteiro and van de Winkel 2003). SIgA in external secretions can bind and cross-link pathogens, thereby slowing their mobility and inhibiting their ability to adhere to epithelial cells (Lamm 1997). SIgA can also intercept and neutralize pathogens, primarily viruses, intracellularly during transepithelial transport, assuming the pathogen and SIgA go through the same intracellular compartment (Mazanec et al. 1992). Furthermore, dIgA can bind bacteria and viruses that have already invaded target cells at the basolateral surface of the protective epithelial layer, and pIgR can shuttle the antibody-antigen complex to the apical surface, safely removing the pathogen (Kaetzel et al. 1991; Lamm et al. 1992). Finally, free SC has been shown to bind to pathogens and bacterial toxins, even in the absence of association with IgA (Dallas and Rolfe 1998; de Oliveira et al. 2001).

3.2
pIgR D1 Structure

The N-terminal ligand-binding domain of pIgR (D1) is necessary and sufficient to bind pIgs in the absence of the other pIgR domains (Frutiger et al. 1986; Bakos et al. 1994). pIgR D1, regardless of its glycosylation state, binds dIgA with an equilibrium dissociation constant of 300 nM but does not bind to monomeric forms of IgA1-Fc (Hamburger et al. 2004). The crystal structure of pIgR D1 (Fig. 2c) confirmed a folding topology similar to immunoglobulin variable domains. D1 has two disulfide bonds, one of which is the conserved disulfide bond found within the hydrophobic core of Ig domains, and an additional disulfide bond linking the C and C' strands. There are significant differences between D1 and antibody variable domains in the counterparts of the CDRs, which display highly noncanonical conformations (Hamburger et al. 2004). CDR1, the primary determinant in dIgA binding, contains a single helical turn composed of residues that are highly conserved across different species. An interesting consequence of the helical turn in pIgR D1 is that a hydrophobic residue (Val29), whose counterpart is normally buried in the extended structure of the CDR1 loops in antibody variable Ig domains, is solvent exposed and may be located at the pIg-binding interface. The crystal structure also clarified the roles of other residues that had been implicated in pIg binding by earlier peptide binding and mutagenesis studies, suggesting that some provide direct contacts with pIgs (Fig. 2d) and others serve as anchors to stabilize structural features within D1. CDR2, the main structural element conferring binding specificity for pIgM, is a very short, tightly turning loop with a glutamic acid likely required for pIgM binding. Interestingly, only human and bovine pIgR bind pIgM with high affinity (Socken and Underdown 1978), and these are the only two species that contain a charged residue in their CDR2 loops. The main difference between pIgR D1 and variable Ig domains is seen in the position of the CDR3 loop, which is in an unusual orientation, pointing away from the other CDRs. The position of the CDR3 loop is stabilized by hydrogen bonds between highly conserved residues in the loop and the adjacent β-sheet, resulting in the burial of a highly conserved tyrosine residue. In antibody variable domains, the CDR3 loop is typically found extending outward from the Fab core and contributes to both the antigen-binding site and the dimer interface between adjacent variable (V_L and V_H) domains. The pIgR D1 CDR3 conformation instead resembles that of camel single-chain antibodies, in which the CDR3 folds back and covers the hydrophobic surface that would form a dimer interface in human Fabs (Desmyter et al. 1996).

Although no structural information has been reported for other domains of pIgR, significant sequence similarity between D1 and the remaining domains indicates that D2 through D5 adopt a similar fold. In particular, the buried disulfide bond common to Ig domains is conserved in each pIgR domain, and the secondary disulfide bond linking the C and C' strands in D1 is also conserved in domains D3 through D5. However, the sequences corresponding to the CDR loops of D1 are divergent in D2 through D5, consistent with their ligand-binding role in D1. The sequence of pIgR D1 also shows 43% sequence identity with the N-terminal domain of Fcα/μR, an IgA- and IgM-specific Fc receptor expressed on most B lymphocytes and macrophages (Shibuya et al.

2000). It is not yet known whether Fcα/μR recognizes IgA or IgM using the same mechanism as pIgR, although the high sequence identity suggests the possibility.

3.3
IgA–Receptor Interactions: Implications for Signaling

Whereas pIgR is responsible for transcytosis of pIgs across the mucosal epithelium, the IgA-specific Fc receptor FcαRI (also known as CD89) mediates inflammatory responses to pathogens in the serum. FcαRI is a type I transmembrane receptor with two extracellular Ig domains, a transmembrane anchor and a cytoplasmic tail lacking typical signaling motifs (Maliszewski et al. 1990; Monteiro and van de Winkel 2003). Although FcαRI is a member of the Ig superfamily of Fc receptors like FcγRIII and FcεRI, it shares higher sequence similarity with members of the leukocyte receptor cluster on chromosome 19, such as the killer cell Ig-like receptors (KIRs) and the leukocyte Ig-like receptors (LIRs) (Wende et al. 1999). FcαRI is expressed on the surface of monocytes, eosinophils, neutrophils, and macrophages and binds both monomeric and dimeric forms of IgA (Monteiro and van de Winkel 2003). FcαRI mediates immune effector responses such as phagocytosis, ADCC, respiratory burst, and cytokine release (Monteiro et al. 1990). Monomeric and polymeric IgA, but not SIgA, can bind FcαRI to trigger phagocytosis through the clustering of the receptor (van Egmond et al. 2000; Vidarsson et al. 2001).

Recent crystal structures of the FcαRI ectodomain (Ding et al. 2003; Herr et al. 2003) and its complex with IgA1-Fc (Fcα) have shed some light on IgA-mediated immune responses (Herr et al. 2003). The FcαRI ectodomain is comprised of two Ig domains oriented at approximately right angles to one another (Ding et al. 2003; Herr et al. 2003). Although the FcγRs (Maxwell et al. 1999; Sondermann et al. 1999; Sondermann et al. 2000) and FcεRI (Garman et al. 1998) also have overall bent structures, D1 of FcαRI is rotated in the opposite direction to resemble the KIR and LIR folds (Fan et al. 1997; Chapman et al. 2000). In contrast to the 1:1 interaction between FcR and antibody hinge region observed in the FcγRIII:Fcγ (Sondermann et al. 2000) and FcεRI:Fcε (Garman et al. 2000) complexes, two molecules of FcαRI bind to one Fcα homodimer, one at each Cα2-Cα3 interface (Fig. 2f) (Herr et al. 2003), consistent with analytical ultracentrifugation experiments in solution (Herr et al. 2003). This binding surface is analogous to the Cγ2-Cγ3 interface of Fcγ, where a number of proteins, including FcRn, bind to IgG (DeLano et al. 2000; Martin et al. 2001). The FcαRI:Fcα interface is made up of residues from D1 of FcαRI binding primarily to the Cα3 domain of Fcα as well as a few residues from the Cα2 domain. A significant percentage of the buried surface area in the interface is contributed by residues in the FG loop of the Cα3 domain of Fcα (Herr et al. 2003). This loop was shown to be one of the binding sites for pIgR D1 (White and Capra 2002) (Fig. 2e). Furthermore, the FG loop is only ~10 Å away from Fcα Cys311 (Herr et al. 2003), which forms a disulfide bond with pIgR D5 (Fallgreen-Gebauer et al. 1993). The overlapping FcαRI and pIgR binding sites on Fcα, combined with the close proximity of the pIgR D5 disulfide bridge, have been suggested (Herr et al. 2003) to explain why SIgA does not bind to or activate FcαRI in the absence of an integrin coreceptor (van Egmond et al. 2000; van Spriel et al. 2001; Vidarsson et al. 2001).

Comparison of the FcαRI:Fcα complex to other complexes involving related receptors from the leukocyte receptor complex on chromosome 19 illustrates divergence of the ligand binding sites on these receptors. FcαRI binds Fcα using the N-terminal portion of D1 (Herr et al. 2003) (Fig. 2f), in contrast to the KIR receptors, whose binding site for MHC class I molecules is located at the D1-D2 junction (Boyington et al. 2000). Interestingly, LIR-1 uses residues in both the D1-D2 interface and the N-terminal region of D1 to recognize HLA-A2 (Willcox et al. 2003). This suggests that FcαRI and KIR receptors have evolved divergently from a common LIR-1 precursor, which uses both binding modes to recognize its target ligand (Willcox et al. 2003).

4
Pathogen Evasion of Host Mucosal Immunity

4.1
IgA1 Proteases

Bacteria have evolved several mechanisms for evading immune responses in the gut. These approaches include interfering with passive and active immunity by specifically cleaving secretory IgA1, preventing FcαRI activation by sterically occluding the receptor-binding site on IgA, and even hijacking the transcytotic pathway via interaction with pIgR to invade the mucosal epithelium. The first two avenues for immune evasion have not yet been fully elucidated through high-resolution crystal structures, although we can gather some insight from knowledge of the solution structure of intact IgA1 and the crystal structure of IgA1-Fc. IgA1 proteases are secreted by a number of bacterial genera, including *Neisseria*, *Streptococcus*, and *Haemophilus* species (Plaut et al. 1975; Male 1979). These proteases share a common feature of specificity for Pro-Thr or Pro-Ser dipeptides in the hinge region of IgA1 (Kilian et al. 1980), although the IgA1-Fc region has also been implicated in substrate recognition (Chintalacharuvu et al. 2003). As described above, IgA1 has an elongated hinge region that is found in an extended conformation, due to both its amino acid sequence and its high levels of O-linked glycosylation (Fig. 1a). These characteristics render the IgA1 hinge a suitable substrate for the IgA1 proteases. Given that IgA2 has a 13-residue truncation in the hinge region, this subclass is not susceptible to proteolysis. Cleavage of the hinge region of IgA1 would leave only the Fab regions specifically bound to the bacterial surface, thus significantly minimizing steric occlusion arising from an intact secretory IgA1 (Reinholdt and Kilian 1987). Furthermore, in *Streptococcus pneumoniae*, anticapsular Fab fragments remaining after cleavage of IgA1 facilitate adhesion to epithelial cells, apparently by minimizing the negative charge of the bacterial capsule (Weiser et al. 2003).

4.2
IgA-Binding Proteins

Bacteria that have already managed to breach the mucosal epithelium can prevent inflammatory responses via FcαRI by secreting IgA-binding proteins that sterically block the receptor-binding site. These include Sir22 and Arp4 from *Streptococcus pyogenes*, β-protein secreted by group B Streptococcus (Pleass et al. 2001), and the superantigen-like protein 7 (SSL7) of *Staphylococcus aureus* (Langley et al. 2005). Sir22 has been shown to bind tightly to serum and secretory IgA1 and IgA2, with a K_D of 4 nM. The binding domain was localized to a 29-residue predicted α-helical region. A 50-residue construct incorporating this region that was cross-linked by an N-terminal cysteine retained specific IgA-binding activity, with a K_D of 20 nM (Sandin et al. 2002). Each of the streptococcal IgA-binding proteins interacts with the Cα2-Cα3 region of IgA (Pleass et al. 2001), which corresponds to the FcαRI-binding site, as described above (see Fig. 2f) (Herr et al. 2003). As would be expected, these streptococcal proteins inhibit the ability of IgA to bind FcαRI, and Arp4 can inhibit respiratory burst from neutrophils triggered by FcαRI (Pleass et al. 2001). Like Sir22, the staphylococcal protein SSL7 binds IgA with low nanomolar affinity but also binds avidly to the complement protein C5 and inhibits complement-mediated bacterial cell lysis (Langley et al. 2005). The structure of SSL7 has been determined, revealing a superantigen-like fold composed of an N-terminal OB (oligonucleotide/oligosaccharide binding) domain and a C-terminal "β-grasp" domain consisting of a β-sheet wrapped around an α-helix (Al-Shangiti et al. 2004) (Fig. 2g). Although no direct information is yet available on the IgA- or C5-binding surfaces on SSL7, Langley et al. have mapped conserved residues from several known SSL7 alleles onto the external face of the OB domain, and they suggest that this may correspond to an IgA- or C5-binding site (Langley et al. 2005). Preliminary mutational results indicate that SSL7, like the streptococcal IgA-binding proteins, also binds to the Cα2-Cα3 region of IgA (Langley et al. 2005).

4.3
pIgR-Binding Proteins

In addition to secreting proteins that can cleave IgA1 or block the FcαRI-binding site on IgA, *Streptococcus pneumoniae* can directly mediate invasion of the mucosal epithelium by hijacking the transcytosis pathway via pIgR. *S. pneumoniae* (or pneumococcus) secretes a choline-binding protein A (CbpA) that is anchored to the bacterial surface via a highly conserved choline binding motif (Jedrzejas 2001). CbpA was shown to be important for bacterial adherence (Rosenow et al. 1997), and the human host receptor for *S. pneumoniae* was identified as pIgR (Zhang et al. 2000). Either insertional knockout of *cbp* or antibodies against CbpA or pIgR abolished bacterial adherence and invasion, and two CbpA domains, R1 and R2, were shown to bind to the extracellular domains of human pIgR (Zhang et al. 2000). R1 and R2 share 89% sequence identity and are highly conserved in CbpA from many strains of the bacteria. Peptide mapping and mutagenesis results highlighted the importance of a conserved hexapeptide motif (YRNYPT) within the R domains (Hammerschmidt et al. 2000; Elm et al. 2004). Domain deletion, mutagenesis, and peptide binding studies have recently revealed that domains 3 and 4 of pIgR (D3-4) are necessary and sufficient to bind and uptake CbpA (Lu et al. 2003; Elm et al. 2004). Interestingly, while SIgA and free SC in mucosal secretions inhibit pneumococcal invasion, pneumococci translocate across nasopharyngeal epithelial cells using the pIgR reverse transcytosis pathway (Zhang et al. 2000). Epstein-Barr virus (EBV) complexed with EBV-specific pIgA has also been shown to invade mucosal epithelial cells via pIgR (Sixbey and Yao 1992). However, it is not clear whether this occurs in vivo, because EBV is transcytosed across polarized epithelial cells but only infects single-cell suspensions of epithelial cells (Gan et al. 1997).

The solution NMR structure of the R2 domain of CbpA from *S. pneumoniae* has been reported along with binding studies using the intact protein (Luo et al. 2004). The R2 domain consists of three antiparallel α-helices that are nearly coplanar (Fig. 2h). One face of the domain shows high negative electrostatic potential, whereas the opposite face exhibits strong positive electrostatic potential. The YPT sequence from the conserved hexapeptide motif is found in the loop connecting the first two α-helices. This conserved region extends outward from the domain and forms a highly hydrophobic region flanked by a lysine and an arginine, which together create a zone of neutral electrostatic potential. Mutations in the tyrosine or proline of the YPT motif diminished binding of CbpA to both SIgA and free SC (Luo et al. 2004). The high sequence identity between R1 and R2, along with similarities in their CD and NMR spectra, indicate that R1 and R2 share the same fold. Interestingly, the authors found that R1 and R2 could each independently bind two sites on pIgR with similar affinity and that an R1-R2 construct containing both domains bound with nearly the same affinity as the isolated R1 or R2 domains. The basis for this was revealed by isothermal titration calorimetry experiments, which indicated that loss of conformational freedom of the R1-R2 pair on binding resulted in an unfavorable entropy change that compensated for the more favorable enthalpy change for R1-R2 binding compared to R1 or R2 alone (Luo et al. 2004).

5
Future Directions

In the last few years, several new three-dimensional structures have provided significant insight into mechanisms of mucosal immunity. However, several important issues remain unresolved and await further structural work. In particular, the structure of full-length SC (i.e., D1–D5 of the pIgR ectodomain) would be of great interest in order to better understand its interactions with IgA and CbpA from *S. pneumoniae*. In a similar vein, the structures of dimeric IgA and secretory IgA (or at least structures of the Fcα-J chain-SC core of SIgA) will be important additions to the structural repertoire. Generation of sufficient quantities of pure, homogeneous dIgA or SIgA has been the limiting factor in these types of studies, although expression systems have been described recently for production of specific dIgA and SIgA (Chintalacharuvu and Morrison 1999; Corthesy 2002). Finally, structures of various IgA-binding receptors and bacterial proteins, alone and in complex with IgA, combined with biophysical studies of their interactions will provide important insights into gut immunology and may lead to effective therapeutic strategies. For instance, understanding how the M cell receptor on Peyer's patches recognizes IgA2 could eventually lead to the development of effective oral vaccines, which would be of particular interest in developing regions of the world.

Acknowledgements The authors would like to thank Dr. Steve Perkins (University College London) for providing the coordinates of pentameric IgM.

References

Al-Shangiti AM, Naylor CE, Nair SP, Briggs DC, Henderson B and Chain BM (2004). Structural relationships and cellular tropism of staphylococcal superantigen-like proteins. Infect Immun 72:4261–70.

Armstrong SJ, and Dimmock NJ (1992). Neutralization of influenza virus by low concentrations of hemagglutinin-specific polymeric immunoglobulin A inhibits viral fusion activity, but activation of the ribonucleoprotein is also inhibited. J Virol 66:3823–32.

Asano M, Takenouchi-Ohkubo N, Matsumoto N, Ogura Y, Nomura H, Suguro H and Moro I (2004). Multiple cleavage sites for polymeric immunoglobulin receptor. Immunology 112:583–9.

Atkin JD, Pleass RJ, Owens RJ and Woof JM (1996). Mutagenesis of the human IgA1 heavy chain tailpiece that prevents dimer assembly. J Immunol 157:156–9.

Bakos MA, Widen SG and Goldblum RM (1994). Expression and purification of biologically active domain I of the human polymeric immunoglobulin receptor. Mol Immunol 31:165–8.

Bastian A, Kratzin H, Eckart K and Hilschmann N (1992). Intra- and interchain disulfide bridges of the human J chain in secretory immunoglobulin A. Biol Chem Hoppe Seyler 373:1255–63.

Bastian A, Kratzin H, Fallgren-Gebauer E, Eckart K and Hilschmann N (1995). Intra- and inter-chain disulfide bridges of J chain in human S-IgA. Adv Exp Med Biol 371A: 581–3.

Boehm MK, Woof JM, Kerr MA and Perkins SJ (1999). The Fab and Fc fragments of IgA1 exhibit a different arrangement from that in IgG: a study by X-ray and neutron solution scattering and homology modelling. J Mol Biol 286:1421–47.

Boyington JC, Motyka SA, Schuck P, Brooks AG and Sun PD (2000). Crystal structure of an NK cell immunoglobulin-like receptor in complex with its class I MHC ligand. Nature 405:537–43.

Brandtzaeg P (1974). Presence of J chain in human immunocytes containing various immunoglobulin classes. Nature 252:418–20.

Brandtzaeg P (1975). Human secretory immunoglobulin M. An immunochemical and immunohistochemical study. Immunology 29:559–70.

Brandtzaeg P (1975). Immunochemical studies on free and bound J chain of human IgA and IgM. Scand J Immunol 4:439–50.

Brandtzaeg P (2003). Mucosal immunity: integration between mother and the breast-fed infant. Vaccine 21:3382–8.

Brandtzaeg P, Baekkevold ES, Farstad IN, Jahnsen FL, Johansen FE, Nilsen EM and Yamanaka T (1999). Regional specialization in the mucosal immune system: what happens in the microcompartments? Immunol Today 20:141–51.

Brandtzaeg P, Karlsson G, Hansson G, Petruson B, Bjorkander J and Hanson LA (1987). The clinical condition of IgA-deficient patients is related to the proportion of IgD- and IgM-producing cells in their nasal mucosa. Clin Exp Immunol 67:626–36.

Brewer JW, and Corley RB (1997). Late events in assembly determine the polymeric structure and biological activity of secretory IgM. Mol Immunol 34:323–31.

Cann GM, Zaritsky A and Koshland ME (1982). Primary structure of the immunoglobulin J chain from the mouse. Proc Natl Acad Sci USA 79:6656–60.

Casanova JE, Apodaca G and Mostov KE (1991). An autonomous signal for basolateral sorting in the cytoplasmic domain of the polymeric immunoglobulin receptor. Cell 66:65–75.

Chapman TL, Heikema AP, West AP, Jr. and Bjorkman PJ (2000). Crystal structure and ligand binding properties of the D1D2 region of the inhibitory receptor LIR-1 (ILT2). Immunity 13:727–36.

Chintalacharuvu KR, Chuang PD, Dragoman A, Fernandez CZ, Qiu J, Plaut AG, Trinh KR, Gala FA and Morrison SL (2003). Cleavage of the human immunoglobulin A1 (IgA1) hinge region by IgA1 proteases requires structures in the Fc region of IgA. Infect Immun 71:2563–70.

Chintalacharuvu KR and Morrison SL (1999). Production and characterization of recombinant IgA. Immunotechnology 4:165–74.

Chintalacharuvu KR, Tavill AS, Louis LN, Vaerman JP, Lamm ME and Kaetzel CS (1994). Disulfide bond formation between dimeric immunoglobulin A and the polymeric immunoglobulin receptor during hepatic transcytosis. Hepatology 19:162–73.

Cleary TG (2004). Human milk protective mechanisms. Adv Exp Med Biol 554:145–54.

Corper AL, Sohi MK, Bonagura VR, Steinitz M, Jefferis R, Feinstein A, Beale D, Taussig MJ and Sutton BJ (1997). Structure of human IgM rheumatoid factor Fab bound to its autoantigen IgG Fc reveals a novel topology of antibody-antigen interaction. Nat Struct Biol 4:374–81.

Corthesy B (2002). Recombinant immunoglobulin A: powerful tools for fundamental and applied research. Trends Biotechnol 20:65–71.

Coyne RS, Siebrecht M, Peitsch MC and Casanova JE (1994). Mutational analysis of polymeric immunoglobulin receptor/ligand interactions. Evidence for the involvement of multiple complementarity determining region (CDR)-like loops in receptor domain I. J Biol Chem 269:31620–5.

Crottet P and Corthesy B (1998). Secretory component delays the conversion of secretory IgA into antigen-binding competent F(ab')2: a possible implication for mucosal defense. J Immunol 161:5445–53.

Dallas SD and Rolfe RD (1998). Binding of *Clostridium difficile* toxin A to human milk secretory component. J Med Microbiol 47:879–88.

Davis AC, Roux KH and Shulman MJ (1988). On the structure of polymeric IgM. Eur J Immunol 18:1001–8.

de Oliveira IR, de Araujo AN, Bao SN and Giugliano LG (2001). Binding of lactoferrin and free secretory component to enterotoxigenic *Escherichia coli*. FEMS Microbiol Lett 203:29–33.

Deisenhofer J (1981). Crystallographic refinement and atomic models of a human Fc fragment and its complex with fragment B of protein A from *Staphylococcus aureus* at 2.9- and 2.8-Å resolution. Biochemistry 20:2361–70.

DeLano WL, Ultsch MH, A. M. de Vos and Wells JA (2000). Convergent solutions to binding at a protein-protein interface. Science 287:1279–83.

Desmyter A, Transue TR, Ghahroudi MA, Thi MH, Poortmans F, Hamers R, Muyldermans S and Wyns L (1996). Crystal structure of a camel single-domain VH antibody fragment in complex with lysozyme. Nat Struct Biol 3:803–11.

Ding Y, Xu G, Yang M, Yao M, Gao GF, Wang L, Zhang W and Rao Z (2003). Crystal structure of the ectodomain of human FcαRI. J Biol Chem 278:27966–70.

Eiffert H, Quentin E, Decker J, Hillemeir S, Hufschmidt M, Klingmuller D, Weber MH and Hilschmann N (1984). The primary structure of human free secretory component and the arrangement of disulfide bonds. Hoppe Seylers Z Physiol Chem 365:1489-95.

Elm C, Braathen R, Bergmann S, Frank R, Vaerman JP, Kaetzel CS, Chhatwal GS, Johansen FE and Hammerschmidt S (2004). Ectodomains 3 and 4 of human polymeric Immunoglobulin receptor (hpIgR) mediate invasion of *Streptococcus pneumoniae* into the epithelium. J Biol Chem 279:6296-304.

Elm C, Rohde M, Vaerman JP, Chhatwal GS and Hammerschmidt S (2004). Characterization of the interaction of the pneumococcal surface protein SpsA with the human polymeric immunoglobulin receptor (hpIgR). Indian J Med Res 119 Suppl: 61-5.

Erlandsson L, Andersson K, Sigvardsson M, Lycke N and Leanderson T (1998). Mice with an inactivated joining chain locus have perturbed IgM secretion. Eur J Immunol 28:2355-65.

Fallgreen-Gebauer E, Gebauer W, Bastian A, Kratzin HD, Eiffert H, Zimmermann B, Karas M and Hilschmann N (1993). The covalent linkage of secretory component to IgA. Structure of sIgA. Biol Chem Hoppe Seyler 374:1023-8.

Fan QR, Mosyak L, Winter CC, Wagtmann N, Long EO and Wiley DC (1997). Structure of the inhibitory receptor for human natural killer cells resembles haematopoietic receptors. Nature 389:96-100.

Feinstein A, Munn EA (1969). Conformation of the free and antigen-bound IgM antibody molecules. Nature 224:1307-9.

Feinstein A, Munn EA and Richardson NE (1971). The three-dimensional conformation of M and A globulin molecules. Ann NY Acad Sci 190:104-21.

Fernandez MI, Pedron T, Tournebize R, Olivo-Marin JC, Sansonetti PJ and Phalipon A (2003). Anti-inflammatory role for intracellular dimeric immunoglobulin a by neutralization of lipopolysaccharide in epithelial cells. Immunity 18:739-49.

Frutiger S, Hughes GJ, Hanly WC, Kingzette M and Jaton JC (1986). The amino-terminal domain of rabbit secretory component is responsible for noncovalent binding to immunoglobulin A dimers. J Biol Chem 261:16673-81.

Frutiger S, Hughes GJ, Paquet N, Luthy R and Jaton JC (1992). Disulfide bond assignment in human J chain and its covalent pairing with immunoglobulin M. Biochemistry 31:12643-7.

Furtado PB, Whitty PW, Robertson A, Eaton JT, Almogren A, Kerr MA, Woof JM and Perkins SJ (2004). Solution structure determination of monomeric human IgA2 by X-ray and neutron scattering, analytical ultracentrifugation and constrained modelling: a comparison with monomeric human IgA1. J Mol Biol 338:921-41.

Gan YJ, Chodosh J, Morgan A and Sixbey JW (1997). Epithelial cell polarization is a determinant in the infectious outcome of immunoglobulin A-mediated entry by Epstein-Barr virus. J Virol 71:519-26.

Garcia-Pardo A, Lamm ME, Plaut AG and Frangione B (1981). J chain is covalently bound to both monomer subunits in human secretory IgA. J Biol Chem 256:11734-8.

Garman SC, Kinet JP and Jardetzky TS (1998). Crystal structure of the human high-affinity IgE receptor. Cell 95:951-61.

Garman SC, Wurzburg BA, Tarchevskaya SS, Kinet JP and Jardetzky TS (2000). Structure of the Fc fragment of human IgE bound to its high-affinity receptor FcεRIα. Nature 406:259–66.

Geneste C, Iscaki S, Mangalo R and Pillot J (1986). Both Fcα domains of human IgA are involved in in vitro interaction between secretory component and dimeric IgA. Immunol Lett 13:221–6.

Halpern MS, Koshland ME (1970). Novel subunit in secretory IgA. Nature 228:1276–8.

Hamburger AE, West AP, Jr. and Bjorkman PJ (2004). Crystal structure of a polymeric immunoglobulin binding fragment of the human polymeric immunoglobulin receptor. Structure (Camb) 12:1925–35.

Hammerschmidt S, Tillig MP, Wolff S, Vaerman JP and Chhatwal GS (2000). Species-specific binding of human secretory component to SpsA protein of *Streptococcus pneumoniae* via a hexapeptide motif. Mol Microbiol 36:726–36.

Harris LJ, Larson SB, Hasel KW, Day J, Greenwood A and McPherson A (1992). The three-dimensional structure of an intact monoclonal antibody for canine lymphoma. Nature 360:369–72.

Harris LJ, Skaletsky E and McPherson A (1998). Crystallographic structure of an intact IgG1 monoclonal antibody. J Mol Biol 275:861–72.

Hendrickson BA, Conner DA, Ladd DJ, Kendall D, Casanova JE, Corthesy B, Max EE, Neutra MR, Seidman CE and Seidman JG (1995). Altered hepatic transport of immunoglobulin A in mice lacking the J chain. J Exp Med 182:1905–11.

Hendrickson BA, Rindisbacher L, Corthesy B, Kendall D, Waltz DA, Neutra MR and Seidman JG (1996). Lack of association of secretory component with IgA in J chain-deficient mice. J Immunol 157:750–4.

Herr AB, Ballister ER and Bjorkman PJ (2003). Insights into IgA-mediated immune responses from the crystal structures of human FcαRI and its complex with IgA1-Fc. Nature 423:614–20.

Herr AB, White CL, Milburn C, Wu C and Bjorkman PJ (2003). Bivalent binding of IgA1 to FcαRI suggests a mechanism for cytokine activation of IgA phagocytosis. J Mol Biol 327:645–57.

Hexham JM, White KD, Carayannopoulos LN, Mandecki W, Brisette R, Yang YS and Capra JD (1999). A human immunoglobulin (Ig)A cα3 domain motif directs polymeric Ig receptor-mediated secretion. J Exp Med 189:747–52.

Huber R, Deisenhofer J, Colman PM, Matsushima M and Palm W (1976). Crystallographic structure studies of an IgG molecule and an Fc fragment. Nature 264:415–20.

Janeway CA, Travers P, Walport M and Capra JD (1999). Immunobiology: the immune system in health and disease. New York, Garland Publishing.

Jedrzejas MJ (2001). Pneumococcal virulence factors: structure and function. Microbiol Mol Biol Rev 65:187–207.

Johansen FE, Braathen R and Brandtzaeg P (2001). The J chain is essential for polymeric Ig receptor-mediated epithelial transport of IgA. J Immunol 167:5185–92.

Kaetzel CS, Robinson JK, Chintalacharuvu KR, Vaerman JP and Lamm ME (1991). The polymeric immunoglobulin receptor (secretory component) mediates transport of immune complexes across epithelial cells: a local defense function for IgA. Proc Natl Acad Sci USA 88:8796–800.

Kerr MA (1990). The structure and function of human IgA. Biochem J 271:285–96.

Kett K, Brandtzaeg P, Radl J and Haaijman JJ (1986). Different subclass distribution of IgA-producing cells in human lymphoid organs and various secretory tissues. J Immunol 136:3631–5.

Kilian M, Mestecky J, Kulhavy R, Tomana M and Butler WT (1980). IgA1 proteases from *Haemophilus influenzae, Streptococcus pneumoniae, Neisseria meningitidis,* and *Streptococcus sanguis*: comparative immunochemical studies. J Immunol 124:2596–600.

Krugmann S, Pleass RJ, Atkin JD and Woof JM (1997). Structural requirements for assembly of dimeric IgA probed by site-directed mutagenesis of J chain and a cysteine residue of the α-chain CH2 domain. J Immunol 159:244–9.

Lamm ME (1997). Interaction of antigens and antibodies at mucosal surfaces. Annu Rev Microbiol 51:311–40.

Lamm ME, Robinson JK and Kaetzel CS (1992). Transport of IgA immune complexes across epithelial membranes: new concepts in mucosal immunity. Adv Exp Med Biol 327:91–4.

Langley R, Wines B, Willoughby N, Basu I, Proft T and Fraser JD (2005). The staphylococcal superantigen-like protein 7 binds IgA and complement C5 and inhibits IgA-FcαRI binding and serum killing of bacteria. J Immunol 174:2926–33.

Lu L, Lamm ME, Li H, Corthesy B and Zhang JR (2003). The human polymeric immunoglobulin receptor binds to *Streptococcus pneumoniae* via domains 3 and 4. J Biol Chem 278:48178–87.

Luo R, Mann B, Lewis WS, Rowe A, Heath R, Stewart ML, Hamburger AE, Sivakolundu S, Lacy ER, Bjorkman PJ, Tuomanen E and Kriwacki RW (2004). Solution structure of choline binding protein A, the major adhesin of *Streptococcus pneumoniae*. EMBO J.

Male CJ (1979). Immunoglobulin A1 protease production by *Haemophilus influenzae* and *Streptococcus pneumoniae*. Infect Immun 26:254–61.

Maliszewski CR, March CJ, Schoenborn MA, Gimpel S and Shen L (1990). Expression cloning of a human Fc receptor for IgA. J Exp Med 172:1665–72.

Mantis NJ, Cheung MC, Chintalacharuvu KR, Rey J, Corthesy B and Neutra MR (2002). Selective adherence of IgA to murine Peyer's patch M cells: evidence for a novel IgA receptor. J Immunol 169:1844–51.

Martin WL, West AP, Jr., Gan L and Bjorkman PJ (2001). Crystal structure at 2.8 Å of an FcRn/heterodimeric Fc complex: mechanism of pH-dependent binding. Mol Cell 7:867–77.

Matsushima M, Marquart M, Jones TA, Colman PM, Bartels K and Huber R (1978). Crystal structure of the human Fab fragment Kol and its comparison with the intact Kol molecule. J Mol Biol 121:441–59.

Max EE, Korsmeyer SJ (1985). Human J chain gene. Structure and expression in B lymphoid cells. J Exp Med 161:832–49.

Maxwell KF, Powell MS, Hulett MD, Barton PA, McKenzie IF, Garrett TP and Hogarth PM (1999). Crystal structure of the human leukocyte Fc receptor, FcγRIIa. Nat Struct Biol 6:437–42.

Mazanec MB, Kaetzel CS, Lamm ME, Fletcher D and Nedrud JG (1992). Intracellular neutralization of virus by immunoglobulin A antibodies. Proc Natl Acad Sci USA 89:6901–5.

Mestecky J, McGhee JR (1987). Immunoglobulin A (IgA): molecular and cellular interactions involved in IgA biosynthesis and immune response. Adv Immunol 40:153–245.

Mestecky J, Zikan J and Butler WT (1971). Immunoglobulin M and secretory immunoglobulin A: presence of a common polypeptide chain different from light chains. Science 171:1163–5.

Monteiro RC, Kubagawa H and Cooper MD (1990). Cellular distribution, regulation, and biochemical nature of an Fcα receptor in humans. J Exp Med 171:597–613.

Monteiro RC, van de Winkel JG (2003). IgA Fc receptors. Annu Rev Immunol 21:177–204.

Mosmann TR, Gravel Y, Williamson AR and Baumal R (1978). Modification and fate of J chain in myeloma cells in the presence and absence of polymeric immunoglobulin secretion. Eur J Immunol 8:94–101.

Mostov KE (1994). Transepithelial transport of immunoglobulins. Annu Rev Immunol 12:63–84.

Mostov KE, de Bruyn A, Kops A, Deitcher DL (1986). Deletion of the cytoplasmic domain of the polymeric immunoglobulin receptor prevents basolateral localization and endocytosis. Cell 47:359–64.

Mostov KE, Deitcher DL (1986). Polymeric immunoglobulin receptor expressed in MDCK cells transcytoses IgA. Cell 46:613–21.

Moura IC, Arcos-Fajardo M, Sadaka C, Leroy V, Benhamou M, Novak J, Vrtovsnik F, Haddad E, Chintalacharuvu KR and Monteiro RC (2004). Glycosylation and size of IgA1 are essential for interaction with mesangial transferrin receptor in IgA nephropathy. J Am Soc Nephrol 15:622–34.

Natvig IB, Johansen FE, Nordeng TW, Haraldsen G and Brandtzaeg P (1997). Mechanism for enhanced external transfer of dimeric IgA over pentameric IgM: studies of diffusion, binding to the human polymeric Ig receptor, and epithelial transcytosis. J Immunol 159:4330–40.

Niles MJ, Matsuuchi L and Koshland ME (1995). Polymer IgM assembly and secretion in lymphoid and nonlymphoid cell lines: evidence that J chain is required for pentamer IgM synthesis. Proc Natl Acad Sci USA 92:2884–8.

Norderhaug IN, Johansen FE, Schjerven H and Brandtzaeg P (1999). Regulation of the formation and external transport of secretory immunoglobulins. Crit Rev Immunol 19:481–508.

Outlaw MC, Dimmock NJ (1990). Mechanisms of neutralization of influenza virus on mouse tracheal epithelial cells by mouse monoclonal polymeric IgA and polyclonal IgM directed against the viral haemagglutinin. J Gen Virol 71:69–76.

Pasquier B, Launay P, Kanamaru Y, Moura IC, Pfirsch S, Ruffie C, Henin D, Benhamou M, Pretolani M, Blank U and Monteiro RC (2005). Identification of FcαRI as an inhibitory receptor that controls inflammation: dual role of FcRγ ITAM. Immunity 22:31–42.

Perkins SJ, Nealis AS, Sutton BJ and Feinstein A (1991). Solution structure of human and mouse immunoglobulin M by synchrotron X-ray scattering and molecular graphics modelling. A possible mechanism for complement activation. J Mol Biol 221:1345–66.

Plaut AG, Gilbert JV, Artenstein MS and Capra JD (1975). *Neisseria gonorrhoeae* and *neisseria meningitidis*: extracellular enzyme cleaves human immunoglobulin A. Science 190:1103–5.

Pleass RJ, Areschoug T, Lindahl G and Woof JM (2001). Streptococcal IgA-binding proteins bind in the Cα2-Cα3 interdomain region and inhibit binding of IgA to human CD89. J Biol Chem 276:8197–204.

Randall TD, King LB and Corley RB (1990). The biological effects of IgM hexamer formation. Eur J Immunol 20:1971–9.

Reinholdt J, Kilian M (1987). Interference of IgA protease with the effect of secretory IgA on adherence of oral streptococci to saliva-coated hydroxyapatite. J Dent Res 66:492–7.

Roe M, Norderhaug IN, Brandtzaeg P and Johansen FE (1999). Fine specificity of ligand-binding domain 1 in the polymeric Ig receptor: importance of the CDR2-containing region for IgM interaction. J Immunol 162:6046–52.

Rojas R, Apodaca G (2002). Immunoglobulin transport across polarized epithelial cells. Nat Rev Mol Cell Biol 3:944–55.

Roos A, Bouwman LH, van Gijlswijk-Janssen DJ, Faber-Krol MC, Stahl GL and Daha MR (2001). Human IgA activates the complement system via the mannan-binding lectin pathway. J Immunol 167:2861–8.

Rosenow C, Ryan P, Weiser JN, Johnson S, Fontan P, Ortqvist A and Masure HR (1997). Contribution of novel choline-binding proteins to adherence, colonization and immunogenicity of *Streptococcus pneumoniae*. Mol Microbiol 25:819–29.

Russell MW, Reinholdt J and Kilian M (1989). Anti-inflammatory activity of human IgA antibodies and their Fab alpha fragments: inhibition of IgG-mediated complement activation. Eur J Immunol 19:2243–9.

Sandin C, Linse S, Areschoug T, Woof JM, Reinholdt J and Lindahl G (2002). Isolation and detection of human IgA using a streptococcal IgA-binding peptide. J Immunol 169:1357–64.

Satow Y, Cohen GH, Padlan EA and Davies DR (1986). Phosphocholine binding immunoglobulin Fab McPC603. An X-ray diffraction study at 2.7 Å. J Mol Biol 190:593–604.

Shibuya A, Sakamoto N, Shimizu Y, Shibuya K, Osawa M, Hiroyama T, Eyre HJ, Sutherland GR, Endo Y, Fujita T, Miyabayashi T, Sakano S, Tsuji T, Nakayama E, Phillips JH, Lanier LL and Nakauchi H (2000). Fcα/μ receptor mediates endocytosis of IgM-coated microbes. Nat Immunol 1:441–6.

Shimada S, Kawaguchi-Miyashita M, Kushiro A, Sato T, Nanno M, Sako T, Matsuoka Y, Sudo K, Tagawa Y, Iwakura Y and Ohwaki M (1999). Generation of polymeric immunoglobulin receptor-deficient mouse with marked reduction of secretory IgA. J Immunol 163:5367–73.

Sixbey JW, Yao QY (1992). Immunoglobulin A-induced shift of Epstein-Barr virus tissue tropism. Science 255:1578–80.

Socken DJ, Underdown BJ (1978). Comparison of human, bovine and rabbit secretory component-immunoglobulin interactions. Immunochemistry 15:499–506.

Sondermann P, Huber R and Jacob U (1999). Crystal structure of the soluble form of the human Fcγ-receptor IIb: a new member of the immunoglobulin superfamily at 1.7 A resolution. EMBO J 18:1095–103.

Sondermann P, Huber R, Oosthuizen V and Jacob U (2000). The 3.2-Å crystal structure of the human IgG1 Fc fragment-FcγRIII complex. Nature 406:267-73.

Song W, Bomsel M, Casanova J, Vaerman JP and Mostov K (1994). Stimulation of transcytosis of the polymeric immunoglobulin receptor by dimeric IgA. Proc Natl Acad Sci USA 91:163-6.

Suh SW, Bhat TN, Navia MA, Cohen GH, Rao DN, Rudikoff S and Davies DR (1986). The galactan-binding immunoglobulin Fab J539: an X-ray diffraction study at 2.6-Å resolution. Proteins 1:74-80.

Svehag SE, Bloth B (1970). Ultrastructure of secretory and high-polymer serum immunoglobulin A of human and rabbit origin. Science 168:847-9.

Tamer CM, Lamm ME, Robinson JK, Piskurich JF and Kaetzel CS (1995). Comparative studies of transcytosis and assembly of secretory IgA in Madin-Darby canine kidney cells expressing human polymeric Ig receptor. J Immunol 155:707-14.

Tomasi TB, Jr., Tan EM, Solomon A and Prendergast RA (1965). Characteristics of an immune system common to certain external secretions. J Exp Med 121:101-24.

Vaerman JP, Langendries A, Giffroy D, Brandtzaeg P and Kobayashi K (1998). Lack of SC/pIgR-mediated epithelial transport of a human polymeric IgA devoid of J chain: in vitro and in vivo studies. Immunology 95:90-6.

Vaerman JP, Langendries A and C. van der Maelen (1995). Homogenous IgA monomers, dimers, trimers and tetramers from the same IgA myeloma serum. Immunol Invest 24:631-41.

Vaerman JP, Langendries AE, Giffroy DA, Kaetzel CS, Fiani CM, Moro I, Brandtzaeg P and Kobayashi K (1998). Antibody against the human J chain inhibits polymeric Ig receptor-mediated biliary and epithelial transport of human polymeric IgA. Eur J Immunol 28:171-82.

Van de Perre P (2003). Transfer of antibody via mother's milk. Vaccine 21:3374-6.

van Egmond M, van Garderen E, van Spriel AB, Damen CA, van Amersfoort ES, van Zandbergen G, van Hattum J, Kuiper J, van de Winkel JG (2000). FcαRI-positive liver Kupffer cells: reappraisal of the function of immunoglobulin A in immunity. Nat Med 6:680-5.

van Spriel AB, Leusen JH, van Egmond M, Dijkman HB, Assmann KJ, Mayadas TN, van de Winkel JG (2001). Mac-1 (CD11b/CD18) is essential for Fc receptor-mediated neutrophil cytotoxicity and immunologic synapse formation. Blood 97:2478-86.

Vidarsson G, van Der Pol WL, van Den Elsen JM, Vile H, Jansen M, Duijs J, Morton HC, Boel E, Daha MR, Corthesy B, van De Winkel JG (2001). Activity of human IgG and IgA subclasses in immune defense against Neisseria meningitidis serogroup B. J Immunol 166:6250-6.

Wan T, Beavil RL, Fabiane SM, Beavil AJ, Sohi MK, Keown M, Young RJ, Henry AJ, Owens RJ, Gould HJ and Sutton BJ (2002). The crystal structure of IgE Fc reveals an asymmetrically bent conformation. Nat Immunol 3:681-6.

Weiser JN, Bae D, Fasching C, Scamurra RW, Ratner AJ and Janoff EN (2003). Antibody-enhanced pneumococcal adherence requires IgA1 protease. Proc Natl Acad Sci USA 100:4215-20.

Wende H, Colonna M, Ziegler A and Volz A (1999). Organization of the leukocyte receptor cluster (LRC) on human chromosome 19q13.4. Mamm Genome 10:154-60.

White KD, Capra JD (2002). Targeting mucosal sites by polymeric immunoglobulin receptor-directed peptides. J Exp Med 196:551–5.

Wiersma EJ, Chen F, Bazin R, Collins C, Painter RH, Lemieux R and Shulman MJ (1997). Analysis of IgM structures involved in J chain incorporation. J Immunol 158:1719–26.

Wiersma EJ, Collins C, Fazel S and Shulman MJ (1998). Structural and functional analysis of J chain-deficient IgM. J Immunol 160:5979–89.

Willcox BE, Thomas LM and Bjorkman PJ (2003). Crystal structure of HLA-A2 bound to LIR-1, a host and viral major histocompatibility complex receptor. Nat Immunol 4:913–9.

Wilson IA, Rini JM, Fremont DH, Fieser GG and Stura EA (1991). X-ray crystallographic analysis of free and antigen-complexed Fab fragments to investigate structural basis of immune recognition. Methods Enzymol 203:153–76.

Wold AE, Mestecky J, Tomana M, Kobata A, Ohbayashi H, Endo T and Eden CS (1990). Secretory immunoglobulin A carries oligosaccharide receptors for *Escherichia coli* type 1 fimbrial lectin. Infect Immun 58:3073–7.

Wurzburg BA, Garman SC and Jardetzky TS (2000). Structure of the human IgE-Fc Cε3-Cε4 reveals conformational flexibility in the antibody effector domains. Immunity 13:375–85.

Yoo EM, Coloma MJ, Trinh KR, Nguyen TQ, Vuong LU, Morrison SL and Chintalacharuvu KR (1999). Structural requirements for polymeric immunoglobulin assembly and association with J chain. J Biol Chem 274:33771–7.

Zhang JR, Mostov KE, Lamm ME, Nanno M, Shimida S, Ohwaki M and Tuomanen E (2000). The polymeric immunoglobulin receptor translocates pneumococci across human nasopharyngeal epithelial cells. Cell 102:827–37.

Zikan J, Mestecky J, Kulhavy R and Bennett JC (1986). The stoichiometry of J chain in human secretory dimeric IgA. Mol Immunol 23:541–4.

Zikan J, Novotny J, Trapane TL, Koshland ME, Urry DW, Bennett JC and Mestecky J (1985). Secondary structure of the immunoglobulin J chain. Proc Natl Acad Sci USA 82:5905–9.

Subject Index

activation-induced cytidine
    deaminase (AID) 160
adhesion molecule 19, 28–30, 44
affinity maturation 168
AID 63, 67, 140, 160
aly 32
aly/aly 25, 33, 40, 142
- mutation 31
alymphoblastic (aly/aly)
    mouse 122
anaerobic expansion 145
APRIL 123
Arp4 193

B cell antigen receptor (BCR) 157
B cells 155
- B-1 cells 157
- B-2 cells 157
- marginal zone (MZ) 159
- proliferation 156
bacteria 60, 67, 73, 75, 77, 156
- commensal 156
- pathogenic 156
BAFF 123
BCR
- high-affinity 167
- specificity 162
biofilm 119

CCL19 62
CCL21 62
CCR 7-deficient mice 129
CCR7 62
CCR9 67

CD1 165
CD3⁻ cells 28, 29, 34–36
CD40 167
- CD40L interaction 167
- deficient mice 167
CD4⁺ cells 28, 29, 34–36
chemokine 22, 28–30, 33, 42–44,
    62, 75, 76
cholera toxin 127
class switch recombination 160
Clostridium difficile 119
colonic lymphoid patch 26
commensal 59, 60, 67, 73
commensal bacteria 77, 155
commensal intestinal bacteria 121
complement 163
- activation 163
- fragment 163
- receptor 163
Cre/loxP 158
cryptopatch (CP) 26, 36, 40, 42
crypts 65, 70, 73, 78
crystal structure
- FcαRI 183
- IgA (or Fcα) 177
- IgE (or Fcσ) 177
- IgG (or Fcγ) 177
- IgM 177
- pIgR D1 183
- SSL7 183
CSR 140
CX$_3$CR1 73
CXCL13 62, 77
CXCR5 62
cytokine 19, 22, 40–42, 44

DC-SIGN 75, 76
dendritic cell (DC) 126, 128, 157
diversity of $V_{H\alpha}$ sequence 123

Enterobacter cloacae 121
epithelial-mesenchymal cell
  interaction 30
Epstein-Barr virus (EBV) 158

Fas 160
FcαRI 175
- complex with IgA1-Fc 180
FcR γ chain 178
- ITAM of 178
follicle-associated epithelium (FAE)
  23, 26, 30, 31, 36
follicular dendritic cell (FDC) 155

gene conversion 156
germ-free 162
germ-free mice 127
germinal center (GC) 21, 22, 65–67, 155
germline transcription 167
gut homing receptor 67
gut-associated lymphoid tissue
  (GALT) 155

HIV 75–77
hyperplasia 147

ICAM-1 62, 63
Id2 62, 64
IgA 121, 156
- deficiency 130
- Fab 179
- Fc 179
- hinge 178
- induction protocol 127
- N-glycan 181
- O-linked glycosylation 179
- plasma cells 138
- receptor 131
- secreting cells 120
- tailpieces 178
IgA1 protease 175

IgM
- Fab 184
- Fc 177
- tailpieces 184
Ikaros 35
IL-7 28, 40–43
- receptor α 29
IL-7R 28, 29, 40–42
- signaling 40, 41
- signaling pathway 34, 41
IL-7Rα 29, 31, 40
immune evasion 192
immune exclusion 175
immune response 167
- T cell-dependent 167
immunoglobulin 156
- rearrangement 156
- receptor 156
- repertoire 156
immunoreceptor tyrosine activation
  motif (ITAM) 158
inducer cells 28, 29, 36, 39, 41–44
inducible lymphoid tissue 25
inflammatory bowel disease 60, 77, 78
intestinal epithelial lymphocyte
  subset 120
intestinal loop 129
intestinal microflora 163
intestinal permeability barrier 124
isolated lymphoid follicle (ILF) 21, 26, 31, 32, 36, 40, 139, 155

J chain 178
$J_H^{-/-}$ strain 130

lamina propria (LP) 138, 156
latent membrane protein
  (LMP) 158
LIGHT 37
LTαβ 44
LTβR 44
lymph node (LN) 22, 25–27, 29, 30, 32–37, 39–44
- development 37
- organogenesis 34
lymphatic vessel 27

Subject Index

lymphoid tissue inducer cells 29, 34, 35, 39, 41–44
lymphonodular hyperplasia 131
lymphotoxin (LT) 25, 28–33, 36, 37, 40, 41, 43, 62, 72
lymphotoxin α-deficient mouse 122
LYVE-1 27

M cells 64–67
macrophage 125
MAdCAM 33, 34
mesenchymal organizer cells 44
mesenteric lymph node (MLN) 19, 21, 24–26, 124, 155
MHC Class II-deficient mouse 123
mice without MLN 129
microbiocidal mechanism 125
microbiota 138
microflora 60, 61, 67, 68, 72, 73
microfold (M) cells 156
MR1 166
mucosa-associated invariant T (MAIT) cells 166
MyD88 163

natural killer-T (NK-T) cells 164
NF-κB1 28
NF-κB2 28
NKX 2.3 33, 34
NKX homeodomain protein 33
nuclear factor-κB (NF-κB) 30, 32, 33, 62
nuclear factor-κB-inducing kinase (NIK) 32, 33, 40, 142
– deficient 32
nutrition 120

organizer cells 28–30, 41, 43, 44

Peyer's patch (PP) 19, 21, 23–26, 29–37, 39–42, 44, 125, 155
plasma cells 156
plasmablast 168
polymeric Ig receptor (pIgR)
– carbohydrates of 178
– transcytosis of 175

polymeric IgA (pIgA) 178
polymeric IgM (pIgM) 184
polymeric immunoglobulin receptor 130
polyspecific IgA binding 122
probiotic 119
Prox 1 27

reverse transcytosis 183

secretory IgA (sIgA) 67, 68, 73, 175
secretory IgM (SIgM) 175
segmented filamentous bacteria (SFB) 145
self-ligand 165
serum IgA 178
Sir22 193
solution structure
– choline binding protein A (CbpA) 183
– IgA1 177
– IgA2 177
– IgM 177
somatic hypermutation 156
specific pathogen-free (SPF) 119
Staphylococcus saprophyticus 127
stroma 62, 72, 75
stromal 29
stromal cells 142
subepithelial DC 125
superantigen 167
systemic immune ignorance 123

T cells 164
– αβ 164
– antigen-specific 160
– bystander 160, 166
– cell-dependent (TD) antigen 160
– γδ 164
term parabiosis 143
terminal ileum 73
tertiary lymphoid structures 60, 63, 77
TGF-β 167
thymus 166
TNF 29, 33, 36, 37, 40, 44

TNF$^{-/-}$ 36
TNFR   39
TNFRI   36, 37, 40
TNFRI$^{-/-}$ 33
TNFRII   36
TNFRp55   37
Toll-like receptor (TLR)   121, 126, 163
TRANCE   28–30, 40, 41, 62
TRANCE$^{+/-}$ 40

TRANCER   39
transcription factor   33, 36
transgenic   162

ulcerative colitis   77

VCAM-1   62, 63
VEGF   27
vertebrate   21, 22

Current Topics in Microbiology and Immunology

Volumes published since 1989 (and still available)

Vol. 264/I: **Hacker, Jörg; Kaper, James B. (Eds.):** Pathogenicity Islands and the Evolution of Microbes. 2002. 34 figs. XVIII, 232 pp. ISBN 3-540-42681-7

Vol. 264/II: **Hacker, Jörg; Kaper, James B. (Eds.):** Pathogenicity Islands and the Evolution of Microbes. 2002. 24 figs. XVIII, 228 pp. ISBN 3-540-42682-5

Vol. 265: **Dietzschold, Bernhard; Richt, Jürgen A. (Eds.):** Protective and Pathological Immune Responses in the CNS. 2002. 21 figs. X, 278 pp. ISBN 3-540-42668X

Vol. 266: **Cooper, Koproski (Eds.):** The Interface Between Innate and Acquired Immunity, 2002. 15 figs. XIV, 116 pp. ISBN 3-540-42894-X

Vol. 267: **Mackenzie, John S.; Barrett, Alan D. T.; Deubel, Vincent (Eds.):** Japanese Encephalitis and West Nile Viruses. 2002. 66 figs. X, 418 pp. ISBN 3-540-42783X

Vol. 268: **Zwickl, Peter; Baumeister, Wolfgang (Eds.):** The Proteasome-Ubiquitin Protein Degradation Pathway. 2002. 17 figs. X, 213 pp. ISBN 3-540-43096-2

Vol. 269: **Koszinowski, Ulrich H.; Hengel, Hartmut (Eds.):** Viral Proteins Counteracting Host Defenses. 2002. 47 figs. XII, 325 pp. ISBN 3-540-43261-2

Vol. 270: **Beutler, Bruce; Wagner, Hermann (Eds.):** Toll-Like Receptor Family Members and Their Ligands. 2002. 31 figs. X, 192 pp. ISBN 3-540-43560-3

Vol. 271: **Koehler, Theresa M. (Ed.):** Anthrax. 2002. 14 figs. X, 169 pp. ISBN 3-540-43497-6

Vol. 272: **Doerfler, Walter; Böhm, Petra (Eds.):** Adenoviruses: Model and Vectors in Virus-Host Interactions. Virion and Structure, Viral Replication, Host Cell Interactions. 2003. 63 figs., approx. 280 pp. ISBN 3-540-00154-9

Vol. 273: **Doerfler, Walter; Böhm, Petra (Eds.):** Adenoviruses: Model and Vectors in VirusHost Interactions. Immune System, Oncogenesis, Gene Therapy. 2004. 35 figs., approx. 280 pp. ISBN 3-540-06851-1

Vol. 274: **Workman, Jerry L. (Ed.):** Protein Complexes that Modify Chromatin. 2003. 38 figs., XII, 296 pp. ISBN 3-540-44208-1

Vol. 275: **Fan, Hung (Ed.):** Jaagsiekte Sheep Retrovirus and Lung Cancer. 2003. 63 figs., XII, 252 pp. ISBN 3-540-44096-3

Vol. 276: **Steinkasserer, Alexander (Ed.):** Dendritic Cells and Virus Infection. 2003. 24 figs., X, 296 pp. ISBN 3-540-44290-1

Vol. 277: **Rethwilm, Axel (Ed.):** Foamy Viruses. 2003. 40 figs., X, 214 pp. ISBN 3-540-44388-6

Vol. 278: **Salomon, Daniel R.; Wilson, Carolyn (Eds.):** Xenotransplantation. 2003. 22 figs., IX, 254 pp. ISBN 3-540-00210-3

Vol. 279: **Thomas, George; Sabatini, David; Hall, Michael N. (Eds.):** TOR. 2004. 49 figs., X, 364 pp. ISBN 3-540-00534X

Vol. 280: **Heber-Katz, Ellen (Ed.):** Regeneration: Stem Cells and Beyond. 2004. 42 figs., XII, 194 pp. ISBN 3-540-02238-4

Vol. 281: **Young, John A. T. (Ed.):** Cellular Factors Involved in Early Steps of Retroviral Replication. 2003. 21 figs., IX, 240 pp. ISBN 3-540-00844-6

Vol. 282: **Stenmark, Harald (Ed.):** Phosphoinosites in Subcellular Targeting and Enzyme Activation. 2003. 20 figs., X, 210 pp. ISBN 3-540-00950-7

Vol. 283: **Kawaoka, Yoshihiro (Ed.):** Biology of Negative Strand RNA Viruses: The Power of Reverse Genetics. 2004. 24 figs., IX, 350 pp. ISBN 3-540-40661-1

Vol. 284: **Harris, David (Ed.):** Mad Cow Disease and Related Spongiform Encephalopathies. 2004. 34 figs., IX, 219 pp. ISBN 3-540-20107-6

Vol. 285: **Marsh, Mark (Ed.):** Membrane Trafficking in Viral Replication. 2004. 19 figs., IX, 259 pp. ISBN 3-540-21430-5

Vol. 286: **Madshus, Inger H. (Ed.):** Signalling from Internalized Growth Factor Receptors. 2004. 19 figs., IX, 187 pp. ISBN 3-540-21038-5

Vol. 287: **Enjuanes, Luis (Ed.):** Coronavirus Replication and Reverse Genetics. 2005. 49 figs., XI, 257 pp. ISBN 3-540-21494-1

Vol. 288: **Mahy, Brain W. J. (Ed.):** Foot-and-Mouth-Disease Virus. 2005. 16 figs., IX, 178 pp. ISBN 3-540-22419X

Vol. 289: **Griffin, Diane E. (Ed.):** Role of Apoptosis in Infection. 2005. 40 figs., IX, 294 pp. ISBN 3-540-23006-8

Vol. 290: **Singh, Harinder; Grosschedl, Rudolf (Eds.):** Molecular Analysis of B Lymphocyte Development and Activation. 2005. 28 figs., XI, 255 pp. ISBN 3-540-23090-4

Vol. 291: **Boquet, Patrice; Lemichez Emmanuel (Eds.)** Bacterial Virulence Factors and Rho GTPases. 2005. 28 figs., IX, 196 pp. ISBN 3-540-23865-4

Vol. 292: **Fu, Zhen F (Ed.):** The World of Rhabdoviruses. 2005. 27 figs., X, 210 pp. ISBN 3-540-24011-X

Vol. 293: **Kyewski, Bruno; Suri-Payer, Elisabeth (Eds.):** CD4+CD25+ Regulatory T Cells: Origin, Function and Therapeutic Potential. 2005. 22 figs., XII, 332 pp. ISBN 3-540-24444-1

Vol. 294: **Caligaris-Cappio, Federico, Dalla Favera, Ricardo (Eds.):** Chronic Lymphocytic Leukemia. 2005. 25 figs., VIII, 187 pp. ISBN 3-540-25279-7

Vol. 295: **Sullivan, David J.; Krishna Sanjeew (Eds.):** Malaria: Drugs, Disease and Post-genomic Biology. 2005. 40 figs., XI, 446 pp. ISBN 3-540-25363-7

Vol. 296: **Oldstone, Michael B. A. (Ed.):** Molecular Mimicry: Infection Induced Autoimmune Disease. 2005. 28 figs., VIII, 167 pp. ISBN 3-540-25597-4

Vol. 297: **Langhorne, Jean (Ed.):** Immunology and Immunopathogenesis of Malaria. 2005. 8 figs., XII, 236 pp. ISBN 3-540-25718-7

Vol. 298: **Vivier, Eric; Colonna, Marco (Eds.):** Immunobiology of Natural Killer Cell Receptors. 2005. 27 figs., VIII, 286 pp. ISBN 3-540-26083-8

Vol. 299: **Domingo, Esteban (Ed.):** Quasispecies: Concept and Implications. 2006. 44 figs., XII, 401 pp. ISBN 3-540-26395-0

Vol. 300: **Wiertz, Emmanuel J.H.J.; Kikkert, Marjolein (Eds.):** Dislocation and Degradation of Proteins from the Endoplasmic Reticulum. 2006. 19 figs., VIII, 168 pp. ISBN 3-540-28006-5

Vol. 301: **Doerfler, Walter; Böhm, Petra (Eds.):** DNA Methylation: Basic Mechanisms. 2006. 24 figs., VIII, 324 pp. ISBN 3-540-29114-8

Vol. 302: **Robert N. Eisenman (Ed.):** The Myc/Max/Mad Transcription Factor Network. 2006. 28 figs. XII, 278 pp. ISBN 3-540-23968-5

Vol. 303: **Thomas E. Lane (Ed.):** Chemokines and Viral Infection. 2006. 14 figs. XII, 154 pp. ISBN 3-540-29207-1

Vol. 304: **Stanley A. Plotkin (Ed.):** Mass Vaccination: Global Aspects -- Progress and Obstacles. 2006. 40 figs. IX, 268 pp. ISBN 3-540-29382-5

Vol. 305: **Radbruch, Andreas; Lipsky, Peter E. (Eds.):** Current Concepts in Autoimmunity. 2006. 29 figs. IIX, 276 pp. ISBN 3-540-29713-8

Vol. 306: **William M. Shafer (Ed.):** Antimicrobial Peptides and Human Disease. 2006. 12 figs. XII, 262 pp. ISBN 3-540-29915-7

Vol. 307: **John L. Casey (Ed.):** Hepatitis Delta Virus. 2006. 22 figs. XII, 228 pp. ISBN 3-540-29801-0

Printing: Krips bv, Meppel
Binding: Stürtz, Würzburg